Steroids and Brain Edema

Edited by

H. J. Reulen · K. Schürmann

Editorial Board

J. W. F. Beks · I. Klatzo · D. M. Long
H. M. Pappius · J. Ransohoff

With 60 Figures

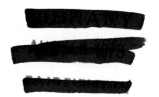

Springer-Verlag
New York · Heidelberg · Berlin 1972

Proceedings of an International Workshop held in Mainz, W. Germany, June 19 to 21, 1972

Sponsor: Sharp & Dohme GmbH., München, subsidiary of Merck & Co., Inc., Rayway, NJ/USA

ISBN 0-387-05958-X Springer-Verlag New York · Heidelberg · Berlin
ISBN 3-540-05958-X Springer-Verlag Berlin · Heidelberg · New York

© by Springer-Verlag Berlin · Heidelberg 1972. Library of Congress Catalog Card Number 72-91334.
Printed in Germany.

Typesetting, printing and binding: Universitätsdruckerei Mainz GmbH

Preface

The control of brain edema is still one of the major problems in surgical and conservative treatment of various cerebral lesions. Many attempts have been made to develop methods for reducing the high mortality associated with brain edema. After many years of using hypertonic solutions it can be stated that this type of therapy has not yielded satisfactory results. During recent years increasing evidence has been accumulated on the efficacy of steroids on brain edema. Steroids were reported to result in rapid relief of signs and symptoms of increased intracranial pressure and neurological dysfunction accompanying cerebral edema.

It was the aim of this workshop to evaluate the effect of corticosteroids on brain edema as an advance in therapy. It was hoped that this could be achieved by a multidisciplinary approach. Though, the volume contains the contributions of various experts – internists, neurochemists, neurologists, neuropathologists, neurosurgeons, pharmacologists, physiologists – who have added considerable experimental and clinical evidence on the action of steroids on brain edema. New pathophysiological aspects regarding the mechanisms underlying the formation and resolution of brain edema are presented. The effectiveness of corticosteroid therapy in various forms of clinical and experimental brain edema, e.g. accompanying brain tumors, head injury, spinal cord injury, cerebrovascular lesions, etc. as well as dosage and duration of treatment are critically discussed.

Workshops, although eminently suited to explore specific problems and to interpret the value of new data, have the disadvantage that the information remains confined to a small group. This book, therefore, is thought to be a vehicle for the spreading of this information to all persons interested in the subject clinically or experimentally.

The rapid publication of the proceedings could be realized by the excellent cooperation of the authors, the editorial board, and the Springer-Verlag. We take great pleasure to express our thanks to their invaluable help. Dr. William Meinert helped in compiling and revising of the discussions. We also wish to thank for the generosity of the sponsor, Sharp & Dohme GmbH, München, who supplied the financial basis for the meeting and especially Dr. Helmut F. Hofmann and his staff for their support in the organization of the symposium and their constant attention to our many requests.

Mainz, Dezember 1972

Hans J. Reulen · Kurt Schürmann

Contents

VIII

List of Contributors

Baethmann, A.   Institut für Chirurgische Forschung, Chirurgische Klinik der Universität, 8000 München und Division of Biology, California Institute of Technology, Pasadena, CA 91109, USA

Barker, M.   H. C. Naffziger Laboratories for Neurosurgical Research, University of California, School of Medicine, San Francisco, CA 94122, USA

Barlow, Ch. F.   Department of Neurology, Harvard Med. School and the Children's Hospital, Medical Center, Boston, MA 02115, USA

Bartko, D.   Neurological Clinic, Comenius University, Bratislava, Mickiewczova 13, CSSR, and Universität Mainz, Neurochirurgische Universitätsklinik, 6500 Mainz, Langenbeckstraße 1, W. Germany

Beks, J. W. F.   Department of Neurosurgery, University Hospital, Groningen, Netherland

Bouzarth, W.   Department of Neurosurgery, Episcopal Hospital, Centennial Building, Front Street and Lehig Avenue, Philadelphia, PA 19125, USA

Brendel, W.   Institut für Chirurgische Forschung, Chirurgische Klinik der Universität, 8000 München, W. Germany

Brock, M.   Neurochirurgische Klinik der Med. Hochschule Hannover, 3000 Hannover-Kleefeld, Roderbruchstr. 101, W. Germany

Brodersen, P.   Bispebjerg Hospital, Dept. Neurology, Bispebjerg-Bakke, Copenhagen, Denmark

Clasen, R. A.   Univ. of Illinois, College of Med., Presbyterian St. Luke's Hospital, 1753 West Congress Parkway, Chicago, IL 60612, USA

Demopoulos, H. B.   Department of Pathology, New York University Medical Center, 550 First Ave., New York, NY 10016, USA

Hadjidimos, A.   Neurochirurgische Universitätsklinik Mainz, 6500 Mainz, Langenbeckstr. 1, W. Germany

Hager, H.

Pathologisches Institut der Universität Gießen, 6300 Gießen, Klinikstr. 37, W. Germany

Hansebout, R. R.

Department of Neurosurgery, Montreal Neurological Inst., McGill University, 3801 University Street, Montreal 112, Canada

Harrison, M. J. G.

University Department of Clinical Neurology, The National Hospital, Queen Square, London WCI, Great Britain

Herrmann H. D.

Neurochirurgische Universitätsklinik, 6650 Homburg/Saar, W. Germany

Hossmann, K. A.

Max-Planck-Institut für Hirnforschung, 5000 Köln-Merheim, Ostmerheimer Straße 200, W. Germany

Klatzo, I.

Laboratory of Neuropathology and Neuroanatomical Sciences, National Institute of Neurological Diseases and Stroke, National Inst. of Health, Bethesda, MD 20014, USA

Krück, F.

II. Med. Klinik der Universitätskliniken, 6650 Homburg/ Saar, W. Germany

Kullberg, G.

Neurokirurgiska Kliniken, Lanslasarettet, Lund, Sweden

Landoldt, A.

Kantonsspital Zürich, Neurochirurgische Universitätsklinik Zürich, Rämistr. 80, Switzerland

Lassen, N. A.

Department of Clinical Physiology, Bispebjerg-Hospital, Bispebjerg Bakke, Copenhagen, Denmark

Long, D. M.

University of Minnesota, Dept. of Neurosurgery, Medical School, B-590 Mayo Memorial Building, Minneapolis, MN 55455, USA

Lundberg, N.

University of Lund, Dept. of Neurosurgery, Univ. Hospital, Lund, Sweden

Maxwell, R. E.

University of Minnesota, Department of Neurosurgery, Medical School, B-590 Mayo Memorial Building, Minneapolis, MN 55455, USA

Miller, D.

Department of Neurosurgery, Institute of Neurological Sciences, Glasgow, Scotland

Overgaard, J.

Odense Sygehus, Neurokirurgiska afdeling U, Odense, Denmark

Pappius, H. M.

The Donner-Lab. for Experimental Neurochemistry, The Montreal Neurological Institute, McGill University, Montreal 112, Canada

Patten, M. B.

Medical Neurology Branch, Dept. of Health, Education and Welfare, National Inst. of Health, Bethesda, MD, USA

Ransohoff, J.   Department of Neurosurgery, New York University, Medical Center, School of Medicine, 550 First Ave., New York, NY 10016, USA

Reulen, H. J.   Neurochirurgische Universitätsklinik Mainz, 6500 Mainz, Langenbeckstr. 1, W. Germany

Sano, K.   Department of Neurosurgery, University of Tokyo, Henze, Bun Kyo-ku, Japan

Schmiedek, P.   Institut für Chirurgische Forschung, Chirurgische Universitätsklinik und Neurochirurgische Universitätsklinik, 8000 München, W. Germany

Schürmann, K.   Neurochirurgische Universitätsklinik Mainz, 6500 Mainz, Langenbeckstr. 1, W. Germany

Siegel, B. A.   The Edward Mallinckrodt Inst. of Radiology, Washington Univ., School of Medicine, 510 South Kingshighway, St. Louis, MO 63110, USA

Spatz, M.   Laboratory of Neuropathology and Neuroanatomical Sciences, National Institute of Neurological Diseases and Stroke, National Institutes of Health, Bethesda, MD 20014, USA

Taylor, A. R.   Dept. of Neurological Surgery, Royal Victoria Hospital, Grosvenor Road, Belfast, B. T., Northern Ireland

Withrow, C. D.   Department of Pharmacology, College of Medicine, University of Utah, Salt Lake City, UT 84112, USA

Zwetnow, N.   University of Gothenburg, Department of Neurosurgery, Sahlgrenska Sjukhuset, Gothenburg, Sweden

Chapter I

Experimental Aspects of Brain Edema and Therapeutic Approach

Pathophysiological Aspects of Brain Edema

Igor Klatzo

Laboratory of Neuropathology and Neuroanatomical Sciences, National Institute of Neurological Diseases and Stroke, National Institute of Health, Bethesda, MD 20014, USA

With 2 Figures

The subject of brain edema (BE) has been burdened for many years by confusion with regard to understanding the essential pathophysiological aspects of the process. Various classifications were based mainly either on some gross characteristics, such as Reichardt's [29] Hirnödem v. Hirnschwellung, or on etiological factors involved (e.g. traumatic, inflammatory, necrotic, hemorrhagic, etc.), which contributed only some limited descriptive value.

Accepting the definition of edema as an *abnormal accumulation of a fluid in a tissue* it follows that there are basically two possibilities for location of such a fluid i.e. it can be intra- or extracellular and in general pathology one finds examples of such basic type of edema according to intra- or extracellular location of edema fluid. Pursuing further this basic division of edema into two types, one can postulate that in intracellular edema the crucial pathogenic event is related to a disturbance in cell membrane permeability of individual cells resulting in cellular imbition, whereby in the second type an increased vascular permeability allows an increased passage of fluid of hematogenous origin leading to extracellular inundation of the tissue.

Assuming that a similar situation must also exist in the brain, I proposed the terms *vasogenic* and *cytoxic* types of BE as describing best two basic different pathomechanisms which may be involved in abnormal fluid accumulation in the brain [14]. At that time there were still forthcoming electron microscopic (EM) reports claiming that BE is always intracellular and that large extracellular spaces occasionally observed were created by rupture of cell membrane, either *in vivo* or during EM processing. This misconception persisted until a sizeable, functional extracellular space allowing a free diffusion of even large protein molecules in the normal brain, as well as, an extracellular spread of edema fluid deriving from injured blood vessels have been unequivocally demonstrated in numerous EM studies [4, 6, 9, 10, 16, 17, 19]. These findings have thus validated one of the main tenets of the vasogenic edema concept, namely – the predominantly extracellular spread of edema fluid.

The other main tenet, – increase in cerebrovascular permeability, is invariably associated with alterations of the blood-brain barrier (BBB) and has been the subject of several investigations in our laboratory. The morphological site of the BBB for protein has been previously established to be the tight junctions formed by membrane fusion of adjacent endothelial cells lining the cerebral vasculature [4, 28]. Since pinocytotic transport across the endothelium does not appear to play a major role [3] disturbances of the BBB resulting in extravascular leakage of serum proteins and spread of edema fluid must be due either to physical destruction of endothelium, creating discontinuity of the vascular lining or to opening of endothelial tight junctions. The latter is of special interest since it can be assumed that non-destructive, temporary opening of tight junctions may be operative in a variety of neuropathological conditions associated with BE.

A model for a reversible opening of tight junctions was established by application of hypertonic solutions to cerebral vasculature. It was demonstrated that various electrolytes and non-electrolytes which have little or no lipid solubility but differ in chemical and ionic properties produce a similar BBB breakdown, the intensity of which depends directly on the osmotic concentration of the solutions [27]. The effect of these hypertonic solutions was initially studied by topical application of a circular filter paper pledget soaked with a test solution to the exposed pial surface of the rabbit brain. The breakdown of the BBB was manifested by the blue staining of underlying brain tissue due to extravasation of systemically injected Evans Blue (EB) indicator. With this approach the threshold values for BBB damaging osmotic concentrations were established, as well as, the reversibility of BBB injury was determined by administering the EB indicator at different time intervals following topical application of hypertonic solutions.

In order to observe ultrastructurally the osmotic effect on the cerebral vasculature in another series of experiments, hypertonic solutions were applied to a cerebral hemisphere of the rabbit by unilateral internal carotid artery perfusion. Similarly, the osmotic concentration thresholds and reversibility of BBB injury were established. Ultrastructural behaviour of the BBB was assessed using horseradish peroxidase as the EM tracer. The EM observations revealed unequivocal pictures of the tracer passing *between* the tight junctions without evidence of cellular damage to endothelial cells themselves. Especially, the occasionally observed pictures of the tracer seemingly entrapped between two points of junctional fusion strongly imply an intravital existence of a patent for proteins route between the adjacent endothelial cells since it appears inconceivable that such pictures could be produced by lateral spreading of the tracer from some distant point of cellular disruption of the endothelial lining.

Beside the described above reversible BBB injury due to osmotic effect, there are, undoubtedly, other mechanisms for the opening of interendothelial tight junctions. Endothelial contraction induced by histamin-type mediators has been demonstrated by Majno et al. [21]. An interesting alteration of the BBB, which potentially could be of great significance for the problem of BE, has been observed with regard to serotonin. A traumatic serotonin release into the cerebro-spinal fluid was originally demonstrated by Sachs [30]. Later, Misra et al. [22] reported serotonin in CSF following acute cerebrovascular accidents and quadriplegia. Most recently, Osterholm et al. [26] have shown serotonin elevation in CSF, as well as in various parts of the brain after experimental head trauma. The production of BE itself by intracerebral injection of serotonin was first described by Bulle [5]. This finding was confirmed by Osterholm et al. [26] who reported that minute amounts of serotonin induced a marked edema of the injected cat hemisphere. Concerning the mode of action it has been shown in tissues other than brain that serotonin 1) acts on endothelial cellular cement loosening

2

up intercellular junctions [20] and 2) it produces a constriction of the venules [8]. The mechanism of serotonin action on cerebrovascular permeability is being currently investigated in our laboratory by Westergaard and Brightman (unpublished). In this study, since serotonin does not penetrate the BBB, is has been introduced into the brain parenchyma by intraventricular perfusion, whereas horseradish peroxidase tracer has been injected systemically.

The preliminary EM observations indicate that in regions of the brain penetrated by serotonin from ventricular lumen the capillary permeability to peroxidase remains unaffected; on the other hand, there is s striking presence of peroxidase showing invasion of vascular walls of blood vessels larger than capillaries. Thus it can be concluded that in the brain serotonin does not act on endothelial tight junctions themselves but when it reaches from outside a blood vessel endowed with cellular elements more than endothelium it conceivably produces a contraction of these elements resulting in a secondary opening of endothelial tight junctions allowing a penetration of proteins such as peroxidase tracer. This observation alone, on ability of serotonin to affect the permeability of cerebral blood vessels, should justify more extensive studies on other biogenic amines with regard to their potential role in dynamics of vasogenic BE.

An interesting behaviour of cerebrovascular permeability has been observed in cerebral ischemia. In experiments by Olsson and Hossmann [24], after a period of ischemia produced by clamping major arterial supply, an application of strongly damaging BBB agents failed to produce an increased vascular permeability. It almost appears that ischemia leads to some physicochemical alterations resulting in a "tighter" adherence of the interendothelial tight junctions. Such postischemic resistance of the BBB may persist for several days. Eventually, the ischemic necrosis of the tissue disrupts physically the continuity of the blood vessels and the resulting leakage persists until there is reconstitution of new vascular channels with normally functioning BBB. This invariably occurs after an elapse of approximately 3 weeks irrespective of the size of the ischemic infarct [25].

In general, the observations presented above emphasize the *diversity of mechanisms* which may be operative in inducing increased cerebrovascular permeability – a crucial pathogenic event in vasogenic BE.

After penetration of the endothelial barrier the serum contents are free to migrate through the extracellular spaces. Their spreading, however, shows a striking predilection for the white matter, regardless of the etiology of primary vascular damage. How much structural features of the CNS may account for this predilection can only be speculated. It is conceivable that an advancing front of vasogenic edema encounters less resistance by migrating through extracellular cannels between rather straight and orderly arranged nerve fiber tracts than by pushing through a jungle of tangled cellular structures of the grey matter.

As the area of actual vascular damage and increased permeability in vasogenic edema is usually limited and progression of edema occurs by extravascular migration through extracellular spaces [15], an ultimate extent of edema territory is largely influenced by two factors: 1) the level of systolic blood pressure (SBP) and 2) the duration of vascular injury and opening of the BBB. Simplistically, this resembles a situation with a broken main where the size of the resulting flood will depend mostly on:

3

a) the *pressure* in the pipe system and b) the *time* the flooding remains unchecked.

The effect of SBP on the extent of vasogenic edema has been clearly demonstrated [15]. Thus, elevating SBP about 100 mm of mercury from initial levels in the experimental cold lesion model results in edema reaching its maximal 24 hours peak within a few hours. Conversely, lowering the SBP produces a dramatic inhibition of edema development. The latter should be kept well in mind when evaluating various therapeutic measures. For example, it is still uncertain to what extent the seemingly beneficial effect of hypothermia can be attributed to the lowering of the tissue metabolic rate or to the lowering of the SPB. Also, in recent investigations on controlling edema by administration of substances interfering with catecholamines synthesis their pharmacological effect could be confused with the effect of severe hypotension which some of these compounds produce.

The duration of leakage from the injured blood vessels is of unquestionable relevance for the ultimate extent of vasogenic edema. Several situations in this regard might be pertinent. A brief, reversible disturbance of the BBB, which otherwise can be conspicuously demonstrated with dye indicators, will not allow escape of serum contents in amounts to term the involved brain tissue edematous. Such transitional BBB disturbances we have encountered, in addition to the osmotic injury mentioned, mostly in experimental conditions in which a vascular spasm appeared to be significantly involved. A reversible BBB opening without appreciable edema was observed in acute elevation of SBP [12], air embolism, acute asphyxia [23], etc. When the BBB opening persists for a longer time edema invariably develops and consistently its spread shows a conspicuous predilection for the white matter, even though the primary vascular injury is frequently located within the grey matter. If the vascular damage is associated with destruction of endothelial lining, its repair and reestablishment of the BBB will depend on how massive and how completely necrotic was the lesion, as well as, on the persistence of pathogenic factors of a primary lesion. For example, in our experimental cold lesion model the abnormal vascular leakage within the necrotized upper layers of the cortex persists for about two days, and restoration of the normal vascular permeability in this area coincides with beginning of edema resolution [15]. The duration of increased cerebrovascular permeability in an ischemic infarct has been described above. It can be assumed that in conditions such as brain tumors, abscesses, etc. where the pathogenic factors are of persistent nature the abnormal cerebrovascular permeability may stay equally chronic.

The vasogenic type of BE is, unquestionably, clinically most important and common. As much as we presently know about the dynamics of its development, the aspects of its resolution remain obscure. The only conspicuous finding from our studies pertains to a morphological evidence of uptake of extravasated protein tracers by cells of mesodermal origin (pericytes, microglia) with suggestion of a transport towards blood vessels, subarachnoidal and ventricular spaces.

The *cytotoxic* type of BE remains much less explored and understood than the vasogenic type. As stated previously [14], the basic mechanism in cytotoxic edema is related to an effect of a pathogenic factor *directly* on cellular elements of brain parenchyma causing their swelling. Since in this case the crucial event is the intracellular shift of water, which itself passes freely through the BBB, the status of cerebrovascular permeability is of no significance here and the BBB may remain entirely intact.

4

However, it is now generally accepted that the BBB phenomenon involves more than impairment to the passage of substances at the tight junction level and that BBB function includes also complex mechanisms for homeostatic regulation of chemical environment of brain parenchyma, among them active and facilitated transport systems. The latter could be easily affected in conditions where a cytoxic agent, in addition to inducing intracellular fluid uptake, is also responsible for alteration of brain tissue metabolic requirements.

A typical picture of cytotoxic BE can be observed in an area of ischemic infarction, where EM observations reveal an extreme swelling of cellular elements of the parenchyma, frequently associated with rupture of cell membranes. Of special interest in this connection are the observations of Hossmann and Olsson [11] who reported a remarkable suppression of mentioned tissue changes and a recovery of neuronal function if during the period of ischemia the brain was continuously perfused with a saline solution. These findings seem to indicate that it is not the deficiency of oxygen supply *per se* but an accumulation of metabolic waste products, such as lactic acid, which may be responsible for acute hydropic and destructive alterations of the brain tissue cellular elements in ischemia. This interpretation is also supported by the fact that our own efforts, as well as, of Dr. Pappius and her coworkers (personal communication) to induce experimentally a BE in anoxic conditions with retained blood circulation were persistently unsuccessful, whereas Bakay and Bendixen [12] reported that only when hypoxia was associated with considerable hypercapnia was there evidence of increased cerebrovascular permeability to proteins and incipient BE.

Until recently the triethyl tin poisoning has been one of the most typical examples of cytotoxic BE. In this condition triethyl tin, bypassing the BBB, specifically affects the myelin sheaths inducing a splitting of myelin lamellae, intramyelinic vacuole formation and a general, striking edema of the white matter [1, 18].

Most recently our laboratory became involved in investigations on a similarly interesting condition, namely – the effect of hexachlorophene on the brain. This substance has been extensively used as a germicidal agent and also has been recommended as a broad spectrum fungicide and bactericide [7]. In one investigation reported so far concerning the effect of this substance on the brain Kimbrough and Gaines [13] found a severe edema limited to the white matter which showed an intense vacuolization of myelin. In our current studies on the effect of hexachlorophene all tested animals (rats, rabbits and monkeys) proved to be susceptible to this compound. In addition to white matter involvement (Fig. 1), edematous changes were also apparent in the basal ganglia (Fig. 2). The cerebral cortex appeared at first to be resistant, however, in the monkey we have found a conspicuous swelling of subpial unmyelinated nerve fibers. Clinically, the animals given hexachlorophene showed tremors, ataxia and paralyses, especially of the lower extremities; in monkeys it was possible to observe a definite papilloedema. There were no changes in cerebrovascular permeability to protein tracers; on the other hand glucose transport was strikingly elevated. Since with proper manipulation of the dosage the edematous hexachlorophene changes can be made chronic or reversible, the study of this model appears to be especially suitable for the elucidation of various biochemical events in hydropic alteration and for studying the ways of reducing or preventing the cytotoxic edema.

The foregoing review summarizes briefly some progress in understanding basic pathophysiological aspects of BE. The amount of this new data appears rather unim-

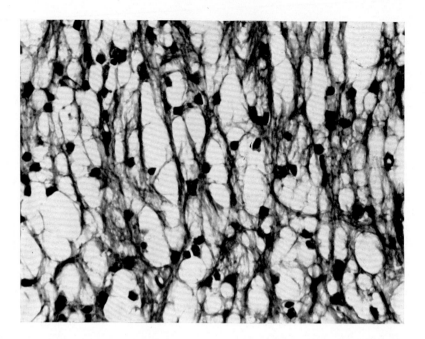

Fig. 1. Rat given 15 mgm/kg of hexachlorophene daily for 2 weeks. The extreme vacuolization of the white matter. Hematoxylin and eosin; × 260

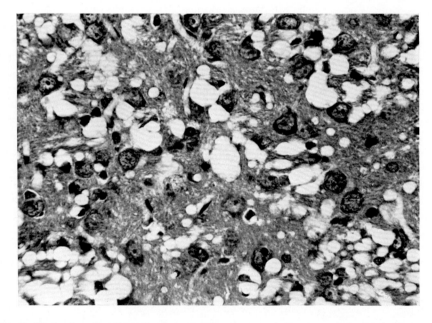

Fig. 2. Thalamic region from the same rat. Numerous vacuoles are conspicuous in the neuropil. The nerve cells appear well preserved. Hematoxylin and eosin; × 460

6

pressive, especially in view of undiminished urgent need for clinical management of this condition. Undoubtedly, some empirical approaches and clinical trials may bring some spectacularly beneficial results. Nonetheless, our efforts towards understanding the basic mechanisms must continue as this offers solid promise for eventual comprehensive control of BE.

References

1. Aleu, F. P., Katzman, R., Terry, R. D.: Fine structure and electrolyte analyses of cerebral edema induced by alkyl tin intoxication. J. Neuropath. exp. Neurol. **22**, 403 (1963).
2. Bakay, L., Bendixen, H. H.: Central nervous system vulnerability in hypoxic states: Isotope uptake studies. *In:* Selective Vulnerability of the Central Nervous System in Hypoxaemia. McMenemey, W. H., Schade, J. F. (Eds.), Oxford: Blackwell Scient. Publ. p. 63, 1963.
3. Brightman, M. W.: The intracerebral movement of proteins injected into blood and cerebrospinal fluid of mice. *In:* Brain Barrier Systems. Lajtha, A., Ford, D. H. (Eds.) Progress in Brain Research, Vol. 29, pp. 19–37, Amsterdam: Elsevier 1968.
4. — Reese, T. S.: Junctions between intimately apposed cell membranes in the vertebral brain. J. Cell Biol. **40**, 648–677 (1969).
5. Bulle, P. H.: Effects of reserpine and chlorpromazine in prevention of cerebral edema and reversible cell damage. Proc. Soc. exp. Biol. **94**, 553–556 (1957).
6. Gonatas, N. K., Zimmerman, H. M., Levine, S.: Ultrastructure of inflammation with edema in the rat brain. Amer. J. Path. **42**, 455–469 (1963).
7. Gump, W. S.: Toxicological properties of hexachlorophene. J. Soc. Cosmetic Chemists **20**, 173–184 (1969).
8. Haddy, F. J.: The mechanism of edema production by acetylcholine, serotonin, histamine and norepinephrine. Fed. Proc. **19**, 93 (1960).
9. Hirano, A., Zimmerman, H. M., Levine, S.: The fine structure of cerebral fluid accumulation. III. Extracellular spread of cryptococcal polysaccharides in the acute stage. Amer. J. Path. **45**, 1–19 (1964).
10. — Zimmerman, H. M., Levine, S.: Fine structure of cerebral fluid accumulation. X. A review of experimental edema in the white matter. *In:* Klatzo, I., Seitelberger, F. (Eds.) Brain Edema. pp. 569–589, Berlin-Heidelberg-New York: Springer 1967.
11. Hossmann, K. A., Olsson, Y.: Suppression and recovery of neuronal function in transient cerebral ischemia. Brain Res. **22**, 313–325 (1970).
12. Johansson, B., Li, C. L., Olsson, Y., Klatzo, I.: The effect of acute arterial hypertension on the blood-brain barrier to protein tracers. Acta neuropath. (Berl.) **16**, 117–124 (1970).
13. Kimbrough, R. D., Gaines, T. B.: Hexachlorophene effects on the rat brain. Study of high doses by light and electron microscopy. Arch. Environmental Health **23**, 114–118 (1971).
14. Klatzo, I.: Neuropathological aspects of brain edema; Presidential address. J. Neuropath. exp. Neurol. **26**, 1–14 (1967).
15. — Wisniewski, H., Steinwall, O., Streicher, E.: Dynamics of cold injury edema. *In:* Klatzo, I., Seitelberger, F. (Eds.) Brain Edema, pp. 554–563, Berlin–Heidelberg–New York: Springer 1967.
16. Lampert, P., Carpenter, S.: Electron microscopic studies on the vascular permeability and the mechanism of demyelination in experimental allergic encephalomyelitis. J. Neuropath. exp. Neurol. **24**, 11–24 (1965).
17. — Garro, F., Pentschew, A.: Lead encephalopathy in suckling pigs. *In:* Klatzo, I. Seitelberger, F. (Eds.) Brain Edema, pp. 413–425, Berlin-Heidelberg New York: Springer 1967.
18. Lee, J. C., Bakay, L.: Ultrastructural changes in the edematous central nervous system. I. Triethyl tin edema. Arch. Neurol **13**, 48–57 (1965).
19. — Bakay, L.: Ultrastructural changes in the edematous central nervous system. II. Cold induced edema. Arch. Neurol. **14**, 36–49 (1966).

7

20. Majno, G., Palade, G. E.: Studies on inflammation. I. The effect of histamine and serotonin on vascular permeability: An electron microscopic study. J. biophys. biochem. Cytol. **11**, 571–605 (1961).
21. — Shea, S. M., Leventhal, M.: Endothelial contraction induced by histamin-type mediators; an electron microscopic study. J. Cell Biol. **42**, 647–672 (1969).
22. Misra, S. S., Singh, K. S. P., Ghargava, K. P.: Estimation of 5-hydroxytryptamine (5 HT) level in cerebrospinal fluid of patients with intracranial or spinal lesions. J. Neurol. Neurosurg. Psychiatr. **30**, 163–165 (1967).
23. Mossakowski, M. J., Long, D. M., Myers, R. E., Rodriguez, H., Klatzo, I.: Early histochemical changes in perinatal asphyxia. J. Neuropath. exp. Neurol. **27**, 500–516 (1968).
24. Olsson, Y., Hossmann, K. A.: Vulnerability of the blood-brain barrier (BBB) to proteins after cerebral ischemia. J. Neuropath. exp. Neurol. **29**, 125 (1970).
25. — Crowell, R. M., Klatzo, I.: The blood-brain barrier to protein tracers in focal cerebral ischemia and infarction caused by occlusion of the middle cerebral artery. Acta Neuropath. (Berl.) **18**, 89–102 (1971).
26. Osterholm, J. L., Bell, J., Myer, R., Pyenson, J.: Experimental effects of free serotonin on the brain and its relation to brain injury. Part I: The neurological consequences of intracerebral serotonin injections. Part 2: Trauma induced alterations in spinal fluid and brain. Part 3: Serotonin induced cerebral edema. J. Neurosurg. **31**, 408–421 (1969).
27. Rapoport, S. T., Hori, M., Klatzo, I.: Reversible osmotic opening of the blood-brain barrier. Science **173**, 1026–1028 (1971).
28. Reese, T. S., Karnovsky, M. J.: Fine structural localization of the blood-brain barrier to exogenous peroxidase. J. Cell. Biol. **34**, 207–217 (1967).
29. Reichardt, M.: Zur Entstehung des Hirndrucks. Dtsch. Z. Nervenheilk. **28**, 306 (1904).
30. Sachs, E., Jr.: Acetylcholine and serotonin in the spinal fluid. J. Neurosurg. **14**, 22–27 (1957).

Functional Aspects of Abnormal Protein Passage Across the Blood-Brain Barrier

K.-A. Hossmann and Y. Olsson*

Max-Planck-Institute for Brain Research, Cologne-Merheim, W. Germany, and Institute of Pathology, University of Upsala, Sweden

With 3 Figures

Summary. The influence of functional disturbances of the brain to the passage of circulating protein tracers in a standardized chemical blood-brain barrier lesion was studied in cats subjected to different periods of global cerebral ischemia. Ischemia was produced by arterial clamping, and the chemical lesion by intracarotid injection of mercuric chloride. When ischemia was long enough to cause depolarization of the cell membranes, the chemical lesion failed to provoke extravasation of the protein tracers. In normal animals and in those which functionally had recovered from ischemia, the tracer passed through the endothelial lining of the cerebral vessels and spread into the intercellular spaces. It is concluded that abnormal passage of circulating proteins in vasogenic brain edema depends not only on the vascular lesion but also on the functional state of the brain.

Introduction

The recent finding of Rapoport *et al.* [9] on the reversible opening of tight junctions and its relation to brain edema has thrown a new light on the pathomechanism of abnormal protein passage across the blood-brain barrier (BBB). It appears from this investigation that in vasogenic brain edema macromolecules may leak between the endothelial cells of the brain capillaries which in the normal state are fused together by tight junctions [1]. This implies that tight junctions are not static contacts between endothelial cells but may be formed and released by cellular changes, e.g. cytoplasmic contractions [9].

The possibility of changes in the properties of interendothelial cell junctions has also been discussed in another experimental condition [7]. Extravasation of serum proteins caused by standardized chemical and hemodynamic lesions was inhibited by a period of transient ischemia which was severe enough to completely suppress neuronal function. The inhibition was reversible and disappeared when neuronal function returned. It is obvious that both the changes in the behaviour of the blood-brain barrier and the suppression of neuronal function were related to the metabolic disorder in ischemia. The reason for the inhibition of abnormal protein passage, however, remains unclear as long as the exact pathomechanism of protein exudation in vasogenic edema has not been solved.

---

* The experiments reported here were performed in the Laboratory of Neuropathology and Neuroanatomical Sciences, N. I. H., Bethesda Md., and in the Cologne laboratory.

9

A precondition for the study of this question is the precise morphological localization of protein tracers by which the route of exudation from the vessel lumen into the brain parenchyma can be determined. In the present investigation the protein tracers Evans blue and peroxidase were used for this purpose. Evans blue has a strong affinity to serum proteins and can be traced macroscopically and on the cellular level by fluorescence microscopy [11]. Small amounts of horseradish peroxidase are demonstrated enzymatically by the method of Graham and Karnovsky [5], and can be localized by both light and electron microscopy.

With this technique protein exudation was investigated in a standardized chemical blood-brain barrier lesion which was produced by intracarotid injection of mercuric chloride [3]. The lesions were preceeded by different periods of global cerebral ischemia and the functional impact on the cerebral cortex was controlled by neurophysiological methods.

Material and Methods

Animal preparation. The experiments were performed in adult cats. The animals were anaesthetized by a single intraperitoneal injection of 30 mg/kg sodium pentobarbital, immobilized with 10 mg/kg gallamine triethiodide and mechanically ventilated with room air. Body temperature, arterial blood pressure and end-tidal CO_2 were monitored and kept within physiological limits.

Production of Increased Cerebrovascular Permeability. Increased vascular permeability was produced by intracarotid injection of a 6×10^{-5} solution of mercuric chloride in saline according to the technique of Flodmark and Steinwall [3]. The right carotid artery was exposed and cannulated with a polyethylene tube. The solution of mercuric chloride was injected in 30 sec through the carotid catheter under a pressure high enough to expel the blood from the pial vessels. This was controlled microscopically by observing the cortical surface through a window in the skull. The volume of the injected solution depended on the blood pressure and varied between 30 and 50 ml.

Production of ischemia. The chest was opened from the left dorsolateral side and the innominate and the left subclavian arteries were exposed close to their origin at the aortic arch. Global cerebral ischemia was produced by clamping these vessels without blocking the venous outflow from the brain. In some animals the resulting increase in arterial blood pressure was counterbalanced by infusion of a ganglion blocking agent (camphor sulfonate). At the end of the ischemic period the clamps were removed and a vasoactive agent (Novadral or norepinephrine) was infused to prevent postischemic hypotension.

Neurophysiological methods. The functional impact of ischemia was assessed by recording the electrocorticogram and the response in the pyramidal tract following an electrical stimulation of the motor cortex, as has been described elsewhere [7]. In some animals cortical impedance was assessed by a four electrodes technique [6]. The electrodes were inserted in a row 1.5 mm under the surface of the right suprasylvian gyrus. A constant current pulse was passed through the outer electrodes and impedance was calculated from the voltage drop across the inner electrodes.

10

Tracers and morphological techniques. The protein tracers Evans blue and horseradish peroxidase were injected intravenously immediately before the production of the blood-brain barrier lesion, and the animals were allowed to survive about 30 min. Evans blue was localized macroscopically and fluorescence microscopically according to the technique of Steinwall and Klatzo [11]. Peroxidase was traced light and electron microscopically according to the technique of Reese and Karnovsky [10].

Results

An arrest of the cerebral blood flow by arterial clamping causes a rapid suppression of the energy producing metabolism which is reflected by typical changes in the functional state of the neurons (Fig. 1). When ischemia is complete, the EEG is suppressed within 15 sec, synaptic transmission – as evidenced by the suppression of the I waves in the pyramidal response (PR) – is abolished in 2–4 min, and the cell membranes start to depolarize after 4–6 min. When ischemia is incomplete, these times may be considerably longer.

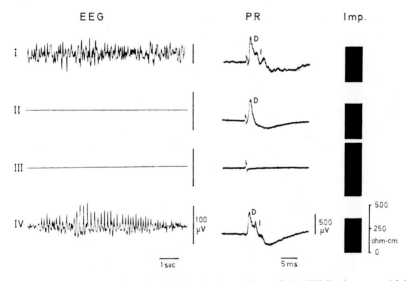

Fig. 1. Functional sequel of cerebral ischemia. Recording of the EEG, the pyramidal response (PR) and cortical impedance (Imp.). The stages I–IV correspond to the four experimental groups. I. normal EEG, PR and impedance prior to ischemia. II. Suppression of the EEG and the I-waves of the PR after 3 min ischemia; cortical impedance has not yet changed. III. Suppression of both the EEG and the PR, and increase in impedance after 20 min ischemia. IV. Return of the EEG and normalization of the PR and impedance 1 h after ischemia

The depolarization of the cell membranes can be precisely evaluated by neurophysiological means. It is reflected by a sudden negative shift in the cortical steady potential (terminal depolarization, [2]), and by the suppression of electrical nerve cell excitability such as the D wave of the pyramidal response. At the same time cerebral impedance begins to rise because ions and fluid shift from the extracellular into the intracellular compartment [12].

When the cerebral blood circulation is restored recovery of neuronal function occurs in reverse order. The restoration of the energy metabolism causes a repolarisation of the cell membranes accompanied by a decrease in cerebral impedance and a gradual return of neuronal excitability. Synaptic transmission and EEG activity return as soon as cerebral impedance and the cortical steady potential have normalized [6].

Intracarotid infusion of mercuric chloride was timed in relation to the functional sequel of ischemia (Tab. 1, Fig. 1). One group, serving as the controls, was not subjected to cerebral ischemia. In the second group, ischemia was long enough to suppress the EEG and the I waves of the pyramidal response (PR), but not the D wave. The third group was subjected to ischemia long enough to suppress both the EEG and the pyramidal response. The fourth group had functionally recovered from the preceding ischemia before the chemical lesion was performed.

Table 1. Summary of the results on the effect of ischemia on the exudation of protein tracers produced by intracarotid infusion of mercuric chloride

Group	Total nr of cats	Nr of cats with exudation
I. No ischemia (Controls)	6	6
II. Ischemia without suppression of PR	10	9
III. Ischemia with suppression of PR	13	2
IV. Ischemia with recovery of PR	4	4

I. BBB Damage without Preceding Ischemia

Exudation of protein tracers, Evans blue and horseradish peroxidase, occurred already 5–10 min after the intracarotid injection of mercuric chloride. It was clearly defined on the side of injection (Fig. 2). Macroscopically, there were multiple rounded areas with abnormal blue staining due to exudated Evans blue. The extent of these areas varied among the individual animals; in some animals there was an extensive confluent staining of predominantly grey matter, in other animals the blue areas were confined to smaller parts of the cortex.

Light microscopically, Evans blue and horseradish peroxidase were identified in the walls of the vessels, sometimes forming distinct lines which apparently outlined the margins of individual cells. Such a penetration occurred either isolated or in combination with a diffuse exudation of the tracer around the vessels involved.

By electron microscopy, peroxidase was found to be localized in the basement membranes of the vascular walls, surrounding the pericytes and smooth muscle cells (when present) in the media (Fig. 2).

When the tracer was washed out of the vessel lumen by the fixative, the luminal part of the cleft between the endothelial cells did not contain peroxidase; nor did we observe any column of peroxidase through the junctions. The contraluminal part of

12

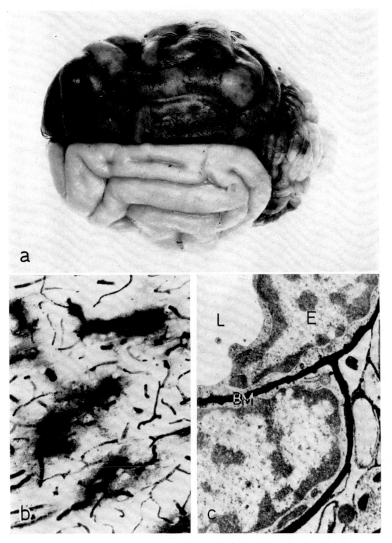

Fig. 2. Vasogenic brain edema following injection of mercuric chloride into the right carotid artery without preceding ischemia (Group I). a) Gross view of the brain after intravenous injection of Evans blue; note the extensive staining of the right hemisphere. b) Light microscopical demonstration of multiple foci of peroxidase extravasation in the cerebral cortex. c) Electron microscopical localization of peroxidase in the basement membrane of a cortical capillary (L: vessel lumen; BM: basement membrane; E: endothelial cell)

the cleft, on the other hand, frequently was filled with the tracer extending from the basement membrane. An opening of the tight junctions and a separation of the endothelial cells was observed only in a very few instances. Since there was no solid column of tracer in these gaps, their intravital origin remains unclarified.

The cytoplasm of the endothelial cells occasionally contained pinocytotic vesicles filled with peroxidase. These vesicles were predominantly confined to the contraluminal part of the endothelial cell cytoplasm close to the basement membrane. A diffuse infiltration of peroxidase into the endothelial cell cytoplasm was rarely observed.

In numerous vessels large amounts of the tracer were found in the cytoplasm of the pericytes where they filled multiple membrane bound vesicles of varying size. These cytoplasmic inclusions appeared under the light microscope as the "perivascular globules" which previously have been described by Steinwall and Klatzo [11] in the same type of edema.

In those areas in which the tracer diffusely penetrated the perivascular tissue ("parenchymatous" type of exudation), there was an extensive spread of the tracer into the intercellular spaces between glial and neuronal processes. Generally, there was no invasion into cells; the tracer penetrated only some neurons in circumscribed areas where it completely filled the cell body and extended into the axon and the dendrites.

The electrophysiological findings depended on the extent of the edema. In those animals in which only small circumscribed areas were stained with the tracer, the EEG and the impedance remained normal. Only during the injection of the mercuric chloride did a transient reduction of the amplitude of the EEG occur and presumably was due to the expelling of the blood by the injected solution.

In other animals in which the staining was extensive and diffuse, EEG amplitude after a free intervall of 5–10 min gradually decreased and occasionally became isoelectric. In these instances impedance continuously rose up to more than twofold the control value.

II. Ischemia without Suppression of the Pyramidal Response

In this group of animals cerebral blood flow was stopped until EEG became isoelectric and until synaptic transmission was abolished, but care was taken to restore the cerebral circulation before changes in the electrical excitability of the pyramidal tract neurons occurred. Consequently, the cell membranes remained polarized and cerebral impedance did not increase.

Immediately after the end of ischemia, mercuric chloride was injected into the carotid artery, and extravasation of the circulating protein tracers was observed as in the first group. In 9 out of 10 animals exudation of the tracer occurred in the hemisphere on the side of the injection. In 8 animals exudation was already macroscopically visible by the blue staining of the brain, and in one animal numerous small areas were detected under the dissection microscope. The fluorescence and the electron microscopic localization of the tracer was the same as that in nonischemic animals subjected to the same lesion.

III. Ischemia with Suppression of the Pyramidal Response

The experimental situation was similar to that of the second group, but the arterial blood supply to the brain was interrupted until both the EEG and the pyramidal response were completely suppressed, and ischemia was then continued for another 2–20 min (total duration of ischemia 10–30 min). Cerebral impedance in this group was increased up to twice the pre-ischemic value before the blood flow was restored.

In 13 out of 15 animals in this group, injection of mercuric chloride immediately after the end of ischemia did not produce any abnormal exudation of the circulating protein tracers (Fig. 3). Although in some animals severe morphological changes were

14

observed in the endothelial cells, neither a diffuse nor a pinocytotic uptake of the tracer occurred and the interendothelial tight junctions remained intact. In only 2 animals, a few vessels showed an abnormal permeability microscopically, however these changes were so discrete that no staining was observed under the dissection microscope.

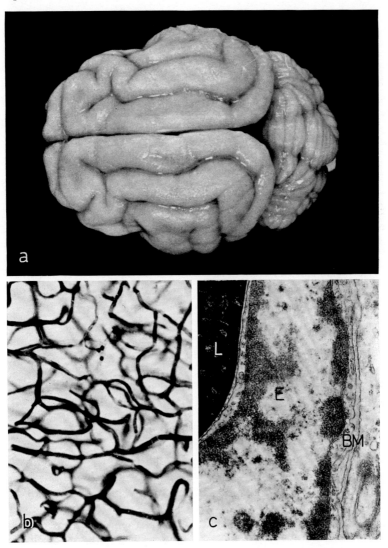

Fig. 3. Absence of protein exudation following intracarotid injection of mercuric chloride in animals subjected to ischemia with suppression of the pyramidal response (Group III). a) Gross view of the brain; Evans blue was injected intravenously and the brain was fixed by perfusion. Note the absence of Evans blue exudation. b) Light microscopical distribution of peroxidase in a brain which has been fixed by immersion. The tracer remains confined to the vessel lumen. c) Electron micrograph of a cortical capillary: the tracer is visible in the vessel lumen but does not penetrate the vascular endothelium (L: vessel lumen; BM: basement membrane; E: endothelial cell)

IV. Ischemia with Recovery of Neuronal Function

The close time relationship between the suppression of the pyramidal response and the failure of protein exudation following the chemical lesion led to the question: would extravasation occur when the pyramidal response has recovered after a period of transient ischemia? Four animals were subjected to an ischemia of 15–20 min, and the intracarotid injection of mercuric chloride was performed about 1 h later when the pyramidal response had fully recovered and when cerebral impedance had normalized.

In all of these cases marked exudation of the tracers occurred as in nonischemic cats subjected to the same lesion. The electrophysiological alterations were also similar to those of the first group. In the cats with extensive staining of the cerebral cortex cerebral impedance increased and EEG secondarily was suppressed, whereas in one animal with discrete lesions no EEG changes were observed.

Discussion

It appears from the presented material that during and after ischemia the blood-brain barrier undergoes vulnerability changes to the injection of mercuric chloride which chronologically correlate with the changes in the functional state of the brain. The most prominent finding is the failure of abnormal protein passage through the endothelial lining of the vessels when the cell membranes depolarize.

Van Harreveld and Ochs [12] have shown that asphyctic depolarization of the cell membranes (due to the breakdown of the sodium pump) causes a swelling of the cells and a decrease in the size of the extracellular space because ions and fluid shift from the extracellular into the intracellular compartment. Our own calculations on the reduction of the extracellular space in ischemia suggest that the fluid which is shifted into the intracellular compartment amounts to about 10% of the total brain volume [6].

When the osmotic shrinkage of the endothelial cells can cause an opening of the tight junctions [9], ischemic cell swelling, in reverse, may lead to a particularly close contiguity of the barrier cells. This may be the reason that even after prolonged cerebral ischemia the blood-brain barrier does not break down [7].

It should be noted in this context, that global cerebral ischemia regularily is combined with a hemodynamic lesion, because blood pressure in the cerebral vessels suddenly rises from 0 to more than 150 mmHg when the blood flow is restored. Even in the normal brain an induced acute hypertension with an increase of arterial blood pressure of less than 100 mmHg consistently causes vasogenic brain edema [8] which seems to be due to the separation of the barrier cells [4]. An opening of the tight junctions may be prevented by an ischemic swelling of the endothelial cells, and this phenomenon may explain the fact that the even higher blood pressure increase after global ischemia does not cause any abnormal protein passage across the blood-brain barrier.

An argument against the separation of endothelial cells in edema produced by mercuric chloride is the failure of morphological evidence for the interendothelial passage of the circulating tracers. Instead, pinocytotic vesicles in the endothelial cytoplasm containing the protein tracer have been observed, making it impossible to exclude a transendothelial route of exudation. Consequently, both the interendothelial and the transendothelial mode of exudation remain under discussion.

A period of ischemia would interfere with any of the two routes of exudation either indirectly by ischemic cell swelling, or directly by the suppression of an active transport mechanism. An abnormal protein passage in vasogenic brain edema therefore does not depend on the vascular lesion alone, but also on the functional state of the brain.

References

1. Brightman, M. W., Reese, T. S.: Junctions between intimately apposed cell membranes in the vertebrate brain. J. Cell Biol. **40**, 648–677 (1969).
2. Bureš, J., Burešová, O.: Die anoxische Terminaldepolarisation als Indicator der Vulnerabilität der Großhirnrinde bei Anoxie und Ischämie. Pflügers Arch. ges. Physiol. **264**, 325–334 (1957).
3. Flodmark, S., Steinwall, O.: Differentiated effects on certain blood-brain barrier phenomena and on the EEG produced by means of intracarotidally applied mercuric dichloride. Acta physiol. scand. **57**, 446–453 (1963).
4. Giacomelli, F., Wiener, J., Spiro, D.: The cellular pathology of experimental hypertension. V. Increased permeability of cerebral arterial vessels. Amer. J. Path. **59**, 133–160 (1970).
5. Graham, R. C., Karnovsky, M. J.: The early stages of absorption of injected horseradish peroxidase in the proximal tubules of mouse kidney; ultrastructural cytochemistry by a new technique. J. Histochem. Cytochem. **14**, 291–302 (1966).
6. Hossmann, K.-A.: Cortical steady potential. Impedance and excitability changes during and after total ischemia of cat brain. Exp. Neurol. **32**, 163–175 (1971).
7. Hossmann, K.-A., Olsson, Y.: Influence of ischemia on the passage of protein tracers across capillaries in certain blood-brain barrier injuries. Acta neuropath. (Berl.) **18**, 113–122 (1971).
8. Johansson, B., Li, C. L., Olsson, Y., Klatzo, I.: The effect of acute arterial hypertension on the blood-brain barrier to protein tracers. Acta neuropath. (Berl.) **16**, 117–124 (1970).
9. Rapoport, S. I., Hori, M., Klatzo, I.: Reversible Osmotic Opening of the Blood-Brain Barrier. Science **173**, 1026–1028 (1971).
10. Reese, T. S., Karnovsky, M. J.: Fine structural localization of a blood-brain barrier to exogenous peroxidase. J. Cell Biol. **34**, 207–217 (1967).
11. Steinwall, O., Klatzo, I.: Selective vulnerability of the blood-brain barrier in chemically induced lesions. J. Neuropath. exp. Neurol. **25**, 542–559 (1966).
12. Van Harreveld, A., Ochs, S.: Cerebral impedance changes after circulatory arrest. Amer. J. Physiol. **187**, 180–192 (1956).

The Effects of Hypertonic Urea on the Blood-Brain Barrier and on the Glucose Transport in the Brain

Maria Spatz, Zbigniew M. Rap, Stanley I. Rapoport, and Igor Klatzo

Laboratory of Neuropathology and Neuroanatomical Sciences, National Institute of Neurological Diseases and Stroke, Bethesda, MD, USA, and Laboratory of Neurophysiology, National Institute of Mental Health, Bethesda, MD, USA

With 6 Figures

Summary. The effects of hypertonic urea on the blood-brain barrier (BBB) were studied in rabbits perfused through the internal carotid artery. Hypertonic urea solution produced two groups of barrier damage. In the first group, damage was irreversible and was associated with brain edema and hyperemia. These animals had an increased uptake of glucose which could not be self-inhibited as determined by a double-tracer technique. The second group of animals had reversible or partially reversible BBB damage without edema or hyperemia. Glucose uptake was increased also in those animals but could be self-inhibited. These results suggest that when hypertonic urea produces reversible or partially reversible barrier damage it also stimulates brain uptake of glucose by facilitated diffusion.

Introduction

Intravenous hypertonic solutions have been used as treatment for the reduction of intracranial pressure in cerebral edema [1, 2]. Recently, a different aspect concerning the effect of hypertonic solutions on the brain was described by Rapoport, Hori, and Klatzo [17, 18]. They demonstrated a reversible blood-brain barrier (BBB) breakdown when some concentrated solutions of electrolytes and relatively lipid insoluble non-electrolytes, such as urea, were applied to the surface of the pia-arachnoid of the rabbit brain. They suggested that these solutions open the tight junctions between endothelial cells by osmotically shrinking the cells, as has been confirmed recently with electron microscopy [3]. Theses observations have been extended by studying the effect of hypertonic solutions by the intracarotid route in order to relate the opening of BBB to brain function and possibly to brain edema.

In this paper, we present a part of our study on barrier breakdown by hypertonic urea and on the effect of this treatment on uptake of glucose analogues by the brain. Perfusion of hypertonic urea produced two distinct groups of animals of which one was associated with brain edema. The common denominator for both groups was the BBB injury which permitted a free passage of protein tracers, but showed a differential effect for the diffusion of glucose from blood to brain.

Methods

Young adult rabbits weighing 1.5–3.0 kg were used in groups of 3–9 animals for these experiments. Under sodium pentobarbital anesthesia (in concentration 25 mg/ml/kg

19

body weight), a polyethylene tube was inserted into the left common carotid artery just below the bifurcation of the external and internal carotid arteries. The external carotid was ligated in order to perfuse directly into the left internal carotid artery according to Steinwall and Steinwall and Klatzo [21, 22]. The solutions used were 2 and 3 molar urea, normal saline and Ringer. Their pH was adjusted to 7.4 with a few drops of NaH_2PO_4 solution. All solutions were warmed to 37° C before injection.

I. Reversibility of BBB breakdown in rabbits perfused with urea solutions was studied with sequential use of two barrier tracers. Na fluorescein (10% in isotonic saline) was injected intravenously (0.5 ml/kg) preceding perfusion and Evans blue (2% in isotonic saline) was administered intravenously (2 ml/kg) immediately or at 15, 30, 45 min, 1, 3, 6, 12 or 24 h after perfusion. Evans blue was allowed to circulate either for 15 min or for 30–60 min before sacrificing the animals. Rabbits injected with isotonic saline or with Ringer solution via the internal carotid artery served as controls.

II. To evaluate some functional aspects of osmotic breakdown, the brain uptake of glucose analogues was studied 10 min after intracarotid urea perfusion. A modified Oldendorf double-isotope technique was applied to measure differential brain uptake of tracers injected as a mixture intracarotidally 15 sec prior to the decapitation of the rabbit [12]. In this method, ^3H_2O is used as reference, with which the uptake of a ^{14}C labeled substance, such as ^{14}C 2-deoxy-D-glucose or ^{14}C 3-0-methyl-D-glucose, is compared. The isotopes were purchased from the New England Nuclear Corporation, Boston, Massachusetts. For the inhibition studies, the injected mixture contained both labeled and unlabeled 2-deoxy-D-glucose or D-glucose. Each brain was removed quickly and carefully examined for the presence or absence of hyperemia. The samples were taken from the temporo-latero-occipital regions of the left and right hemispheres and from the underlying basal ganglia. The tissues were homogenized, weighed and solubilized for radioisotope counting in a Beckman liquid scintillation counter (Model LS-250). The same procedures were used for the study of control rabbits which received saline or Ringer's solution instead of urea. The brain uptake index (BUI) was calculated as follows:

$$BUI = \frac{\text{Tissue } ^{14}C/\text{Tissue } ^3H}{\text{Injected Mixture } ^{14}C/\text{Injected Mixture } ^3H} \times 100$$

Additional details will be published elsewhere.

III. The histological examination was performed on hematoxylin and eosin stained sections of tissue taken from paraformaldehyde perfused brains. The number, size and shape of brain capillaries were evaluated with the benzidine method of Pickworth on brain sections fixed in 10% buffered formalin [14].

Results

I. Breakdown of the BBB was produced in all rabbits perfused with 2 or 3 molar urea solution via the internal carotid artery. BBB injury was irreversible in those rabbits listed in the Table 1 as Group I rabbits, and reversible in Group II rabbits. In Group I rabbits the left hemisphere was markedly hyperemic and edematous (Fig. 1 and 3). Irreversible BBB injury was demonstrated by the extravasation of both Na fluorescein

(Fig. 2) and Evans blue (Fig. 3) throughout the left hemisphere, ipsilateral to the side of perfusion.

Table 1. The Effect of Hypertonic Urea on the Brain

Group I	Group II
Hyperemia	No Hyperemia
Edema	No Edema
Irreversible BBB[a] Injury	Partially Reversible BBB[a] Injury
Increase Glucose Uptake	Increase Glucose Uptake
No Competitive Inhibition of Glucose Uptake	Competitive Inhibition of Glucose Uptake

[a] BBB – Blood-Brain Barrier

Hyperemia and edema of the brain were absent in Group II animals. The BBB was opened reversibly in these rabbits. Na fluorescein injected prior to urea perfusion was demonstrated by deep green fluorescence in the temporo-latero-occipital region of the left hemisphere. However, no blue staining was found in the brain when Evans blue dye was injected 30 min after urea perfusion and allowed to circulate for 15 min. Even for Group II animals, reversibility of BBB opening was not absolute since some infiltration of Evans blue dye was seen if the dye remained in the circulation for 30–60 min. In summary, it appeared that brain edema was usually associated with irreversible barrier opening and hyperemia which were the characteristics of Group I rabbits.

II. An increased brain uptake of glucose analogues was found in both groups of animals 10 min after intracarotid urea perfusion. The 2-deoxy-D-glucose BUI was 2–3 times greater in hyperemic (Group I) than in control brains. The BUI for 2-deoxy-D-glucose/100 mg tissue was 98.53 ± 3.4 S.E. (n = 3) in moderate and 159.14 ± 13.1 S.E. (n = 4) in severe hyperemia as compared to normal 49.29 ± 2.08 S.E. (n = 9). The uptake of 2-deoxy-D-glucose, as measured by the BUI in 7 rabbits, was not significantly different ($P > 0.05$) if 40 mM of the unlabeled compound was injected with the isotope tracer.

In the nonhyperemic brains of Group II, uptake of 2-deoxy-D-glucose was increased by 50 % above control levels. The BUI/100 mg tissue was 73.65 ± 2.46 S.E. (n = 9) for the urea-perfused animals, and 49.65 ± 2.08 S.E. (n = 9) for the controls. In both control and experimental animals of Group II, self-inhibition of 2-deoxy-D-glucose brain uptake was demonstrated when unlabeled 2-deoxy-D-glucose in different concentrations was injected with ^{14}C labeled 2-deoxy-D-glucose (Figs. 4 and 5). As may be seen from Figure 5, the percent of inhibited 2-deoxy-D-glcuose uptake in brain was the same or higher in the urea -perfused animals than in the Ringer perfused controls. In the experimental animals, K_m for 2-deoxy-D-glucose was 22.5 mM while in the controls it was 37.5 mM. K_m is defined as the concentration required to reduce the BUI of 2-deoxy-D-glucose to one-half its uninhibited BUI (Fig. 5). The control value is not significantly different from the value of 55 ± 12.9 S.E. (n = 5) found by Prather and Wright for the frog choroid plexus, where facilitated diffusion

21

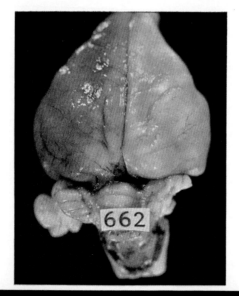

Fig. 1. Hyperemia and edema of left hemisphere. Brain from a rabbit perfused with 3 molar urea via left internal carotid artery

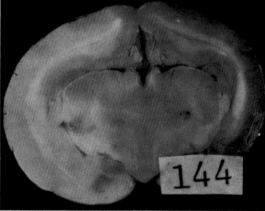

Fig. 2. BBB damage and edema of left hemisphere. Diffuse penetration of Na fluorescein of the cerebral cortex with extention to the basal ganglia. Cross section of a brain from a rabbit perfused with 3 molar urea via left internal carotid artery

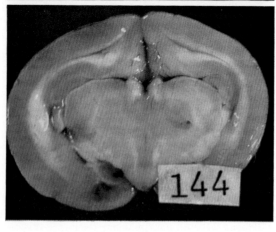

Fig. 3. The same section as in Fig. 2. Note the extravasation of Evans blue dye confined to the same regions as Na fluorescein

of glucose also occurs [15]. Similar findings were observed in animals in which the brain uptake of the nonmetabolizable 3-O-methyl-D-glucose was studied. The BUI for 3-O-methyl-D-glucose was 63.75 ± 1.85 S.E. (n = 4) in urea-treated animals and 30.39 ± 2.88 S.E. (n = 4) in normal. In both experimental and control animals, a 79 % inhibition of 3-O-methyl glucose brain uptake was found with 60 mM glucose.

III. The percent of survivals was 25 with 3 molar and 50 with 2 molar urea 24 h after intracarotid perfusion. Histologically, most of the edematous brains in Group I showed infarcts of variable size with scattered focal hemorrhages. In the nonedematous brains occasional intravascular tiny thrombi were seen too.

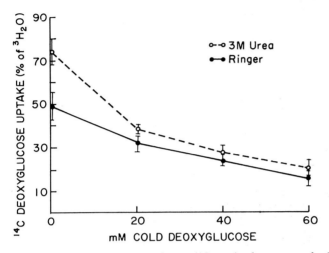

Fig. 4. Self-inhibition of brain 2-deoxy-D-glucose-^{14}C uptake demonstrated with simultaneous injection of unlabeled (cold) 2-deoxy-D-glucose in progressively greater concentrations. Each point of inhibition represents the mean of 4 observations with bars indicating $\pm$ S.D.

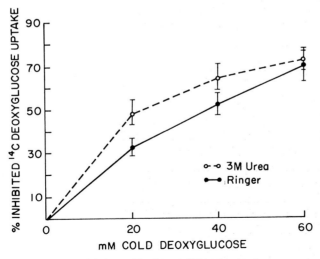

Fig. 5. Percentage of inhibited 2-deoxy-D-glucose-^{14}C brain uptake in experimental and control rabbits. The same experiments as in Fig. 4

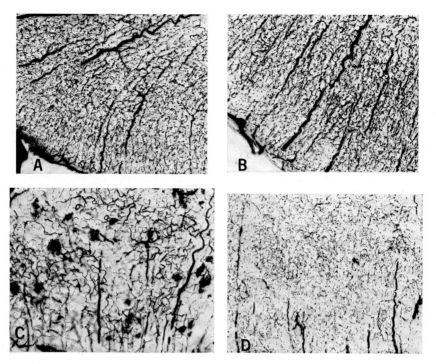

Fig. 6. Brain capillaries in the cerebral cortex: A, B and C ipsilateral to the carotid perfusion; D opposite to the site of perfusion. A with Ringer's solution; B, C and D with 3 molar urea solution. In C severe hyperemia was seen grossly. See text

Ten minutes after intracarotid perfusion with urea, isotonic saline or Ringer, capillaries in both grey and white matter of the left ipsilateral hemisphere were found to be dilated. However, the most striking changes were seen in the urea-treated animals. The number of visible capillaries was increased and many were found also to be markedly tortuous. In the hyperemic brains of Group I, webs of vascular spirals were found adjacent to or surrounding circumscribed areas showing an absence of capillaries. In addition, these brains showed a great number of capillaries bursting with diapedesis of red corpuscles (Fig. 6).

Discussion

The cerebral edema observed in urea-treated rabbits (Group I) was primarily vasogenic in nature as suggested by 1) irreversibly increased permeability to protein and glucose tracers, 2) focal capillary hemorrhages as evident by RBC diapedesis and 3) cerebral infarcts. This type of edema is not unique for urea since it is frequently seen in cerebrovascular, inflammatory and neoplastic diseases, and following head injury [9, 10]. It has been also found in some rabbits following intracarotid perfusion of hypertonic glucose and NaCl [16].

It is likely that the reversibility concept of BBB breakdown by hypertonic solutions by the intracarotid route is correct, but urea turned out not to be the best compound to demonstrate reversibility due to complicating factors. Incomplete reversibility may have been due to 1) a toxic effect of urea in addition to its hypertonic effect on the BBB, 2) a possible incomplete closing of tight junctions in focal regions of the brain, 3) slowing of cerebral circulation and possible anoxia. Although a threshold of 2 molar urea was found when Evans blue was permitted to remain in the brain 15 min, some Evans blue extravasation did appear at any urea concentration if the dye was allowed to circulate longer than 30 min, suggesting an additional toxic effect of urea. The role of other factors might be clarified by electronmicroscopic and circulatory studies of brain of urea-injected animals. We have recently found also that lactamide, which acts reversibly like urea on the pia-arachnoid vessels, gives complete reversibility when perfused intracarotidly [16, 17].

In spite of these limitations, intracarotid hypertonic urea perfusion provided a good model for studying glucose transport and offered new insight into the problem of glucose transfer from blood to brain. In Group I rabbits, irreversible BBB injury was associated with increased entry of [14]C 2-deoxy-D-glucose, and this increase was not inhibited by unlabeled substance. The lack of self-inhibition indicates that increased entry is not by facilitated diffusion, as defined by Crone [6] and Oldendorf [13]. In Group II rabbits, which also showed an increase in BUI for 2-deoxy-D-glucose, self-inhibition was proportional to the concentration of unlabeled material injected with the tracer. This indicates that the increase in BUI represents an increase in facilitated diffusion from blood to brain. These conclusions were supported by similar results obtained with nonmetabolized 3-O-methyl-D-glucose.

The increase in both BUI and facilitated diffusion following urea perfusion could be due to an increased number and size of brain capillaries. However, increased BUI did not occur following perfusion of Ringer or of isotonic saline which also produced moderate increases in capillary size and number. Furthermore, BUI would not be expected to increase if only capillary number increased since brain uptake of ^3H_2O and ^{14}C tracer would be expected to change proportionately. Therefore, it appears unlikely that increased capillary number or size produced the observed increases in BUI and facilitated diffusion.

Since BUI represents the ^{14}C tracer taken up with reference to ^3H_2O, it is possible that the increase is due not to an increased tracer uptake but to a decreased ^3H_2O uptake due to brain dehydration and a smaller compartment for water exchange. While we cannot rule out this possibility, it seems unlikely because the quantity (Tissue ^3H_2O/Injected Mixture ^3H_2O), was not significantly different in urea-treated animals from its value in control animals.

Another possibility is that hypertonic urea stimulated glucose transport by a direct osmotic action at the capillary endothelium. BUI was not increased by intracarotid perfusion of isotonic solutions of NaCl and urea but was increased by hypertonic, 3% NaCl, which opens the blood-brain barrier reversibly [20]. The hypertonic solutions may stimulate glucose uptake by osmotically shrinking capillary endothelium or other glucose transporting or metabolizing cells in the brain. Although hypertonic stimulation has not been demonstrated previously in the brain, it has been found in fat, muscle and yeast cells. [4, 5, 8, 11].

The mechanism for this stimulation is obscure. If glucose transport is chemically coupled to transport of an intracellular constituent, such as Na^+, as was suggested to occur in amino acid transport [19], then cellular dehydration would increase the concentration of the constituent and thereby the driving force for glucose transport. In-

25

creasing external glucose concentration, which also increases the driving force on transport, has an effect similar to dehydration in fat and muscle cells [11]. Another possibility is that the concentration of the glucose carrier in the membrane is changed by dehydration, or that the membrane permeability for glucose is otherwise changed. Dehydration also may stimulate metabolism in cells as reported by Clausen and Kuzuya et al. [4, 11], and therefore increased glucose transport may be associated with its increased cellular utilization.

Recently, Ussing and Diamond elaborated models for transport across epithelial layers with tight junctions and showed that such transport could be modified by osmotically shrinking the cells and increasing the interspace between them [7, 23]. It is possible that the osmotic effects of urea may be due to an increase in diameter of the tight junctions between capillary endothelial cells. The mechanism for the increase in BUI and facilitated diffusion deserves further investigation.

Acknowledgments. The authors are indebted to Miss Madora E. Swink, Mr. Joseph T. Walker, Jr., and Miss Jo Ann Holmes for skillful technical assistance.

References

1. Beks, J. W. F., Groen, A., Huizinga, T., Noordhoek, K. H. N., Smit, J. M., Walter, W. G.: Effects of intravenously administered hypertonic urea solution. Acta neurochir. **13**, 1–10 (1965).
2. — ter Weeme, C. A.: The influence of urea and mannitol on increased intraventricular pressure in cold-induced cerebral oedema. Acta neurochir. **16**, 97–107 (1967).
3. Brightman, M. W., Reese, T. S., Rapoport, S. I., Hori, M., Klatzo, I.: (unpublished observation).
4. Clausen, T.: The relationship between the transport of glucose and cations across cell membranes in isolated tissues. III. Effect of Na^+ and hyperosmolarity on glucose metabolism and insulin responsiveness in isolated rat hemidiaphragm. Biochim. biophys. Acta. (Amst.) **150**, 56–65 (1968).
5. — Gliemann, J., Vinten, J., Kohn, P. G.: Stimulating effect of hyperosmolarity on glucose transport in adipocytes and muscle cells. Biochim. biophys. Acta. (Amst.) **211**, 233–243 (1970).
6. Crone, C.: Facilitated transfer of glucose from blood into brain tissue. J. Physiol. **181**, 103–113 (1965).
7. Diamond, J. M.: Standing gradient model of fluid transport in epithelia. Fed. Proc. **30**, 6–13 (1971).
8. Harden, A., Paine, S. G.: Action of dissolved substances upon the autofermentation of yeast. Proc. Roy. Soc. (Lond.). Series B. **84**, 448–459 (1911–1912).
9. Klatzo, I.: Presidential address. Neuropathological aspects of brain edema. J. Neuropath. exp. Neurol. **26**, 1–14 (1967).
10. — Some early reactions of brain tissue to injury. In: Proc. Int. Symposium on Head Injuries, p. 214–221. Edinburgh, London: Churchill Livingstone 1971.
11. Kuzuya, T., Samols, E., Williams, R. H.: Stimulation by hyperosmolarity of glucose metabolism in rat adipose tissue and diaphragm in vitro. J. biol. Chem. **240**, 2277–2283 (1965).
12. Oldendorf, W. H.: Measurement of brain uptake of radiolabeled substances using a tritiated water internal standard. Brain Res. **24**, 372–376 (1970).
13. — Brain uptake of radiolabeled amino acid, amines and hexoses after arterial injection. Amer. J. Physiol. **221**, 1629–1639 (1971).
14. Pickworth, F. A.: A new method of study of the brain capillaries and its application to the regional localisation of mental disorder. J. Anat. (Lond.) **69**, 62–71 (1934).
15. Prather, J. W., Wright, E. M.: Molecular and kinetic parameters of sugar transport across the frog choroid plexus. J. Memb. Biol. **2**, 150–172 (1970).

16. Rap, Z., Spatz, M., Klatzo, I., Rapoport, S. I.: (unpublished observation).
17. Rapoport, S. I., Hori, M., Klatzo, I.: Reversible osmotic opening of the blood-brain barrier. Science **173**, 1026–1028 (1971).
18. — — — Testing of an hypothesis for osmotic opening of the blood-brain barrier. Amer. J. Physiol. **223** (in press) (1972).
19. Schafer, J. A., Heinz, E.: The effect of reversal of Na^+ and K^+ electrochemical potential gradients on the active transport of amino acids in Ehrlich ascites tumor cells. Biochim. biophys. Acta (Amst.) **249**, 15–33 (1971).
20. Spatz, M., Rapoport, S. I., Rap, Z., Klatzo, I.: (unpublished observation).
21. Steinwall, O.: An improved technique for testing the effect of contrast media and other substances on the blood-brain barrier. Acta Radiol. **49**, 281–284 (1958).
22. — Klatzo, I.: Selective vulnerability of the blood-brain barrier in chemically induced lesions. J. Neuropath. exp. Neutrol. **25**, 542–549 (1966).
23. Ussing, H. H.: The interpretation of tracer fluxes in terms of membrane structure. Quart. Rev. Biophys. **1**, 365–376 (1969).

Molecular Aspects of Membrane Structure in Cerebral Edema

Harry B. Demopoulos, Paul Milvy, Sophia Kakari, and Joseph Ransohoff

Departments of Pathology and Neurology, New York University Medical Center, New York, NY 10016, USA

With 2 Figures

Introduction

Cerebral edema, regardless of the inciting cause, and irrespective of the cellular sites e.g., tight junctions of vascular structures, glial processes, etc., ultimately represents a pertubation of membrane biomolecules that maintain water and solute compartments. Furthermore, it is likely that in the highly organized tissues of the central nervous system more than one membrane system is involved in the pathogenesis of cerebral edema and the neural dysfunctions that may accompany this process.

Most cellular processes depend on critically regulated transmembrane transport of substrates and cofactors, as well as on the solid-state functions of membranes [12] i.e., electron transport and neural conduction.

Cerebral edema and the accompanying dysfunctions are benefited by exogenously administered steroids, possibly by effects on separate membrane systems [14]. Steroids function primarily by affecting membrane structure and ultimately their transport and solid-state functions. A better understanding of how the diverse types of membrane biomolecules, which includes the steroids, interact and affect each other may lead to improved therapy and minimization of cerebral edema.

It is possible that some of the agents and processes that lead to cerebral edema may incite a special form of chemical degradation, known as free radical peroxidation, in key membrane lipids. There are several precedents in other pathologic processes for invoking the concept of free radical pathology in membrane biomolecules [4, 6]. A consideration of the rich lipid content of the CNS, the special susceptibility of lipids to radical damage, and the types of agents and processes that incite cerebral edema suggest that the participation of radical mechanisms in edema be tested.

It may be that the intercalation of steroids into membranes, and free radical damage to membrane lipids are inter-related.

Supported by a grant from the New York Foundation, New York, New York

Membrane Structure and Function

Membrane biomolecules include lipids, proteins, and surface mucopolysaccharides, held together by hydrophobic associations and ionic interactions [2]. Various cations, especially calcium, mix intimately with these biomolecules and strongly influence their structure and function.

The cells' limiting membrane, the plasma membrane, while differing in quantitative ways amongst different cell types, is basically a biomolecular leaflet of phospholipid and other amphipathic (one end of molecule is ionic, the other non-polar) substances like cholesterol [5, 10]. The polar, or hydrophilic ends of these lipid molecules are directed to the outer surfaces of the membrane where they are in contact with the aqueous melieux in, and outside the cell. The hydrophobic ends of these amphipathic lipid molecules are directed towards each other, in a double layer, to form the hydrophobic midzone of the membrane (Fig. 1). Proteins interact with membrane lipids by hydrophobic and ionic forces. Segments of proteins composed of aromatic amino acids will form hydrophobic associations with lipids in the non-polar midzone of membranes, whereas ionic groups in proteins will react with the polar head groups of amphipathic lipids at the membrane's surface. Proteins that intertwine with membrane phospholipids may derive some of their structure needed to keep the enzyme, on *or* off, by such associations. Therefore, events that affect membrane lipids may have ramifications extending to the structure and function of the many membrane-bound enzymes. The structural basis for such lipid-protein interactions, as well as lipid-lipid

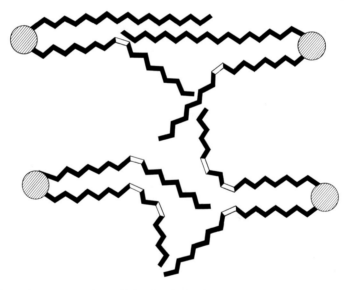

Fig. 1. Schematic representation of bimolecular leaflet of phospholipid molecules, forming the skeleton of a plasma membrane. The circles are the glycerophosphate head groups, which are polar, while the fatty acid tails extend into the hydrophobic midzone. Unsaturated bonds are bent at an angle of 123°, in the cis isomeric configuration, in the fatty acid tails. In the normal membrane there is a saturated carbon separating the two carbons that have unsaturated bonds. This saturated carbon is partly activated and can lose one of its hydrogens quite readily. Note the spaces between the phospholipids. These are the archways for the steroids to intercalate into.

interactions lies in the fact that the fatty acid tails of phospholipids are in the cis (123° bend in chain) isomeric configuration (see Fig. 1). This is quite important because it prevents tight lateral packing of the phospholipids and creates archways and pockets wherein other membrane molecules can insert, e.g., cholesterol, various steroids, and hydrophobic portions of proteins.

Another important feature resulting from the cis configuration of the fatty acids and the lack of tight packing is the maintenance of the fluid state of the membrane. Spin label studies and investigations with freeze-etch fracture methods reveal that the lipids and proteins can have considerable lateral mobility within the membrane [8, 12], analogous to blocks of wood in water. As these pockets, or archways become filled, e.g., by exogenously administered steroids, the membrane becomes less fluid, and more compact. This is sometimes referred to as membrane stabilization [9, 24], but not all steroids do this.

Intercalation of Steroids

Hydrophobic associations, while not in the nature of chemical bonds, nonetheless do serve to keep diverse non-polar molecules close together when they are surrounded by an aqueous melieux. Cellular membranes have water on both sides of their surfaces. It is this aqueous environment that forces the non-polar parts of membrane biomolecules to associate together to form the hydrophobic midzone of membranes. This is the only non-polar area in a cell. When lipoidal materials reach cells after being transported, via complexing to proteins and traveling as serum lipoproteins or other lipid transport mechanisms, they become dissociated from the transport complex and enter the only portions of a cell possible, the membranes. This is true for endogenous and exogenous lipoids, like steroids that are used for various therapies, certain chemical toxins like NO_2, lipoidal chemical carcinogens, etc.

The precise fit of molecules into membranes will depend on their size, shape, and the presence and distribution of charged areas. Many substances are amphipathic, possessing polar and non-polar areas. Examples are the phospholipids, and many steroids. The hydrophobic portion of such substances will enter the midzone, while the charged area will stay close to the membrane surface. Cholesterol supposedly enters and remains perpendicular to the plane of the membrane, while other substances may fit at various angles or to varying degrees of tightness. The association between cholesterol and phospholipids is almost entirely between their hydrophobic portions, and does not involve their charged ends at the membrane surface [18]. The phospholipid fatty acid tails, which are quite loose and "wave" about in the hydrophobic midzone of the membrane, tightly wrap themselves in and about cholesterol molecules and other steroids that may have a similar size, shape, and charge distribution. Because various steroids have different chemical groupings their precise fit into membranes will vary. This is why all steroids do not stabilize membranes.

There are several consequences of steroid-phospholipid interactions. Since membrane bound enzymes may derive some of their structure by hydrophobic associations with the phospholipid tails, anything that will perturb the latter, can have an ultimate affect on the activity of these enzymes. This may be one of the molecular mechanisms whereby steroids affect enzyme activities. The fatty acids that may be dislocated away from a protein and onto steroids may have been playing a structural role to keep the enzyme turned on, *or* off. Another consequence of steroid-phospholipid associations is a degree of protection afforded the fatty acids against their spontaneous chemical degradation by a process known as radical peroxidative damage.

The CNS and Free Radicals

Free radicals are unusually reactive species. Many substances are capable of becoming radicals transiently, and of carrying on the full range of unusual chemical reactions referred to as Kharasch reactions, after the chemist that first described them.

Nerve tissue is most striking chemically because of its enormous lipid content, and biopathologically for its exquisite sensitivities to trauma, hypoxia, and proclivity to undergo *liquefactive* necrosis. Since lipids are the chemical group most prone to free radical damage, the chemical makeup of the CNS and its special pathology may be related by this molecular pathologic mechanism. Other substances like proteins, nucleic acids, carbohydrates, and inorganic molecules can be disarrayed by free radical reactions, but usually require distinctive and powerful physico-chemical agents like ultraviolet light, ionizing radiation, NO_2, chemical carcinogens, etc. Radical production in lipids on the other hand is spontaneous, in the presence of oxygen. Lipid radical reactions can be initiated and catalyzed even in the presence of antioxidants by agents that are common in the central nervous system (heme, cytochromes, cytochrome oxidase, electron transport radicals). It therefore seems that the most important pathologic free radical reactions that may occur in the central nervous system would involve the membrane lipids. In order to test this hypothesis and its role in a variety of neuropathologic situations, including cerebral edema, it is nesessary to have an aquaintenance with free radical chemistry, systems for detecting free radicals and their reactions, and finally to understand how pathologic radical reactions amongst membrane lipids may be prevented or quenched.

Free Radical Reactions

A free radical is any substance that has a lone electron in an outer orbital. Ordinarily electron orbitals are occupied by pairs of electrons, each one of the pair spinning in opposite directions. A lone electron endows the molecule with unusual chemical reactivities and physical properties. Chemically, free radical reactions are different from the typical, so-called Markownikov reactions. The principle reactions are in three categories:

1. Initiation, $X:Y \rightarrow X\cdot + \cdot Y$; A two electron bond is broken to produce two fragments, each of which contains a lone electron. This can occur spontaneously with some substances, like peroxides, $RO:OR \rightarrow 2RO\cdot$, or be facilitated by physical and chemical agents, $Cl_2 \xrightarrow{light} 2\ Cl\cdot$

2. Propagation reactions are one of the main features. These can be in the nature of chain reactions, and are of four types.

a) Atom transfer reactions, usually involving hydrogen, $R\cdot + R'H \rightarrow RH + R'\cdot$; such abstracting is important in lipid radical reactions.

b) Addition reactions, $CH_3\cdot + RCH{=}CH_2 \rightarrow R\overset{\cdot}{C}H{-}CH_2{-}CH_3$

c) Fragmentation reactions

d) Rearrangements.

32

3. Termination, $2R\cdot \rightarrow R:R$. Two free radicals can combine to form a new covalent bond to make a new, larger molecule. These termination reactions, as well as the above addition reactions are important from the point of view of creating anomalous molecular structures in strategic locations, for instance, among the membrane lipids and proteins. Termination reactions are also important with respect to mechanisms for controlling the chain reaction spread of radical reactions. Substances like the thiol amino acids function in this way, cysteine-SH + $R\cdot \rightarrow$ cysteine-S$\cdot$ + RH (hydrogen abstraction first); 2 cysteine-S$\cdot \rightarrow$ cystine (disulfide) (termination reaction) [17].

Physical Detection of Radicals

The unique properties of free radicals allow for their detection and analysis. These physical characteristics derive from the fact that any spinning charged particle will create a magnetic field. Hence protons and electrons generate magnetic fields, albeit weak. When paired electrons occupy an orbital they cancel each others fields because their spins are opposed. A free radical on the other hand, with its unopposed electron, has a weak magnetic field and can thus be detected and analysed by electron paramagnetic resonance (e.p.r.) spectroscopy [16].

The lone electron in a free radical can be represented as a magnetic dipole. When a sample containing free radicals is placed between the pole pieces of an electromagnet, the lone electrons' magnetic dipole acquires two discrete energy levels, about 1 kilocal/mole, apart. If three cm long microwaves are now guided into the radical-containing sample situated between the pole pieces, some of the radical species will absorb the microwave energy and go to the higher energy level. Therefore, e.p.r. spectroscopy can be thought of as a form of induced-microwave absorption spectroscopy, somewhat analogous to U–V and visible light absorption spectroscopy. The e.p.r. signal is plotted by the machine as the first derivative of the absorption signal. The e.p.r. signal acquires a distinctive shape, width and number of lines, depending on the atomic and molecular melieux that the lone electron interacts with. For example, the magnetic field created by a nearby spinning proton will induce two more energy levels in each of the original two that were created for the lone electron, when the sample was first placed between the pole pieces of the electromagnet. With the sample in an electromagnet, a free radical interacting with a single proton will have four energy levels, with two protons, eight energy levels, etc. Therefore, the number of lines in an e.p.r. signal depends on the number of energy levels imposed on the lone electron by its atomic melieux. These lines are referred to as hyperfine structure, and this feature together with the width of the e.p.r. signal, and the g-value (gyromagnetic ratio) provide exact qualitative information. In this way chemically diverse free radicals can not only be identified, but information about the molecular environment of the lone electron can also be obtained.

Antioxidants and Metal Chelators

Antioxidants are agents that can prevent and/or stop radical reactions. They may act at one or multiple points in a complex system of radical reactions. The natural antioxidants are either water soluble or lipid soluble, examples being ascorbic acid and the

33

tocopherols, respectively. Depending on the amount of ascorbic acid present and the specific molecular environment, it may act as a reducing agent to abort radical reactions, or it may act as an oxidant to promote radical reactions.

It has been shown that the antioxidant, diphenylparaphenylene diamine (DPPD), can significantly diminish experimental, cold-induced cerebral edema [13], while another antioxidant, p-ethoxyphenol (EOP), can not. The reason may lie in the different solubilities of the two. DPPD is soluble only in non-polar media, while EOP is water soluble. DPPD would be expected to stop radical reactions occurring in hydrophobic areas, while EOP could only be expected to stop radical reactions that are occurring primarily in an aqueous environment. The naturally occuring antioxidants include both lipid and aqueous acting chemicals. The tocopherols and selenium are probably the main hydrophobic antioxidants, while the thiol amino acids and ascorbic acid act principally in hydrophilic areas. The portion of phospholipids that are liable to free radical damage are the fatty acid tails. The unsaturated ones, and long-chain fatty acids are most sensitive to radical peroxidation, but metal complexes can also start and catalyze this process in the shorter, saturated fatty acids. Many of the metal complexes, like heme, have a preferential solubility in non-polar media, as does oxygen [11, 20]. Thus, the hydrophobic midzone of membranes may be the prime area for radical damage. Oxygen is required for radical reactions [17], and it is 7–8 times more soluble in non-polar media than polar ones [20]. Metal complexes, like heme, increase the rates of spontaneous lipid peroxidation by 5 orders (5,000 times) of magnitude [21]. In view of this enormous catalysis by metals, it may be necessary to use metal chelators to stop undesired radical reactions. Fortunately, some antioxidants have inherent metal chelating properties and this may be an additional factor explaining the differential efficacies of diverse antioxidants.

Free Radical Damage to Membrane Lipids in the CNS

From a chemical point of view, there are only two ways to degrade lipids. One is by free radical reactions, the other by hydrolysis, as with esterases and lipases. In pathologic processes it is possible to activate one, or both mechanisms. Lipid free radical reactions can be initiated, and catalyzed by metal complexes like iron and copper. These are quite powerful and overcome the natural tissue antioxidants that normally can prevent only slow, spontaneous lipid peroxidation. Hence, the presence of heme complexes, as from extravasated blood, cytochromes from ruptured electron transport chains, and copper complexes as found in cytochrome oxidase, can serve to cause free radical damage to membrane lipids. Such initiators also act as catalysts, and are present as part of the picture of traumatic events in the central nervous system (see Table 1 for reactions).

Cerebral edema occurs in a variety of neuropathologic situations. Trauma causes varying degrees of hemorrhage and even without this, there is always enough shearing force to dislocate membrane bound electron transport factors, like the cytochromes, and cytochrome oxidase into critical sites. Normally electron transport is a solid-state function of mitochondrial and endoplasmic reticulum membranes. It takes place along the surfaces of these membranes, just 10–15 Å away from the hydrophobic midzone where the susceptible fatty acid tails are. Trauma can easily cause the dislocation of these metal complexes from the surface, into the middle of the membrane.

34

An additional aspect of this type of mechanism is the fact that the membranes of cell organelles contain far more polyunsaturated fatty acids. This makes them more liable to free radical peroxidation. There is a direct correlation between the degree of unsaturation and rate of peroxidation [7]. Yet another factor that may involve electron transport substances in free radical pathology of membranes is the presence of normally-occurring, controlled radicals within electron transport [22]. There are flavin and coenzyme Q radicals which if dislocated, will start and catalyze abnormal, uncontrolled lipid radical reactions within membranes.

Malignant neoplasms commonly have disordered oxidative and glycolytic metabolic pathways [1, 15]. Recently, it has been shown that tumor mitochondria "leak" electrons because they have poorly structured membranes. These may well produce abnormal radical reactions in tumor cell membranes. Indeed, there are several tumors that have been shown by electron paramagnetic resonance (e.p.r.) spectroscopy to contain high, steady state concentrations of abnormal free radicals, including breast carcinomas, and malignant melanomas [1, 3, 23]. Tumor cells are constantly breaking up, and dying as the tumors grow. This is one simple way whereby the abnormal tumor radicals can be disseminated. Since most of these radicals will be lipoidal they will intercalate into the only possible environment, the membranes of other adjacent cells, be they glial, endothelial, neuronal etc.

Potential Consequences of Radical Damage to Membranes in the CNS

The concept of membrane pathology has developed concomittantly with the aquisition of basic knowledge of normal membrane structure and function. There are several categories of membrane pathology, including surface pertubations, immune damage, direct attack of phospholipids by the phospholipases found in venoms, and damage by hydrolytic enzymes as would be liberated from lysosomes. Lipids in membranes can be degraded by esterases from lysosomes and by lipases. The latter however are not truly within lysosomes [19]. In order to invoke damage to membrane lipids by such enzymes it is necessary to demonstrate their presence in the specific tissue site. Not all lysosomes contain the necessary esterases, and not all cells have the capacity to produce lipases.

Pathologic events like cerebral edema are highly complex in their development and there is probably not one, simple mechanism to explain it. There is evidence that antioxidants can prevent one form of experimentally induced cerebral edema [13], but this does not mean that only free radicals are involved and other processes are excluded. For example, abnormal radical reactions in membranes can lead to leakage of hydrolytic enzymes if lysosomal membranes have been damaged. This leakage may in turn cause more membrane damage, including the proteins if there are proteases in the leaking lysosomes. Tight junctions, which are areas of membrane specialization, may be altered or moved apart by radical reactions in the immediately adjacent membrane biomolecules. Pathologic radical reactions within mitochondria and endoplasmic reticulum may interfere with oxidative metabolism and lower oxidative phosphorylation rates. This will affect ATP production and possibly be reflected in diminished efficiency of the cells' sodium pump, which is ATP dependent.

The series of reactions whereby fatty acids undergo radical damage are shown in Table 1. This is simplified because there are undoubtedly reactions between the pro-

Table 1. Radical Damage to Fatty Acids

A. Peroxidation of fatty acids by hydroperoxide formation

linoleic acid	H H H H H H —C—C = C—C—C = C— H H	+ $\overset{\cdot}{O}$—$\overset{\cdot}{O}$ metal catalyzed	this oxygen molecule is a diradical and abstracts H from carbon # 11, which is partly activated as a result of being in between two carbons with double bonds
carbon atom numbers	8 9 10 11 12 13		

linoleic alkyl radical	H H H H H H —C—C = C—$\overset{\cdot}{C}$—C = C— H	+ $\overset{\cdot}{O}$—OH	there are now two radicals, the hydroperoxy, ·OOH, and the alkyl, R·, on carbon # 11

linoleic hydroperoxide	H H H H H H —C—C = C—C—C = C— H | OOH	metal catalyzed	the two radicals have added together to form a new, two electron covalent bond; this results in some of the molecules shifting their double bonds to become conjugated, and some of the cis bonds to become trans

linoleic alkoxy radical	H H H H H H —C—C = C—C—C = C— H | $\overset{\cdot}{O}$	+ ·OH	hydroperoxides are unstable and schism yields two new radicals, the alkoxy, RO·, and the hydroxyl, ·OH, causing chain reactions

fragments	H H H H —C—C = C—C H || O	+ H H ·C = C—	aldehydes and carboxylic acids are produced from the continued oxidation of the fragments

---

B. Catalysis by metals (R represents the carbon chain)

$Fe^{+3} + ROOH \rightarrow ROO\cdot + H^+ + Fe^{+2}$

$Fe^{+2} + ROOH \rightarrow RO\cdot + OH^- + Fe^{+3}$

C. Some reactions of alkyl, alkoxy and hydroxyl radicals

$2 RO\cdot \rightarrow ROOR$; $RO\cdot + R'H \rightarrow ROH + R'\cdot$;

$R\cdot + RO\cdot \rightarrow ROR$; $RH + \cdot OH \rightarrow R\cdot + HOH$

---

ducts of the different, individual reactions. Fig. 2 contains a schematic representation of how membrane phospholipids may be affected by the reactions of fatty acids in Table 1. It should be compared to Fig. 1.

Therefore, free radical reactions may be an initial pertubation which sets in motion many events at subcellular and cellular levels, all of which may be involved in the neuropathology seen in cerebral edema. The disordered neural behaviour and conduction deficits may not be entirely due to the accumulation of water per se, but to associated membrane pathology occurring in axons and neuronal mitochondria.

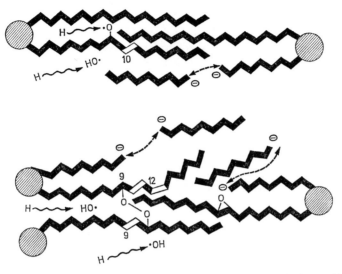

Fig. 2. Schematic representation of free radical peroxidative damage to the fatty acids that formed the hydrophobic midzone seen in Fig. 1. The double bonds are now largely in the non-bent, trans configuration; a saturated carbon no longer separates the carbons with unsaturated bonds and this is referred to as conjugation; alkoxy radicals, RO·, are present and react to form peroxides, ROOR, to join two adjacent fatty acids in an abnormal bond; mobile ·OH radicals are shown as the result of hydroperoxide schism; hydrogens are shown being abstracted, possibly from adjacent lipid and protein molecules; abstracted hydrogens react with hydroxyls to form water in the hydrophobic midzone; fragmentation of fatty acid tails is shown with eventual production of negatively charged carboxylic acid groups, represented as a minus sign inside an oval mark. The numerals, 9, 10, 12, signify the carbon atom number in the carbon chain that makes up the fatty acid

Varying degrees of cell necrosis may be seen with cerebral edema, and this too may not be the direct consequence of the increased water content, but rather may represent membrane pathology that has led to significant leakage of lysosomal hydrolases, resulting in cell death.

Interrelationships of Steroids and Radical Damage to Lipids

The ability of steroids to intercalate into membranes depends in part on the presence of archways, created by the phospholipid fatty acids whose double bonds are in the cis (123° angle bend) configuration. It is precisely these unsaturated areas of the fatty acid tails that are most sensitive to radical damage. If the fatty acids have already been extensively peroxidized, there will be no archways for steroids to fit into. Hence steroids will not stabilize a severely damaged membrane, because they would not have suitable sites.

In instances where peroxidation is progressing at a slow rate, the administration of steroids may serve to prevent the spread of radical chain reactions through the fatty acid tails. This "protection" afforded by steroids is attributable to the fact that the phospholipid fatty acids interact by tight hydrophobic associations with the steroids [18]. The steroid thus serves as a physical barrier to shield the sites of unsaturation in the fatty acids.

Differences in rates of peroxidation may explain the variable beneficial effects of steroids. In situations where cerebral edema has developed as a result of trauma, the presence of relatively large quantities of heme and other metal complexes that would go into solution in the hydrophobic midzone of membranes cause accelerated radical damage. Little benefit might be expected from steroids in this situation. In the case of a brain tumor, the rate of introducing metal complexes into surrounding neural tissue could be expected to be slower than the rate seen with trauma and hemorrhages. The peroxidation would therefore proceed at a slower pace, and be more amenable to prevention by membrane stabilizing steroids.

The concept of the *rate* of free radical damage to membranes is interrelated with the concept of *repair* of membrane damage. At a slow rate of peroxidation, it may be possible for a cell to repair or replace some of the damaged molecules. This can be done individually, analogous to replacing single bricks in a wall, or in small aggregates, or sections of membranes. The repairability of the cells' membranes will depend on whether the Golgi apparatus has been damaged, as this is one of the key sites of membrane biosynthesis.

In summary, the interrelationships of steroids, phospholipids, and membrane bound enzymes suggest that potential experimental therapeutics for cerebral edema might include the conjoint use of steroids, varied antioxidants, and metal chelators.

References

1. Arcos, J. C.: Ultrastructural alteration of the mitochondrial electron transport chain involving electron leak: Possible basis of "Respiratory Impairment" in certain tumors. J. theor. Biol. 30, 533–543 (1971)
2. Dawson, R. M. C.: The nature of the interaction between protein and lipid during the formation of lipoprotein membranes. In: Chapman, D. (Ed.): Biological Membranes, pp. 203–232. New York and London: Academic Press 1968.
3. Demopoulos, H. B., Landgraf, W., Duke, P. S., Tai, H.: Light induced alterations in melanoma related free radicals and the consequences on respiration and growth. Lab. Invest. 15, 1652–1658 (1966).
4. DiLuzio, N. R., Hartman, A. D.: Role of lipid peroxidation in the pathogenesis of the ethanol-induced fatty liver. Fed. Proc. 26, 1436–1442 (1967).
5. Dowben, R. M.: Composition and structure of membranes. In: Dowben, R. M. (Ed.): Biological Membranes, pp. 1–38. Boston: Little, Brown, and Co. 1969.
6. Hartman, A. D., DiLuzio, N. R., Trumbull, M. L.: Modification of chronic carbon tetrachloride hepatic injury by N,N′-Diphenyl-p-Phenylenediamine. Exp. molec. Path. 9, 349–362 (1968).
7. Holman, R. T.: Autoxidation of fats and related substances. In: Holman, R. T., Lundberg, W. O., Malkin, T. (Eds.). Progress in the Chemistry of Fats and Other Lipids. Vol. 2, pp. 51–98. London: Pergamon 1954.
8. Kornberg, R. D., McConnell, H. M.: Inside-outside transitions of phospholipids in vesicle membranes. Biochemistry 10, 1111–1120 (1971).
9. Long, R. A., Hruska, F., Gesser, H. D.: Membrane condensing effect of cholesterol and the role of its hydroxyl group. Biochem. biophys. Res. Commun. 41, 321–327 (1970).
10. Lucy, J. A.: Theoretical and experimental models for biological membranes. In: ibid, 233–288.

11. Mitchell, J. H., Henick, A. S.: Rancidity in Food Products. In: Lundberg, W. O. (Ed.). Autoxidation and antioxidants, Vol. II, pp. 543–592. Interscience: New York 1961.
12. O'Brien, J. S.: Cell Membranes: Composition, Structure, and Function. J. Theor. Biol. **15**, 307–324 (1967).
13. Ortega, B., Demopoulos, H. B., Ransohoff, J.: Effects of antioxidants on experimental brain edema. In: Steroids and Brain Edema. Berlin-Heidelberg-New York: Springer 1972.
14. Pappius, H. M.: Effects of steroids on cold injury edema. In: Steroids and Brain Edema. Berlin-Heidelberg-New York: Springer 1972.
15. Pitot, H. C.: Some biochemical aspects of malignancy. In: Recent Advances in Biochemistry, pp. 335–368, 1966.
16. Poole, C. P.: Electron Spin Resonance. Interscience, New York 1967.
17. Pryor, W. A.: Free Radicals. McGraw-Hill, New York 1966.
18. Rothman, J. E., Engelman, D. M.: Molecular mechanism for the interaction of phospholipid with cholesterol. Nature, **237**, 42–44 (1972).
19. Seligman, M. L., Ueno, H., Hanker, J. S., Kramer, S. P., Wasserkruz, H., Seligman, A. M.: Cytochemical localization of pancreatic lipase with light and electron microscopy. Exp. molec. Path. Suppl. **3**, 21–30 (1966).
20. Stecher, P. G., (Ed.): The Merck Index. p. 775, Merck and Co., Rahway 1968.
21. Tappel, A. L.: Biocatalysis: Lipoxidase and hematic compounds. In: Lundberg, W. O. (Ed.): Autoxidation and antioxidants, Vol. I, pp. 325–366. Interscience, New York 1961.
22. Tollin, G., Fox, J. L.: Free radicals in flavin redox systems. In: Ehrenberg, A., Malmstrom, B. G., Vanngard, T. (Eds.): Magnetic Resonance in Biological Systems, pp. 289–297, Pergamon Press, New York 1967.
23. Wallace, J. D., Driscoll, D. H., Kalomiris, C. G., Neaves, A.: A study of free radicals, occurring in tumorous female breast tissue and their implication to detection. Cancer **25**, 1087–1090 (1970).
24. Weissman, G.: Lysosomes. New Engl. J. Med. **273**, 1084–1090 (1965).

Some Aspects of the Pharmacology of Adrenal Steroids and the Central Nervous System*

C. D. WITHROW and DIXON M. WOODBURY**

Department of Pharmacology, College of Medicine, University of Utah, Salt Lake City, UT 84112, USA

I. Introduction

The pharmacology and biochemistry of adrenal steroids as they relate to the central nervous system (CNS) have been extensively reviewed by Woodbury [76, 77]. In order to reduce redundancy, the present review has been limited to aspects of steroid pharmacology pertinent to their use in the therapy of brain edema. First, the uptake, distribution, exit and metabolism of glucorticoids have been discussed in detail. Second, the effects of both glucocorticoids and mineralocorticoids on CNS electrolyte metabolism in normal and pathological states have been summarized.

II. CNS Uptake, Distribution, Exit and Metabolism of Steroids

A. Uptake

Studies with [14]C- or ^{3}H-labeled steroids have indicated that cortisol [16, 54, 61, 73] and corticosterone [7, 43] readily penetrate the blood-brain barrier (BBB) and enter both brain and cerebrospinal fluid (CSF). Within 2 min after intravenous injection of a single dose of drug, large amounts of hydrocortisone left the blood and entered normal brain tissue. In 10 min after administration, considerably more tissue labeling was observed (61). Other data from experiments in which only single doses of the drug were used also show that tissue uptakes were maximal within 8–15 min after injection [16, 54]. The amount of radioactive cortisol in rat brain was not affected by prior injections of unlabelled cortisol, 1–4 mg, 10 min before administration of radioactive drug [54], but others found betamethasone did appear to affect the distribution of cortisol in brain [16]. On the other hand, the amounts of radioactive cortisol that appeared in brain were directly proportional to the elevation in plasma cortisol [54].

Experiments in eviscerated cats give a slightly different picture of tritiated cortisol uptake in brain. The injection of radioactive cortisol as a bolus resulted in a very high immediate plasma level of drug falling to relatively slowly declining levels during the

* Supported by a United States Public Health Service Program-Project Grant (5-PO1-NS-04553) from the National Institute of Neurological Diseases and Stroke, National Institutes of Health.
** Recipient of a USPHS Research Career Program Award (5-K6-NS-13, 838) from the National Institute of Neurological Diseases and Stroke, National Institutes of Health.

next 2 h. Brain levels were elevated within 10 min, continued to rise during the first hour, and remained constant for the second hour of the experiment. When the cortisol was not injected all at once but rather was given to the animal at a rate such that plasma levels remained almost constant, brain levels were low 10 min after beginning the infusion and continued to rise steadily throughout the 2 h experiment. When eviscerated cats were infused at a constant rate, drug levels in blood and brain continued to rise steadily for 60 min. Elevation of the amount of radioactive cortisol threefold did not affect tissue-blood ratios at 60 min, but did result in much higher absolute radioactivity levels in both blood and brain, and does indicate that any uptake mechanisms are not saturated [73]. Mouse brain levels of corticosterone were found to rise rapidly when endogenous corticosterone levels in plasma were elevated by use of an acute ether stress [10]. Radioactive corticosterone injected into pregnant rats crossed the placenta and entered fetal brain within 30 min after administration [81].

In single-dose experiments in normal dogs, radioactive cortisol injected intravenously rapidly entered the CSF and appeared to peak 60 min after injection [19]. In normal cats given one injection of cortisol, maximum CSF levels were observed 20–40 min after treatment [73]. In eviscerated cats, a bolus injection of cortisol into blood gave peak levels of cortisol in CSF in about 1 h after treatment [73]. The slower peak times in the eviscerated animals was probably a result of the elevated, slowly declining blood levels of cortisol in these animals as contrasted with the rapidly decreasing blood cortisol concentrations in non-eviscerated cats. The maintenance of constant blood cortisol levels in eviscerated cats resulted in constantly rising CSF concentrations of cortisol that gave no indication of leveling off [73]. There is perhaps a slight lag of increases in CSF levels of cortisol behind increases in blood cortisol quantities, but several experiments have shown clearly that CSF concentrations are directly dependent on blood levels of the drug [19, 48].

B. Distribution

Analysis of the brain from humans has shown that cortisol is concentrated in brain to the extent of 27 times the blood level [70]. Henkin *et al.* [33] reported that cat brain has cortisol and corticosterone levels higher than those measured in plasma. It has also been routinely observed in acute experiments that brain levels of cortisol do not decrease as rapidly as do those of blood when single injections of radioactive drug are given to normal animals [20, 54, 73]. Since no evidence exists for active transport of cortisol into brain tissue, the best explanation for elevated tissue/plasma ratios and slow tissue release when blood concentrations are decreased is that binding of cortisol takes place in brain. Direct evidence for binding of corticosterone in rat brain has been published [23, 30, 44, 65], so it appears that steroid binding may be a general characteristic of brain tissue in several species.

The binding of steroids by rat brain has been the subject of several investigations which have yielded some interesting results. First, steroids have been shown to be bound by soluble proteins from cytosol [30, 42] and by proteins in the cell nucleus of neurons [23, 45]. Second, there are differences in the amount of corticosterone bound by either cytosol [30, 42] or nuclear proteins [45] from different regions of the rat brain. Radioactive corticosterone is found concentrated in nuclei from the hippocampus and septum [23, 44], while cytosol proteins from the hippocampus, septum and hypothalamus accumulate corticosterone [65]. Third, the binding shows some specificity in that corticosterone, the important endogenous glucocorticoid in the rat, is bound most avidly [30, 42]. Finally, closely related steroids can interfere with the binding, and the binding sites can be saturated. It is not known whether the selective binding of corticosterone is related to the effects of the steroid on brain function, but the possiblity that the relationship exists is exciting.

The concentration of cortisol in hypothalamic nuclei dissected from dog brain has been reported [16]. The intriguing suggestion that cortisol inhibition of the adrenal-pituitary axis results from selective binding in the hypothalamus was put forth on the basis of these data. Concentration of ^{3}H-corticosterone in purkinje, supraoptic, ventral horn, dorsal root ganglion, and hippocampal pyramidal cells has been observed [20].

Determination of the subcellular distribution of ^{3}H-corticosterone in rat brain showed that the nuclear and supernatant fractions contained most of the steroid, 14 and 69 %, respectively [7]. Direct measurements of corticosterone in mouse brain soluble and particulate fractions showed the distribution of the compound to be as follows (figures are % in each fraction): nuclear, 9.4; myelin, 15.2; synaptic debris, 8.7; nerve endings, 15.4; mitochondria, 7.0; microsomes, 7.3.; and supernatant, 37.0 [10]. The affinity of cortisol and corticosterone for subcellular particles in rat brain apparently varies with age [14]. The high concentrations of hydrocortisone found in choroid plexus may suggest a direct local action in this tissue, perhaps to reduce CSF production [61]. Steroid-sensitive neurons activated by dexamethasone have been identified in the hypothalamus and midbrain, but not in the cortex, dorsal hippocampus or thalamus [64]. The importance of these specific neurons remains to be determined but they may be involved in negative and positive feedback actions of ACTH. Butte et al. [10] have found that endogenous corticosterone levels are lower in rat and mouse brain than in plasma. This finding thus disagrees with those of Touchstone et al. [70] and of Henkin et al. [33] in which tissue-plasma ratios greater than twenty were reported. The studies of Butte et al. [10], however, found that the pituitary, parts of the limbic system, the hypothalamus and the brain stem contained relatively higher concentrations of corticosterone than did the remainder of the brain, an observation in rough agreement with those of others. The binding of steroids in brain and the importance thereof is therefore apparently not settled, so further experiments are necessary before definite conclusions can be reached.

The average level of cortisol in CSF is 0.2–0.4 μg/100 ml, a value that is considerably below the concentration of this steroid in brain and blood [4, 13, 48]. When exogenous cortisol was given, both plasma and CSF concentrations increased, but the CSF/plasma ratios (CSF levels were 6.4 % those in plasma) did not change [48]. In eviscerated cats given single doses or controlled-rate infusions of cortisol, CSF levels were 20–25 % those measured in plasma. When constant rate infusions of different doses of ^{3}H-cortisol were done in eviscerated cats, CSF concentrations followed those in blood, but the CSF concentrations were much less than 25 % of those in blood [73]. Of particular interest in these experiments was the observation that 75 % of CSF cortisol was bound to a protein. Uete et al. [72] found that total corticosteroids in CSF of healthy subjects was 1.26 μg/100 ml, as compared to 15.8 μg/100 ml for blood. Cortisol infused intravenously markedly increased CSF corticosteroids and decreased the blood/CSF steroid ratio. It is not known why CSF and plasma cortisol levels are not the same, but the rapid increase in CSF levels of steroid when blood levels of drug are raised argues strongly against any difficulty in cortisol getting into CSF. Uete *et al.* [72] cite previous studies in which unbound levels of cortisol were the same in CSF and blood. Additional careful studies of the ratios of free drug in plasma and CSF are needed.

C. Exit from CNS

Cortisol given intrathecally rapidly disappears from the CSF and appears in blood [19, 29, 48]. When single doses of a glucocorticoid were given and plasma levels began to decrease as a consequence of drug excretion and metabolism, brain and CSF levels decreased although at a rate slower than that observed in plasma [20, 43, 48, 54, 73]. In washout experiments in which an attempt was made to measure tissue cortisol retention in the cat, it was found that twice as much cortisol was removed from the pituitary as from the whole brain, and that brain retained more cortisol than non-neural tissue [73]. Most data reported thus far are consistent with the notion that the binding of cortisol by brain tissue retards, but does not markedly affect, the loss of steroids from the CNS. It is not known whether cortisol concentrations in CSF are lowered by passage through cerebral capillary membranes into blood, by an active transport system out of the CSF, or by removal by bulk flow of CSF. The low concentrations of cortisol in CSF relative to plasma in normal animals would argue that one of the two last possibilities, or both, are important for the removal of cortisol from CSF.

D. Metabolism of Corticoids by CNS

Incubation of rat brain homogenates with ^{14}C-cortisol results in conversion of this steroid to cortisone to the extent of 15–20 %, but only minimal amounts of tetrahydrocortisol (THF) and tetrahydrocortisone (THE) are produced [27, 40, 55, 63]. Incubation of rat brain homogenates with ^{14}C-cortisone mainly results in its conversion to cortisol to the extent of 20–25 %. Again, very little THF and THE are found. Thus, side-chain reduction and ring-A reduction by brain enzymes do not readily occur. The most common change is in the C-11-keto: hydroxy equilibration, which is a NADP-NADPH-dependent reaction. Not only homogenates, but also nuclei, oxidize cortisol to cortisone. NADP but not NAD enhances this reaction. In brain homogenates of new-born rats, the oxidative process occurs but is very slow; however, it increases rapidly as maturation progresses and becomes maximal at about 21 days after birth. Brain particulate fractions sedimented at 800, 20,000, and 100,000 g are all active in oxidizing cortisol to cortisone, but the 100,000 g supernatant has very little activity [55]. These studies were extended by Grosser and Bliss [27] to other steroids. They observed that NADP-dependent 11-dehydrogenation (11-oxidation) occurs in brain homogenates from rats and dogs, not only with cortisol, but also with corticosterone and 11-β-hydroxyandrost-4-ene-3, 17-dione. The reverse reaction also occurs when cortisone, 11-dehydrocorticosterone, and adrenosterone are used as substrates [27]. Cortex, hypothalamus, subcortex, and cerebellum are all capable of carrying out the conversion of corticosterone to 11-dehydrocorticosterone. Guinea pig brain does not appear to possess 11 β-hydroxysteroid dehydrogenase ac-

44

tivity. Samples from dog hypophysis, cerebral cortex, mammillary body, median eminence and a nucleus supraopticus area all convert cortisol to cortisone *in vitro* [16]. In order to localize the cell type responsible for the hydroxy-keto interconversion, Grosser [24] compared the ability of homogenates of normal mouse brain and of mouse glioma to convert cortisol, corticosterone, and 11 β-hydroxyandrostenedione to their 11-keto derivatives. Glioma homogenates were able to oxidize about 3 times as much steroid as were normal brain homogenates. The acetylation of cortisol by a human astrocytoma has also been reported [28]. These results strongly suggest an involvement of glial cells in steroid metabolism, but further data with normal isolated glial cells are required before definite conclusions are warranted. However, the low ability of brain from new born rats to oxidize steroids and the fact that this activity develops rapidly from the twelfth to twenty-first day after birth, a time when glial cell proliferation begins in rat brain, argues strongly for a role of glial cells in the metabolism of steroids.

Tritiated cortisol is converted by 3-day-old rat brain minces, but not by adult rat brain minces, to cortisol-21-acetate and cortisone-21-acetate [25]. The cerebellum, thalamus-hypothalamus, medulla and cerebral cortex of brains obtained from second trimester, third trimester, newborn and adult baboons also converted cortisol to cortisone, cortisol-21-acetate and cortisone-21-acetate [26]. Again, the adult brain was less active in this regard than were fetal and perinatal brains. The significance of these observations is not clear at present.

The *in vivo* metabolism of ³H-cortisol and ³H-corticosterone by cerebral cortex has been studied by ventriculo-cisternal perfusion techniques. Cortisone and cortisol-21-acetate were detected as conversion products of cortisol metabolism, whereas, 11-dehydrocorticosterone was the sole corticosterone metabolite [29]. Moreover, in *in situ* perfusion experiments with baboon brain tritiated cortisol was converted to cortisone. No recoverable acetate metabolites were found [2].

It is thus clear that CNS tissue can metabolize steroids both *in vitro* and *in vivo*. The predominant reactions appear to be oxidation-reduction at the 11 position and 21-position acetylations. Side-chain reduction and ring-A reductions do not readily occur. The origin of tetrahydrocortisol and 11 β, 17 α, 20 β, 21-tetrahydroxy-pregn-4-ene-3-one in human brain [70] remains to be elucidated.

E. Summary

The pharmacokinetics, metabolism, etc. in the CNS of dexamethasone, the most widely used drug for brain edema therapy, have not been studied. Plasma half-lives of 142 to 367 min [8, 31] and 167 to 368 min [31], however, have been measured for the drug in blood. If the optimal dosage schedule for a drug is repeated administration at intervals equal to its biological half-life, the empirical choice of 4 mg of dexamethasone every 6 h seems reasonable although some patients might have widely fluctuating blood levels. Also, the usual loading dose of 10 mg of dexamethasone, about twice the maintenance dose, is on a pharmacologically sound basis [18]. Therefore, unless there are some surprises in dexamethasone entrance, exit and distribution in the CNS, the usual therapeutic regimen should maintain a reasonably constant level in the brain and CSF. Whether this level is optimal is not known since no dose-effect studies in brain edema therapy have been done.

III. Steroid Effects on CNS Water and Electrolyte Metabolism

A. Introduction

The use of glucocorticoids for the treatment of cerebral edema is well documented. Whether this usefulness is related to effects on electrolyte metabolism is a moot point. The increasing utilization in cerebral edema therapy, however, of steroids and other drugs with known effects on electrolyte balance in blood and other tissues makes it desirable to describe in some detail this particular aspect of steroid pharmacology.

B. Effects on Normal CNS

Desoxycorticosterone (DOC) has been extensively studied with respect to tissue electrolytes, including brain. In tissue other than brain, it has been shown that DOC causes a rise in intracellular Na concentration and a concomitant loss of intracellular K. The effects of DOC on brain electrolytes were studied by Woodbury and Davenport [78] who found that total brain Na and K concentrations and Cl space were not altered by DOC treatment. However, brain intracellular Na concentration, calculated on the assumption that Cl space is a measure of extracellular fluid volume, was markedly decreased. Despite the fact that brain intracellular K concentration remained unchanged, the ratio of intracellular to extracellular K in brain was increased by DOC treatment because plasma K was decreased by the drug. The decrease in brain intracellular Na was associated with an increase in electroshock seizure threshold (EST) – a decrease in brain excitability. The increase in EST was ascribed to possible membrane hyperpolarization caused by enhanced Na transport from brain cells. Gallagher and Glaser [22], however, found that absence of adrenal hormones did not affect rat brain ATPase activity. That a fundamental difference exists in intact rats between the effects of DOC on brain and other tissues is indicated by the fact that only in brain does DOC decrease intracellular Na concentration. Intracellular concentration of Na is increased while that of K is decreased in muscle, heart, liver, and skin of DOC-treated animals. The above-described brain electrolytes effects of DOC have also been reported by Colfer [12], Hoagland [34], and Timiras et al. [68].

The influence of DOC treatment on the turnover of radioactive Na in brain and other tissues of dogs was studied by Overman et al. [51] who found that DOC increased the turnover of brain Na in adrenalectomized but not in intact dogs. However, the measurement of the ^{24}Na uptake was made only 30 min after injection of the isotope and it is difficult to interpret these results since correct analysis of the effects of agents on the uptake of radioelectrolytes by brain requires data on the complete activity-time curves for periods up to 24 h. Although it is likely that DOC actually does increase the turnover of ^{24}Na in brain cells, more convincing information is necessary.

The difficulty with the DOC experiments is that CSF electrolytes were not measured simultaneously with the brain and plasma values. It could be speculated that DOC would have a biphasic effect on brain and CSF electrolytes. Initially it would stimulate Na-K transport, as it does in other tissues, across neuronal cell membranes and across the choroid plexus cells. This would decrease K and increase Na concentrations in the CSF, and increase K and decrease Na concentrations in neuronal cells. The result would be hyperpolarization of the neuronal cells and a decrease in brain excitability. However, DOC has a very powerful effect on the kidney to increase K excretion. Thus, after several days, DOC causes decreased plasma K and total body K depletion. A lowered plasma K would tend to uncouple the Na-K pump in the choroid plexus and thereby inhibit active transport. This effect is known to occur in skeletal muscle when plasma K is decreased. The net effect would be to increase CSF potassium concentration despite the continuing effect of the DOC to stimulate Na-K transport across the choroid plexus. Since the CSF is considered the extracellular fluid of the brain, the increased CSF potassium would stimulate Na-K transport across neuronal cells and add to the DOC-stimulation of this system. The increased CSF potassium, however, would decrease the K ratio across the cell membrane between cell fluid and CSF which is the extracellular environment of the brain cells. This would result in a lower potential than was present earlier and the excitability of the brain would be increased as compared with the initial effect. It has been observed experimentally that excitability decreases initially and then plateaus subsequently on chronic administration at a time when the plasma K has decreased markedly. Thus, the hypothesis fits the experimental findings. It is therefore evident that it is necessary to assess their effects on both CSF and the brain to obtain a complete understanding of the action of steroids on brain electrolytes. This is mandatory because the active transport processes that are influenced by steroids, as well as many other drugs, occur across both the choroid plexus and the nerve cell membrane.

Some unpublished experimental results from our laboratory are of interest in relation to the above-described effects of DOC on brain electrolytes and excitability. DOC administered for days to unilaterally nephrectomized, castrated, adult male rats given 0.9 % sodium chloride solution to drink caused a decrease in brain excitability and in calculated brain intracellular Na concentration (based on chloride space which was not altered by the treatment), an increase in brain extracellular Na concentration, and an increase in the ratio of brain intracellular to extracellular K concentration. Cerebral edema did not occur. However, in *young* rats, who are more vulnerable to the effects of DOC on the kidney, prepared and treated in exactly the same manner, brain excitability was decreased only during the first 11 days of DOC administration. Excitability then increased until the time of sacrifice for electrolyte analyses on the 50th day (the biphasic effect on excitability as discussed above). Large (toxic) doses of DOC caused marked cerebral edema and the extracellular water content of the brain was elevated. In these young rats, instead of the usual pattern of electrolyte changes caused by DOC, intracellular brain Na increased despite the fact that the brain K ratio (relative to plasma and not CSF) was enhanced. If the ratio were related to CSF potassium, it would probably be decreased because of, as described above, the uncoupling effect of the low plasma K on the transport of K across the choroid plexus. Thus, in nontoxic doses in the adult animals, DOC decreased brain excitability and intracellular brain Na concentration, whereas toxic doses in the young animals increased brain excitability and intracellular Na concentration, a change in Na that DOC produces normally in other tissues and which is a result of its effect on the kidney to increase K excretion in urine. The experimental results indicate that DOC in low doses stimulates the active pumping of Na out of brain cells and into CSF; but, as a result of the low plasma K and the presence of excess Na, which enhances the K excretory effects of DOC on the kidney, this effect on both the brain and CSF sodium pump fails, toxicity results and brain excitability increases. The toxic side effects of DOC, such as the convulsions induced in rats in high doses, are probably related to its effects on brain and CSF sodium and potassium.

The changes induced by aldosterone in brain and skeletal muscle electrolytes have been studied in mice [79]. This steroid increases the ratio of plasma to intracellular Na concentration and intracellular to plasma K concentration in both brain and muscle. CSF sodium and potassium values were not measured. Thus, aldosterone and DOC produce similar effects on brain electrolytes but opposite effects on muscle electrolytes. The discrepancy was resolved by Withrow and Woodbury [74] who found that DOC had the same influence as aldosterone on Na and K concentrations in muscle in nephrectomized, partially-eviscerated rats. In this preparation, the marked renal and gastrointestinal losses of K usually caused by DOC were minimized. Thus, the stimulatory effects of DOC on muscle Na-K transport were separated from the inhibitory effects of low extracellular K on Na-K ATPase.

The influence of other adrenocortical steroids and ACTH on brain electrolytes has been studied by Woodbury ([75] and unpublished data) in rats and by Timiras *et al.* [68] in mice. The results may be summarized as follows: In rats, chronic administration of ACTH, cortisone, cortisol, corticosterone, dehydrocorticosterone, and 11-desoxy-17-hydroxycorticosterone had no effect on brain electrolytes in the doses used and for the period administered (28 days). However, they markedly affected brain excitability, and markedly increased brain Na and Cl spaces. The increase in both Na and Cl spaces suggests an effect of cortisol on the permeability of brain cells, such that both Na and Cl enter the cells without a net increase in intracellular Na concentration, or an effect on the glial tissue of brain. The increase in brain Cl space induced by cortisol in mice suggests that extracellular space is influenced by this steroid; an increased permeability may occur, that is, the ground substance and glia may become more fluid. This possibility is borne out by the observation that cortisone inhibits growth and proliferation of glial cells in tissue cultures of cerebral cortex (see [76] for summary). In rats, cortisone causes a slight loss of skeletal muscle Na with little influence on K distribution. ACTH has no effect on muscle (Woodbury, unpublished observations).

The influence of acute administration of cortisol and DOC on brain electrolyte metabolism has also been studied ([80] and unpublished observations). The results for DOC are the same as those obtained with chronic injection of this steroid but relatively greater since sufficient time to allow for lowering of plasma K has not occurred. However, the acute administration of cortisol differed from the chronic in that it increased brain intracellular Na concentration, decreased the Na ratio between brain and plasma, and increased brain excitability. Thus the changes in brain electrolytes induced acutely by cortisol correlate with the observed changes in excitability. The results differ from those noted above for chronic cortisol treatment in which no measurable changes in intracellular brain electrolytes were noted, perhaps because cortisol, like DOC, also increases K excretion. In this particular situation CSF electrolytes were not measured, hence further conclusions as to the lack of effect of chronic cortisol administration on electrolytes are unwarranted. The acute treatment of normal animals with dexamethasone did not change brain Na and H_2O concentrations [53, 66].

An interesting effect of adrenalectomy has been observed on calcium distribution in CSF and probably in brain [21]. Intravenous infusion of calcium markedly elevated the plasma Ca concentration (200 %) to the same extent in intact and adrenalecto-mized rabbits. The CSF level, however, was only slightly elevated (13 %) in the intact animal, whereas it was markedly increased (72 %) in the adrenalectomized animals. When the glucocorticoid dexamethasone was given to adrenalectomized rabbits the rise in CSF calcium concentration (11 %) in response to the infusion of Ca was the same as that measured in intact animals. The adrenalectomized rabbits were also slightly more sensitive to infusion of K than were the intact animals insofar as the elevation of CSF potassium was concerned, but the effect was not nearly as large as with Ca infusion. Intact animals exhibited no change in CSF potassium, whereas those that were adrenalectomized had a 11 % increase in response to K infusion. The adrenalectomized animals were also much more sensitive to the lethal effects of both intravenously and intracisternally administered Ca than were the intact animals. It is evident, therefore, that adrenalectomy compromises the mechanism that regulates Ca movement into the CSF, and that this can be restored by glucocorticoid admini-stration.

C. Effects on Abnormal CNS

The glucocorticoids have been extensively used for the clinical treatment of cerebral edema, and have been shown to be effective for the prevention and/or reduction of cerebral edema in several experimental animal models [3, 6, 36, 39, 41, 59, 66, 67]. Their efficacy, however, is not universally agreed upon [5, 11, 52, 53].

In the experimental and clinical cerebral materials analyzed for electrolyte distor-tions, it is clear that Na and water increase in the edematous areas [52, 53, 58]. K con-centrations reported on a wet-weight basis are lowered in edematous tissues; total K levels calculated on dry weights of tissues are either unchanged or lowered.

Although it is known that in vasogenic edema vascular membrane integrity is compromised so that protein leakage occurs [38], it is not established that the elec-trolyte changes are solely the result of the movement of whole plasma or plasma ultra-filtrate into the tissue. For example, Reulen et al. [58] found that the edematous fluid in white matter had Na concentrations consistent with the fact that edema fluid was a plasma ultrafiltrate; grey matter fluid, however, contained more Na than was present in serum ultrafiltrate. Pappius and Gulati [52], on the other hand, concluded that the in-crease in Na concentration in white matter edema fluid was less than expected if edema fluid contained as much Na as did plasma. The movement of electrolytes in so-called cytotoxic brain edema is not associated with changes in vascular permea-bility [38].

In cases in which steroids have been found to reduce brain edema, and in which electrolytes have been measured, the diminution of brain edema was correlated with a reversal of the pathological water and electrolyte changes [66, 67]. An exception is the work of Pappius and McCann [53] in which it was reported that dexamethasone treatment diminished the increase in brain weight caused by cold injury, but did not change brain water or Na concentrations. As pointed out by Benson et al. [5], how-ever, the findings of Pappius and McCann are difficult to reconcile unless a loss of brain "dry weight" is assumed. Since it has been shown that dexamethasone can restore altered brain vascular permeability [17, 41], at least part of the beneficial ef-fects of the glucocorticoids may be explained on this basis. It may be that the resto-ration of cell wall integrity in cytotoxic edema may account for the decrease of intracellular Na accumulation [66, 69] after steroid treatment. If blood-brain barrier (BBB) changes are important in the production of cerebral edema, the observation of Angel and Burkett [1] that hydrocortisone restores barrier integrity to cocaine may be cited as support for the beneficial effects of steroids in brain edema. The finding, however, that alterations of the BBB by sodium acetrizoate are not affected by methylprednisolone argues that steroids do not affect this barrier [32].

Although dexamethasone has been reported to increase urinary Na output [62], the interpretation that the renal excretion of Na benefits cerebral edema is open to question because much more potent diuretics have little efficacy when compared to dexamethasone.

The electrolyte and H_2O disturbances in cerebral edema might also be explained by compromised Na transport, but this is not well defined. Although some inhibition of Na-K ATPase by triethyltin has been observed [69], others report negative results [37, 49]. The impairment of mitchochondrial ATP formation, purportedly by fatty acids, in balloon compression experiments [60] might disrupt brain fluid balance but this remains to be shown.

If reduced Na transport from cells is responsible for brain edema, reported drug effects are puzzling. It seems reasonable that aldosterone which stimulates Na transport might aid cerebral edema (see Schmiedek, this symposium) despite the fact that it causes systemic Na retention. It also seems reasonable that glucocorticoids might affect Na transport by a "permissive" effect on cell wall integrity, an effect consistent with the arguments of Long et al. [39]. Any beneficial effect of furosemide and ethacrynic acid (see Pappius and Reulen et al., this symposium), both powerful diuretics, on cerebral edema might be explained by their ability to enhance markedly the renal excretion of Na. However, this remains to be proven. The positive responses to spironolactone (see Wesemann and Eggert, and Schmiedek et al., this symposium) are difficult to reconcile with the observation that it has the same therapeutic effects in brain edema as does aldosterone, a drug that is usually antagonized by spironolactone. The effects of acetazolamide on renal Na excretion are minimal, but it does have effects on CSF production that might account for some of its reported efficacy (see Long, this symposium) in brain edema therapy.

As mentioned above, Na transport in the choroid plexus must also be considered when electrolyte distortions on the CNS are being interpreted. In cerebral edema, almost no information is available concerning CSF electrolytes and drug effects thereon. Uete and Nishimura [71] reported an elevation of Na in CSF in some patients after operations for removal of brain tumors and surmised that these patients may have had some brain edema. Cortisol treatment decreased elevated Na concentrations in CSF, but had no effect on normal CSF sodium levels. Hooshmand et al. [35] found that dexamethasone decreased CSF pressure elevated by intracerebral hemorrhage, and also had a slight effect on normal CSF pressure. Ethacrynic acid did not affect elevated CSF pressures. The efficacy of dexamethasone in tuberculous meningitis has been correlated with its effects on CSF pressure [50]. However, Mitus [47] has reported that clinical improvement in some cases of meningeal leukemia occurred in spite of continued elevation of CSF pressure, a finding which suggested that dexamethasone acted by reversal of cerebral edema rather than by a decrease in CSF pressure.

Despite the paucity of information in pathological states, there are several reports that drugs proposed and experimented with (see above) for the therapy of cerebral edema affect CSF production and pressure. Miner and Reed [46] have shown that ethacrynic acid reduces ^{22}Na uptake into CSF and concurrently lowers the rate of formation of CSF. Furosemide has been reported to reduce CSF flow rates by about 45 % [57], and to decrease ^{22}Na uptake into brain and CSF [9]. Acetazolamide reduced CSF flow by 52 % [56]. Domer has reported that mercurial saluretics, thiazides, triamterene, ethacrynic acid, and acetazolamide all reduced CSF formation; furosemide was without effect and spironolactone increased CSF production [15]. Although the reduction of CSF production would certainly be of benefit when intracranial pressure is elevated in cerebral edema, the exact role in the pathological state of drugs that affect CSF parameters remains to be elucidated.

D. Summary

There are some aspects of the effects of steroids and other drugs on CNS electrolyte metabolism that merit additional comment and emphasis.

The fact that glucocorticoids have little effect on electrolyte distribution in normal animals argues against the notion that the beneficial effect of these drugs in brain edema is related to direct effects on electrolyte metabolism. Their effect on ion movements, then, appears to be confined primarily to pathological tissue, and the hypothesis that these drugs decrease abnormal permeability in disturbed membranes seems reasonable from an electrolyte viewpoint.

If a drug, however, is of value in cerebral edema therapy because of a direct effect on electrolyte metabolism, the situation becomes complex. First, consider a drug which enhances Na transport. This would be a desirable effect insofar as the neuron or glial cell is concerned since Na accumulation in cells occurs in brain edema. However, it might be expected that more Na would be pumped into CSF and increase CSF pressure, an undesirable effect. Moreover, renal retention of Na might be enhanced and the expanded extracellular volume with perhaps a rise in blood pressure would not be of benefit.

Next consider the effects of a drug which inhibits Na transport such as the saluretics. Their beneficial effects in brain edema would be expected to result from extracellular Na depletion with a consequent reduction in blood pressure, and perhaps in the reduction of CSF production. Inhibition of Na transport in a cell containing too much Na would be potentially harmful. However, inhibition of transport at the choroid plexus would result in a rise in CSF potassium, and this, as discussed above, might stimulate Na transport in brain cells. On the other hand, most powerful saluretic agents also cause total body K depletion, a factor that could compromise transport in CSF.

Whether a drug exerts effects on brain tissue, choroid plexus and renal tubule at the same time, the net result of any effects depends on several factors. If the enzymes in all sites are equally sensitive to the drug, and they may not be, the amount of enzyme inhibition observed (thinking in terms of ATPase) would be proportional to the amount of drug reaching the site. Since most drugs are given systemically, penetration across the BBB must be a prime consideration. For example, the dose of furosemide given intrathecally which inhibits CSF Na-22 uptake is only 1 mg/kg [9], whereas 10 mg/kg given intravenously was without effect on CSF flow [57]. The dynamics of the system must also be taken into account. If all renal tubular Na transport is inhibited 1 %, the rapid turnover of fluids at this site results in a marked loss of Na from the body. It is doubtful that a 1 % decrease in Na transport in most other cells could be detected. This concept is supported by the observations that effective saluretics do not change tissue electrolyte distribution in animals in which electrolyte loss from the body is prevented. The dynamics of CSF production are between those of tissue plasma membranes and the renal tubule cell. It is therefore not reasonable to expect that a simple explanation for the effects on CNS electrolytes of any drug is forthcoming. Any interpretation of changes in CNS electrolytes caused by drugs must be tentative unless tissue, CSF and renal electrolyte changes are measured at the same time. Thus far, few experiments have been done in which such data have been collected.

Acknowledgements. The authors wish to express special thanks to Mrs. Jill Jones for her library assistance, proof reading and expert typing. We are also grateful to Mrs. Lou Ann Thomas for her help with some of the typing chores.

References

1. Angel, C., Burkett, M. L.: Effects of hydrocortisone and cycloheximide on blood-brain barrier function in the rat. Dis. nerv. Syst. **32**, 53–58 (1971).
2. Axelrod, L. R.: The metabolism of corticosteroids by incubated and perfused brain tissues. In: Influence of Hormones on the Nervous System, pp. 74–84. Ford, D. H. (Ed.), Basel: S. Karger 1971.
3. Bakay, L., Lee, J. C.: Cerebral Edema. Springfield, Illinois: Charles C. Thomas 1965.
4. Baron, D. N., Abelson, D.: Cortisone and hydrocortisone in cerebrospinal fluid. Nature **173**, 174 (1954).
5. Benson, V. M., McLaurin, R. L., Foulkes, E. C.: Traumatic cerebral edema. Arch. Neurol. **23**, 179–186 (1970).
6. Blinderman, E. E., Graf, C. J., Fitzpatrick, T.: Basic studies in cerebral edema. Its control by a corticosteroid (solu-medrol). J. Neurosurg. **19**, 319–324 (1962).
7. Bottoms, G., Goetsch, D. D.: Subcellular distribution of the (^{3}H) corticosterone fraction in brain, thymus, heart, and liver of the rat. Proc. Soc. exp. Biol. **124**, 662–665 (1967).
8. Brooks, S. M., Werk, E. E., Ackerman, S. J., Sullivan, I., Thrasher, K.: Adverse effects of phenobarbital on corticosteroid metabolism in patients with bronchial asthma. New Engl. J. Med. **286**, 1125–1128 (1972).
9. Buhrley, L. E., Reed, D. J.: The effect of furosemide on sodium-22 uptake into cerebrospinal fluid and brain. Exp. Brain Res. **14**, 503–510 (1972).
10. Butte, J. C., Kakihana, R., Noble, E. P.: Rat and mouse brain corticosterone. Endocrinology **90**, 1091–1100 (1972).
11. Clasen, R. A., Cooke, P. M., Pandolfi, S., Carnecki, G., Hass, G. M.: Steroid-antihistaminic therapy in experimental cerebral edema. Arch. Neurol. **13**, 584–592 (1965).
12. Colfer, H. F.: Studies on the relationship between electrolytes of the cerebral cortex and the mechanism of convulsions. Proc. Ass. Res. Nerv. Diseases **26**, 98–117 (1947).
13. Coppen, A., Brooksbank, B. W. L., Noguera, R., Wilson, D. A.: Cortisol in the cerebrospinal fluid of patients suffering from affective disorders. J. Neurol. Neurosurg. Psychiat. **34**, 432–435 (1971).
14. DeVenuto, F., Chader, G.: Interactions between cortisol or corticosterone and fractions of rat thymus, brain and heart cell. Biochim. biophys. Acta (Amst.) **121**, 151–158 (1966).
15. Domer, F. R.: Effects of diuretics on cerebrospinal fluid formation and potassium movement. Exp. Neurol. **24**, 54–64 (1969).
16. Eik-Nes, K. B., Brizzee, K. R.: Concentration of tritium in brain tissue of dogs given [1,2-^{3}H$_2$] cortisol intravenously. Biochim. biophys. Acta (Amst.) **97**, 320–333 (1965).

17. Eisenberg, H. M., Barlow, C. F., Lorenzo, A. V.: Effect of dexamethasone on altered brain vascular permeability. Arch. Neurol. **23**, 18–22 (1970).
18. Fingl, E.: Absorption, distribution, and elimination: practical pharmacokinetics. In: Antiepileptic Drugs, pp. 7–21. Woodbury, D. M., Penry, J. K., Schmidt, R. P. (Eds), New York: Raven Press 1972.
19. Fishman, R. A., Christy, N. P.: Fate of adrenal cortical steroids following intrathecal injection. Neurology **15**, 1–6 (1965).
20. Ford, D. H., Rhines, R. K., Stieg, C.: Hormone localization in the nervous system. In: Influence of Hormones on the Nervous System, pp. 2–16. Ford, D. H. (Ed.), Basel: S. Karger 1971.
21. Fukuda, T., Ui, J.: Breakdown of blood-cerebrospinal fluid barrier for calcium ions in the absence of glucosteroids. Nature **214**, 598–599 (1967).
22. Gallagher, B. B., Glaser, G. H.: Seizure threshold, adrenalectomy and sodium-potassium stimulated ATPase in rat brain. J. Neurochem. **15**, 525–528 (1968).
23. Gerlach, J. L., McEwen, B. S.: Rat brain binds adrenal steroid hormone: radioautography of hippocampus with corticosterone. Science **175**, 1133–1136 (1972).
24. Grosser, B. I: 11β-hydroxysteroid metabolism by mouse brain and glioma 261. J. Neurochem. **13**, 475–478 (1966).
25. — Axelrod, L. R.: Acetylation of cortisol by neonatal rat brain *in vitro*. Steroids **9**, 229–234 (1967).
26. — — Conversion of cortisol to cortisol acetate, cortisone acetate and cortisone by the developing primate brain. Steroids **11**, 827–836 (1968).
27. — Bliss, E. L.: Metabolism of 11-hydroxysteroids by cerebral tissues *in vitro*. Steroids **8**, 915–928 (1966).
28. — Krowas, S. T.: Acetylation of cortisol by a human astrocytoma. J. clin. Endocr. **31**, 589–591 (1970).
29. — Reed, D. J.: Uptake and metabolism of cortisol and corticosterone by rat cerebral cortex *in vivo*. Exp. Neurol. (in press).
30. — Stevens, W., Bruenger, F. W., Reed, D. J.: Corticosterone binding by rat brain cytosol. J. Neurochem. **18**, 1725–1732 (1971).
31. Haque, N., Thrasher, K., Werk, Jr., E. E., Knowles, Jr., H. C., Sholiton, L. J.: Studies on dexamethasone metabolism in man: effect of diphenylhydantoin. J. clin. Endocr. **34**, 44–50 (1972).
32. Harris, A. B.: Steroids and blood-brain barrier alterations in sodium acetrizoate injury. Arch. Neurol. **17**, 282–297 (1967).
33. Henkin, R. I., Casper, A. G. T., Brown, R., Harlan, A. B., Bartter, F. C.: Presence of corticosterone and cortisol in the central and peripheral nervous system of the cat. Endocrinology **82**, 1058–1061 (1968).
34. Hoagland, H.: Studies of brain metabolism and electrical activity in relation to adrenocortical physiology. Recent Progr. Hormone Res. **10**, 29–63 (1954).
35. Hooshmand, H., Dove, J., Houff, S., Suter, C.: Effects of diuretics and steroids on CSF pressure. Arch. Neurol. **21**, 499–509 (1969).
36. Johnson, J. A., Assam, S.: Use of betamethasone in reduction of cerebral edema. Milit. Med. **131**, 44–47 (1966).
37. Katzman, R., Aleu, F., Wilson, C.: Further observations on triethyltin edema. Arch. Neurol. **9**, 178–187 (1963).
38. Klatzo, I.: Presidential address. Neuropathological aspects of brain edema. J. Neuropath. exp. Neurol. **26**, 1–14 (1967).
39. Long, D. M., Hartmann, J. F., French, L. A.: The response of experimental cerebral edema to glucosteroid administration. J. Neurosurg. **24**, 842–854 (1966).
40. Mahesh, V. B., Ulrich, F.: Metabolism of cortisol and cortisone by various tissues and subcellular particles. J. biol. Chem. **235**, 356–360 (1960).
41. Maxwell, R. E., Long, D. M., French, L. A.: The effects of glucosteroids on experimental cold-induced brain edema. J. Neurosurg. **34**, 477–487 (1971).
42. McEwen, B. S., Magnus, C., Wallach, G.: Soluble corticosterone-binding macromolecules extracted from rat brain. Endocrinology **90**, 217–226 (1972).

53

43. McEwen, B. S., Weiss, J. M., Schwartz, L. S.: Selective retention of corticosterone by limbic structures in rat brain. Nature **220**, 911–912 (1968).
44. — — — Uptake of corticosterone by rat brain and its concentration by certain limbic structures. Brain Res. **16**, 227–241 (1969).
45. — — — Retention of corticosterone by cell nuclei from brain regions of adrenalectomized rats. Brain Res. **17**, 471–482 (1970).
46. Miner, L. C., Reed, D. J.: The effect of ethacrynic acid on sodium uptake into the cerebrospinal fluid of the rat. Arch. int. Pharmacodyn. **190**, 316–321 (1971).
47. Mitus, A.: Dexamethasone. Its effectiveness in the treatment of the acute symptoms of meningeal leukemia. Amer. J. Dis. Child. **117**, 307–312 (1969).
48. Murphy, B. E. P., Cosgrove, J. B., McIlquham, M. C., Pattee, C. J.: Adrenal corticoid levels in human cerebrospinal fluid. Canad. med. Ass. J. **97**, 13–17 (1967).
49. Nakazawa, S.: Biochemical studies of cerebral tissues in experimentally induced edema. Neurology **19**, 269–276 (1969).
50. O'Toole, R. D., Thornton, G. F., Mukherjee, M. K., Nath, R. L.: Dexamethasone in tuberculous meningitis. Relationship of cerebrospinal fluid effects to therapeutic efficacy. Ann. intern. Med. **70**, 39–48 (1969).
51. Overman, R. R., Davis, A. K., Bass, A. C.: Effects of cortisone and DCA on radiosodium transport in normal and adrenalectomized dogs. Amer. J. Physiol. **167**, 333–340 (1951).
52. Pappius, H. M., Gulati, D. R.: Water and electrolyte content of cerebral tissues in experimentally induced edema. Acta neuropath. (Berl.) **2**, 451–460 (1963).
53. — McCann, W. P.: Effects of steroids on cerebral edema in cats. Arch. Neurol. **20**, 207–216 (1969).
54. Peterson, N. A., Chaikoff, I. L.: Uptake of intravenously-injected [4-^{14}C] cortisol by adult rat brain. J. Neurochem. **10**, 17–23 (1963).
55. — Jones, C.: The *in vitro* conversion of cortisol to cortisone by subcellular brain fractions of young and adult rats. J. Neurochem. **12**, 273–278 (1965).
56. Reed, D. J.: The effects of acetazolamide on pentobarbital sleep-time and cerebrospinal fluid flow of rats. Arch. int. Pharmacodyn. **171**, 206–215 (1968).
57. — The effect of furosemide on cerebrospinal fluid flow in rabbits. Arch. int. Pharmacodyn. **178**, 324–330 (1969).
58. Reulen, H. J., Medzihradsky, F., Enzenbach, R., Marguth, F., Brendel W.: Electrolytes, fluids, and energy metabolism in human cerebral edema. Arch. Neurol. **21**, 517–525 (1969).
59. Rovit, R. L., Hagan, R.: Steroids and cerebral edema: the effects of glucocorticoids on abnormal capillary permeability following cerebral injury in cats. J. Neuropath. exp. Neurol. **27**, 277–299 (1968).
60. Sato, K., Yamaguchi, M., Mullan, S., Evans, J. P., Ishii, S.: Brain edema. A study of biochemical and structural alterations. Arch. Neurol. **21**, 413–424 (1969).
61. Schwartz, M. L., Tator, C. H., Hoffman, H. J.: The uptake of hydrocortisone in mouse brain and ependymoblastoma. J. Neurosurg. **36**, 178–183 (1972).
62. Shenkin, H. A., Gutterman, P.: The analysis of body water compartments in postoperative craniotomy patients. Part 3: The effects of dexamethasone. J. Neurosurg. **31**, 400–407 (1969).
63. Sholiton, L. J., Werk, Jr., E. E., MacGee, J.: Metabolism of cortisol-4-C^{14} and cortisone-4-C^{14} by rat brain homogenates. Metabolism **14**, 1122–1127 (1965).
64. Steiner, F. A., Ruf, K., Akert, K.: Steroid-sensitive neurones in rat brain: anatomical localization and responses to neurohumours and ACTH. Brain Res. **12**, 74–85 (1969).
65. Stevens, W., Grosser, B. I., Reed, D. J.: Corticosterone-binding molecules in rat brain cytosols: regional distribution. Brain Res. **35**, 602–607 (1971).
66. Taylor, J. M., Levy, W. A., Herzog, I., Scheinberg, L. C.: Prevention of experimental cerebral edema by corticosteroids. Neurology **15**, 667–674 (1965).
67. — — McCoy, G., Scheinberg, L.: Prevention of cerebral edema induced by triethyltin in rabbits by cortico-steroids. Nature **204**, 891–892 (1964).
68. Timiras, P. S., Woodbury, D. M., Goodman, L. S.: Effect of adrenalectomy, hydrocortisone acetate, and desoxycorticosterone acetate on brain excitability and electrolyte distribution in mice. J. Pharmacol. exp. Ther. **112**, 80–93 (1954).

69. Torack, R., Gordon, J., Prokop, J.: Pathobiology of acute triethyltin intoxication. Int. Rev. Neurobiol. **12**, 45–86 (1970).
70. Touchstone, J. C., Kasparow, M., Hughes, P. A., Horwitz, M. R.: Corticosteroids in human brain. Steroids **7**, 205–211 (1966).
71. Uete, T., Nishimura, S.: The effect of the administration of cortisol on the levels of cortisol and electrolytes in blood and cerebrospinal fluid in man. Metabolism **20**, 319–325 (1971).
72. — — Ohya, H., Shimomura, T., Tatebayashi, Y.: Corticosteroid levels in blood and cerebrospinal fluid in various diseases. J. clin. Endocr. **30**, 208–214 (1970).
73. Walker, M. D., Henkin, R. I., Harlan, A. B., Casper, A. G. T.: Distribution of tritiated cortisol in blood, brain, CSF and other tissues of the cat. Endocrinology **88**, 224–232 (1971).
74. Withrow, C. D., Woodbury, D. M.: Direct and indirect effects of desoxycorticosterone (DOC) on skeletal muscle electrolyte and acid-base metabolism. First Int. Congr. Horm. Steroids 1, 503–513 (1964).
75. Woodbury, D. M.: Effects of hormones on brain excitability and electrolytes. Recent Progr. Hormone Res. **10**, 65–107 (1954).
76. — Relation between the adrenal cortex and the central nervous system. Pharmacol. Rev. **10**, 275–357 (1958).
77. — Biochemical effects of adrenocortical steroids on the central nervous system. In: Handbook of Neurochemistry, Vol. 7, Chapter 13, pp. 255–287. Lajtha, A. (Ed.), Plenum Press 1972.
78. — Davenport, V. D.: Brain and plasma cations and experimental seizures in normal and desoxycorticosterone treated rats. Amer. J. Physiol. **157**, 234–240 (1949).
79. — Koch, A.: Effects of aldosterone and desoxycorticosterone on tissue electrolytes. Proc. Soc. exp. Biol. **94**, 720–723 (1957).
80. — Timiras, P. S., Vernadakis, A.: Influence of adrenocortical steroids on brain function and metabolism. In: Hormones, Brain Function and Behavior, pp. 27–54. Hoagland, H. (Ed.), New York: Academic Press 1957.
81. Zarrow, M. X., Philpott, J. E., Denenberg, V. H.: Passage of ^{14}C-4-corticosterone from the rat mother to the foetus and neonate. Nature **226**, 1058–1059 (1970).

Discussion to Chapter I see page 267

Chapter II

Effects of Steroids on Experimental Brain Edema

Effects of Steroids on Cold Injury Edema

Hanna M. Pappius

Montreal Neurological Institute, McGill University, Montreal, Canada

With 2 Figures

Summary. 1. Dexamethasone diminishes total edema which develops in response to a standard freezing lesion.

2. Dexamethasone does not affect the characteristics of the edema that does develop.

3. Dexamethasone drastically diminishes the EEG abnormalities which develop in response to a standard injury to the brain. This effect does not appear to be mediated by the effect of this drug on cerebral edema.

By way of introducing the session on the effects of steroids on experimental brain edema, it would seem appropriate to start by reviewing the work in this field to date. We are indeed fortunate, however, that many of the people whose work would be included in such a review are in fact here. I am sure that they all feel quite able to speak for themselves and would prefer that the interpretation of their experiments be left to them.

I will therefore restrict myself to some general remarks about the criteria for the presence of cerebral edema and the chemical methods that can be used for its quantitative estimation. I will then summarize and up-date our own data on the effects of steroids on changes associated with cold injury edema.

I must point out from the start that, on the basis of the evidence which my collaborators and I have accumulated over the years, it is my personal opinion that the clinically beneficial effects of steroids are not primarily mediated by the effect of these compounds on cerebral edema. I would have preferred to have our workshop entitled "Effects of steroids on injured brain" rather than "on brain edema". I think that if we can come to some concensus on this particular point as a result of our deliberations here, much will have been accomplished.

Edema is an increase in tissue fluid content resulting in an increase in tissue volume. Acceptance of such a definition implies that the one definitive criterion for the presence of cerebral edema is the demonstration of an increased water content of the affected tissues. While application of such a rigid criterion is impossible in clinical situations, in experimental investigations it is essential, even if only in representative experiments.

In our studies, cerebral edema is induced in cats by a freezing lesion, as described originally by Klatzo [3]. Our standard lesion is made by a probe 5 × 10 mm in area, which is cooled to —50° C and applied for 45 sec to the exposed dura over the suprasylvian gyrus of the right hemisphere of the cat.

We determine total edema which develops in response to this standard lesion by the difference in weight between the right, or experimental hemisphere, and the left, or control hemisphere. Since in normal animals average weights of the two hemi-spheres are the same, the increase in weight of the traumatized hemisphere is taken as the weight of the extravasated fluid. This is a rather insensitive, though a direct, method of estimating total edema. Measurement of the increase in water and/or in sodium content of the whole hemisphere represents a similar method of deter-mining total edema and may, in fact, be more sensitive.

Ideally, one would like to label the edema fluid with a marker not normally present in the brain and one which does not normally penetrate into cerebral tissues. This can be done in the case of vasogenic edema, such as the one associated with a freezing le-sion, because the normal barrier to the passage of a variety of substances from brain to blood is broken down or impaired. Serum proteins tagged either with fluorescent or radioactive material have been used in this way [2, 3, 7, 8]. However, as far as quantitative studies are concerned, results so obtained must be interpreted with cau-tion. This is demonstrated in Fig. 1 which illustrates the effect of time following a freezing lesion on the difference in weight and in RISA (radio-iodinated-serum-albumin) content between the hemispheres of cat brain. RISA content of each hemi-sphere was expressed as ml serum which would contain the amount of RISA found in the hemisphere.

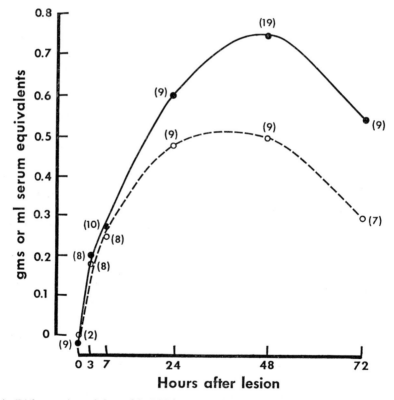

Fig. 1. Difference in weight and in RISA content between the right and left hemispheres of a cat brain after producing a freezing lesion on the right side (from data of Pappius and McCann, 1969). ●——● Difference in weight, o————o Difference in RISA content, ( ) Number of animals.

The difference in weight was measurable within 3 h after the lesion was made and continued to increase for 48 h, decreasing thereafter. At 48 h, the average increase in weight of the experimental hemisphere was about 0.8 gms. Since the average normal cat brain hemisphere in these studies weighed about 10 gms, this increase was equivalent to 8 % increase in weight or volume. Initially, the difference in RISA content of the two hemispheres followed closely the difference in weight, indicating that in edema induced by injury, not only is the so-called blood-brain barrier damaged, but in fact, the fluid which accumulates in cerebral tissues has similar albumin composition to that of plasma. However, a significant discrepancy developed between the two measurements with time. Time precludes a description of further experiments which demonstrated that this discrepancy was at least partly due to the removal of the label and not to repair of the blood-brain barrier at this stage. Thus, while RISA uptake reflects differences in the extent of edema, after the first 24 h it cannot be considered as a quantitative method of estimation of the accumulated edema fluid.

A more sensitive way of measuring edema is to determine the percentage dry weight, which is the reciprocal of the percentage water content of the tissue [1]. In our studies, we have applied this method to representative samples of cerebral cortex and of the white matter thus establishing whether edema was present and obtaining a measure of the extent of edema in the affected tissues. By analyzing edematous tissue samples for sodium and potassium it is possible to obtain information regarding the composition of the edema fluid. In vasogenic edema, the changes in tissue electrolyte content indicate an accumulation of a high-sodium, low-potassium fluid, compatible with its being derived from plasma. Under these conditions there is little, if any, net loss of potassium from the tissue.

But even the demonstration of a decrease in percentage dry weight must be interpreted with caution, and sodium and potassium determinations should be carried out at the same time. Later today, I will present data on the effects of ischemia on water and electrolyte content of cerebral tissues. In those studies, a sharp decrease in percentage dry weight of cerebral cortex was accompanied by a sharp loss of potassium and at least partly represented necrotic loss of tissue mass rather than edematous increase in tissue volume.

We have employed the methods just described to study the effects of steroid treatment on cerebral edema [5, 6, 7].

Our initial, completely unsuccessful attempts to demonstrate effects of cortisone on cerebral edema in the cat [6] were shown later to be due to a lack of biological activity of this particular steroid in that particular species [7]. I mention this here by way of a warning that studies on the effects of steroids, especially the negative ones, should include a demonstration of the biological activity of the substance tested under the experimental conditions used.

Subsequently we showed that pre-treatment with dexamethasone (0.25 mgms or 2.5 mgms/kg/day) diminished total cerebral edema induced in the cat with a freezing lesion [7]. This effect, demonstrable both on the difference in weight between the two hemispheres and on the difference in their RISA content, was statistically significant 48 h following the lesion, but not before.

These earlier results were confirmed in more recent studies [9] which are summarized in Table 1. In the current investigations we compared the effects of dexamethasone with those of furosemide, a renal diuretic whose effect on cerebral edema we also wanted to determine. The latter compound was given in a dose of 3 mgms/kg/day after an initial dose of 5 mgms starting at the time of the lesion. Dexamethasone, 0.25 mgms/kg/day, was started 48 h before the lesion was made and continued for the rest of the experimental period. The untreated and dexamethasone-pretreated groups include results of the earlier experiments.

Table 1. Difference in hemisphere weights in cats with a standard freezing lesion

| Experimental conditions | Time after lesion | |
	24 h	48 h
Untreated	0.65 ± 0.22 (29)	0.72 ± 0.29 (40)
Dexamethasone 0.25 mgms/kg/day	0.53 ± 0.23 (25)	0.56 ± 0.21[a] (28)
Furosemide 3 mgms/kg/day	0.46 ± 0.14[a] (14)	0.48 ± 0.16[a] (14)

Averages in gms $\pm$ S.D. Number of animals in brackets.

[a] Statistically significantly different from untreated, $p < 0.01$.

The effect of dexamethasone on total edema seen at 24 h amounted to a decrease of 18 % and was not statistically significant, despite the relatively large numbers of animals in each group. This is due to a considerable variability between individual animals in both the treated and untreated groups as seen by the size of the standard deviation. At 48 h following the lesion, the decrease was 22 % and was at that stage statistically significant with $p > 0.01$. Furosemide diminished cerebral edema to a greater extent than dexamethasone, the decrease being 29 and 33 % at 24 and 48 h respectively, both representing a significant difference from the untreated group ($p < 0.01$).

Despite their effect on total edema, dexamethasone and furosemide had no effect on the water and electrolyte content of affected tissues. The results for the experimental hemisphere are summarized in Table 2. Data for normal tissues are also included. The typical picture of vasogenic edema is evident: in the cortex no changes in percentage dry weight and electrolyte content; in the white matter, decreased percentage dry weight and potassium content and increased sodium content. I should mention that in some series of our experiments, small changes have been noted in cerebral cortex also. This depends on how close to the lesion the tissue samples are taken.

Two points should be made here. The decreased value for potassium in the white matter does not represent a net loss of potassium from the white matter. Rather it reflects a dilution of potassium originally present by a fluid low in potassium. Secondly, furosemide had no effect on the percentage dry weight of cerebral tissues of either hemisphere in the presence of a freezing lesion, whether given chronically or in a single dose, and it also had no such effect on normal animals indicating that its mechanism of action is different from that of urea [5] and other osmotically active agents.

The lack of effect of dexamethasone and furosemide on the water content of the affected tissues means that the edematous tissues in the treated animals are as edematous as in the untreated ones, but that the volume of the brain affected by edema is smaller, as evidenced by the data on total edema. This is essentially in agreement with the data of other investigators [4, 8]. In particular, I may mention the work of Hagan and Rovit who clearly demonstrated a relative restriction of the spread of edema fluid in dexamethasone-treated cats [8].

Table 2. Percentage dry weight and sodium and potassium content of cerebral tissues of cat after local freezing

Experimental conditions	Experimental hemisphere Time after lesion					
	24 h			48 h		
	DW	Na	K	DW	Na	K
Cerebral cortex						
Normal – no lesion	(19.0)	(58)	(105)			
Untreated (12) (14)	19.6	58	105	19.4	61	100
Dexamethasone (7) (5)	19.6	58	104	20.2	60	105
Furosemide (14) (14)	19.2	58	104	19.7	57	104
White matter						
Normal – no lesion (11)	(32.8)	(50)	(90)			
Untreated (12) (14)	23.0	88	60	23.9	84	64
Dexamethasone (7) (5)	23.8	80	68	23.4	81	67
Furosemide (14) (14)	25.3	86	67	25.3	76	68

Averages. Number of animals for the 24 h and 48 h groups in brackets
Dry weight – mgms%; Na and K – meq/kg wet weight
Dexamethasone, 0.25 mgms/kg/day starting 48 h before lesion
Furosemide, 3 mgms/kg/day starting at the time of lesion, after initial dose of 5 mgms

In our earlier investigations [7], dexamethasone appeared to improve dramatically the EEG abnormalities present in untreated animals 48 h after the lesion. The extent of these abnormalities could not be correlated with the degree of edema and no correlation could be demonstrated between the effects of dexamethasone on edema and on the EEG. These findings were open to two criticisms – they involved a relatively small number of animals and the subjective EEG gradings, although done without knowledge of the treatment which the individual animals received, could not be considered as a quantitative method of estimating brain function. For this reason, a study was initiated by G. J. Ball and H. P. Tutt using computerized frequency analysis of the EEG to re-examine more precisely these effects of dexamethasone. The work is still in progress. One of the investigators (G.J.B.) does the EEG recording and frequency analysis, while the other (H.P.T.) is responsible for treating the animals. Both kindly allowed me access to their respective data so that I could summarize their preliminary results at this time. Cerebral edema was produced in these experiments by our standard freezing lesion as already described. 48 h following the lesion, the monopolar EEG was recorded from the dura of the locally anesthetized cat by eight monopolar electrodes arranged as shown on Figure 2. The frequency spectra of 5 sec of EEG were computed for each channel over 120 sec and the averages of the resulting 24 frequency spectra for each channel were calculated. The area under the curve for each of the delta (0.8–4.0 cycles/sec), theta (4.4–7.2 c/s), alpha (7.6–12.8 c/s) and beta (13.2–20.0 c/s) frequencies was calculated for each averaged frequency spectrum and the ratio of low frequency (delta and theta) to high frequency (alpha and beta) was computed. A high ratio indicates predominance of slow waves in the EEG and is interpreted as abnormal.

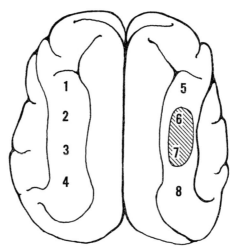

Fig. 2. Placement of electrodes for the electroencephalographic studies in the cat. Shaded area delineates the site of the freezing lesion

The preliminary results are summarized in Table 3. They essentially confirm our earlier findings. The ratio of EEG low frequency to high frequency activity was elevated in all 8 channels in animals with a standard freezing lesion of 48 h duration.

Table 3. Frequency analysis of EEG in cats

Experimental conditions	Left side (control) channel				Right side (experimental) channel			
	1	2	3	4	5	6	7	8
Normal (4)	1.1	1.0	1.0	1.0	1.1	1.0	0.8	2.1
48 h after freezing lesion Untreated (6)	1.8	1.9[a]	1.7	1.9[a]	3.0[a]	3.4[a]	5.0[a]	6.6[a]
Dexamethasone (6) (0.25 mgms/kg/day)	1.5	1.4	1.6	1.6	1.9[a]	2.0[b]	2.1[b]	2.3[a]
Furosemide (6) (3 mgms/kg/day)	2.8[a]	2.9[a]	2.3	3.3	2.6[a]	4.4[a]	7.5[a]	5.7[a]

Averages of ratio of EEG low frequency to high frequency activity. Number of animals in brackets.
[a] Statistically different from normal $p < 0.05$.
[b] Statistically different from untreated $p < 0.05$.
Preliminary data of G. J. Ball and H. P. Tutt.

In dexamethasone-treated animals, the ratios were higher than in normal animals, but in the traumatized hemisphere definitely lower than in untreated animals. Furosemide, which significantly diminished cerebral edema, and to a greater degree than did dexamethasone, had no effect on the EEG abnormality as compared with the untreated group. Although the study is incomplete at this time, the statistical analysis of data to date is included in the Table.

These results suggest, even more strongly than those of Pappius and McCann [7], that the beneficial effects of steroid therapy seen clinically are not fully explained by the effects of dexamethasone on cerebral edema. The functional response to steroids judged here on the basis of the EEG appears to be more striking than the response of cerebral edema, an impression strengthened by the finding that a substance, furosemide, which diminished edema to a greater extent than dexamethasone, had no effect on the EEG abnormality.

Acknowledgements. The author's experimental studies have been supported by the Donner Canadian Foundation and grants from the Medical Research Council of Canada.

References

1. Elliott, K. A. C., Jasper, H.: Measurement of experimentally induced brain swelling and shrinkage. Amer. J. Physiol. **157**, 122–129 (1949).
2. Klatzo, I., Miquel, J., Otenasek, R.: The application of fluorescein-labelled serum proteins (FLSP) to the study of vascular permeability in the brain. Acta neuropath. (Berl.) **2**, 144–160 (1962).
3. Klatzo, I., Piraux, A., Laskowski, E. J.: The relationship between edema, blood-brain-barrier and tissue elements in a local brain injury. J. Neuropath. exp. Neurol. **17**, 548–564 (1958).
4. Long, D. M., Hartmann, J. F., French, L. A.: The response of experimental cerebral edema to glucosteroid administration. J. Neurosurg. **24**, 843–854 (1966).
5. Pappius, H. M., Dayes, L. A.: Hypertonic Urea – its effects on the distribution of water and electrolytes in normal and edematous brain tissues. Arch. Neurol. **13**, 395–402 (1965).
6. Pappius, H. M., Gulati, D. R.: Water and electrolyte content of cerebral tissues in experimentally induced edema. Acta neuropath. (Berl.) **2**, 451–460 (1963).
7. Pappius, H. M., McCann, W. P.: Effects of steroids on cerebral edema in cats. Arch. Neurol. **20**, 207–216 (1969).
8. Rovit, R. L., Hagan, R.: Steroids and cerebral edema: The effects of glucocorticosteroids on abnormal capillary permeability following cerebral injury in cats. J. Neuropath. exp. Neurol. **27**, 277–299 (1968).
9. Tutt, H. P., Pappius, H. M.: In preparation (1972).

The Effects of Glucosteroids upon Experimental Brain Edema

Don M. Long, Robert E. Maxwell, and Lyle A. French

Department of Neurosurgery, University of Minnesota Health Sciences Center, Minneapolis, MN 55455, USA

Summary. Brain edema has been produced in rabbits, cats, dogs, and monkeys by the intracranial implantation of hydrophillic materials, stab wounds, implantation of viable brain tumors, inflation of extradural or subdural balloons, and cortical or spinal cord freezing injury. The temporal course of the evolution and resolution of brain edema in each of these models has been studied by gross photography, the extravasation of fluorescent protein tracers, wet weight/dry weight determinations, light microscopy, histochemistry, and electron microscopy. In a similar series of animals, the effects of glucosteroids given in several ways have been evaluated. Dexamethasone, cortisone, prednisone, and prednisolone have been utilized in dosages varying from 0.25 to 2.5 mg/kg/24 h. Animals have been pre-treated with steroids for 24 and 48 h prior to lesion production, and steroids have then been begun at the time of lesion production and at regular intervals up to 72 h after lesion production. The effects of the administration of glucosteroids upon the same parameters of edema estimation have been assessed. The cold injury model provides the best quantitative data. The administration of glucosteroids to animals in which a cold or spinal cord freezing injury has been inflicted results in a gross reduction in brain edema with reduced extravasation of dye protein complexes. Wet weight/dry weight determinations demonstrate significant retardations in the development of brain edema. At 24 and 48 h there is an approximate 50% reduction in edema, and at 72 h, a reduction of almost 30% persists. Light microscopic and histochemical differences were not striking. Electron microscopic studies revealed definite reduction in astrocytic volume and in white matter extracellular space in treated animals. The resolution of edema appeared to be accelerated. In addition, there was a marked reduction in post-edema astrogliosis in animals receiving glucosteroids.

Introduction

The use of glucosteroids is now commonplace in neurosurgical and neurological practice. Their effectiveness in relieving signs and symptoms of increased intracranial pressure, and improving neurological signs in a variety of clinical problems is unequivocal. Nevertheless, the mechanism by which these improvements are effected remains unclear. The use of steroids for the treatment of brain edema was first introduced by Galicich and French in 1959 [5, 6]. Their subsequent analysis of a series of patients indicated that the steroids were dramatic in relieving signs of increased intracranial pressure, and that the introduction of steroid treatment in conjunction with craniotomy had remarkably reduced post-operative mortality and morbidity in

---

This research was supported by USPHS Grant No. NBO 7341

brain tumor surgery [4]. These initial observations were soon substantiated [7, 28]. Gulati and Rasmussen reported their experience with steroids in brain surgery where no mass lesion was present, and the beneficial effects of the drug therapy were equally dramatic [28].

A few months after the introduction of the drug on a clinical basis, we began a laboratory project to validate the beneficial effect of steroids upon brain edema arising from a variety of causes, and to try to elucidate a mechanism of action for the steroids on brain edema.

The results of the published investigations into the use of steroids with experimental brain edema (both our own and the work of others) can be divided into those demonstrating a positive effect of glucosteroids upon brain edma, and those in which no such effect could be shown. Our initial studies, to be summarized in more detail in this paper, were carried out in rabbits, cats, and dogs in which brain edema had been induced by the intracranial implantation of psyllium seeds, cortical stab wounds, and extradural or subdural inflation of small balloons, or the creation of artificial subdural hematomas. Large doses of steroids administered prior to lesion production or began at the time of brain injury definitely reduced the amount of edema developing as estimated by wet weight/dry weight determination, gross brain appearance, and ultrastructural appearance. Morphometric examination of electron micrographs indicated a statistically significant reduction in volume of astrocyte processes and in the size of the increased extracellular space of edema [16]. At about this same time, Lippert et al., and Blinderman et al., both reported decreased edema in experimental animals after treatment with cortisone. Unfortunately, the number of animals in these reports are such that the results do not contain statistical significance [1, 18]. Taylor and colleagues showed there was a definite decrease in brain water and sodium following dexamethasone administration in triethyl-tin intoxication [33, 34]. Later, Rovit and Hagen studied brain edema and vascular permeability surrounding a radio-frequency lesion produced in cats. The extravasation of radioactive iodinated serum albumin was reduced in animals treated with steroids [29]. On the negative side, Clasen et al., were unable to demonstrate any effect of prednisolone upon cold induced edema in the first 12 h after injury [3, 27]. Pappius and Gulati did not detect significant changes in wet weight/dry weight determinations following local brain freezing, although in a later paper, Pappius and McCann did demonstrate reduced edema at 48 h in similar animals treated with dexamethasone [27, 28]. In addition, the electroencephalographic tracings in treated animals were significantly less abnormal than in their untreated counterparts. Plum et al. found no effect of dexamethasone upon the extravasation of trypan blue into ischemic brain [24, 25]. Kotsilimbas demonstrated an improved survival and increased function in animals treated with dexamethasone after the intracerebral implantation of melanoma. However, the effect appeared to be upon tumor growth and no effect upon brain edema was noted [15].

Because of these somewhat conflicting results, we have recently undertaken a reassessment of this problem utilizing a highly reproducible method of edema production. The effects of glucosteroids upon brain edema resulting from a local cortical freezing lesion have been assessed from time zero to 18 months after lesion production. A summary of the results of this study formed the basis for the majority of this communication, however, a brief summary of previous work in a variety of experimental models will be included for completeness.

66

Methods of Edema Production

1. *Brain Tumors.* The first investigation of edema was carried out in the brain of *rabbits* in which a Brown-Pearce carcinoma had been implanted 2–3 weeks before. Six animals were investigated, three were treated with dexamethasone, 2.0 mg/kg/day, administered intramuscularly from the time the first symptoms of increased pressure appeared in these animals for three days. Animals were then sacrificed following the administration of intravenous sodium fluorescein, and the spread of the fluorescent tracer, gross, light microscopic, and electron microscopic characteristics of the lesions studied. More recently, a primate model of brain edema has been developed by Brown [2]. Human choriocarcinoma is implanted into the hemisphere in an adult *Rhesus monkey.* 16–19 days later the animals develop the first signs of increased intracranial pressure. 12 animals have been employed in this study. Six of the animals received dexamethasone 2.5 mg/kg from the time of the first clinical sign for 4–7 days thereafter. Evaluation of the degree of edema present has been carried out by gross photography, wet weight/dry weight determination, the extravasation of Evans blue albumin, or fluorescein labeled albumin, light microscopy, radioactive brain scanning, and electron microscopy.

Table 1. Animal Models of Edema

1. Rabbits	Brown-Pearce Carcinoma	
	Intracerebral Subdural Psyllium Seeds	
2. Cats	Cortical Cold Lesion	
	Cortical Stab Wound	
3. Dogs	Subdural, Extradural Balloon Inflation	
	Subdural Hematoma	
4. Monkeys	Implanted Choriocarcinoma	
5. Cats	Spinal Cord Cold Lesion	
	Cortical Cold Lesion	

2. *Insertion of intracranial hydrophillic material.* The bulk of our early studies were concerned with the edema developing around a mass of psyllium seed implanted subdurally or intracerebrally in *rabbits.* 125 albino rabbits were utilized in this portion of the study. Fifty of these animals received dexamethasone in doses varying from 0.25 mg/kg of body weight per 24 h to 2.5 mg/kg of body weight per 24 h. One-half of these animals had the drug begun 24 or 48 h prior to lesion production, while in the remaining aimals, drug therapy was begun at the time of lesion production. The development of brain edema was again assessed by gross evaluation, the spread of dye tracers, wet weight/dry weight determinations, and light and electron microscopy.

3. *Intracranial balloon inflation.* The gradual inflation of a small balloon in the subdural or extradural space in *dogs* and the occasional accompanying development of a subdural/extradural hematoma in these animals was also studied. Steroid dose ranges were again from 0.25 to 2.5 mg/kg per 24 h, and drug therapy was begun

both before and with lesion production. Sacrifice was at 48 h, and the same methods for the evaluation of edema were employed.

4. *Cortical or spinal cord freezing lesion.* Upon review of the results of others, and our own results in this diverse group of animal preparations, it was felt that a more precise method for producing a predictable amount of edema would be desirable in order to delineate the effects of glucosteroids upon this edema. For this purpose, the cortical freezing lesion introduced by Klatzo proved to be admirable. Though mechanistically less pleasing than some of the methods more clearly analogous to clinical situations, the method proved to be very reproducible and highly desirable for quantitation. For all purposes, our series now exceeds 300 animals. Of these 168 have been specifically utilized for the study of the effects of glucosteroids. The results in this series of animals make up the bulk of the presentation. All of the animals in this study were anesthetized with intraperitoneal pentobarbital. The skull was exposed by a midline scalp incision and a hand trephine utilized to remove a one-quarter to one-half inch circle of bone. The dura was opened in the cruciate fashion and a metal plate previously cooled to $-50°$ C was applied to the second lateral frontal convolution for 7–10 sec. The adherence of the plate to pia was broken by a wash of physiological saline, the bone button was replaced and the skin closed. All animals were maintained without special care until sacrifice. Ninety-six animals comprised *Group I.* One-half of these animals received dexamethasone, 2.5 mg/kg IM every 12 h starting either 48 h prior to lesion production or at the time of lesion production. One-half the animals received no therapy. Animals were sacrificed at 5 min, 30 min, 1, 6, 12, 48, and 72 h; 5, 7, and 14 days, and 1, 2, 3, 6, 8, 12, and 18 months. All animals received Evan's blue albumin prior to lesion production and sodium fluorescein intravenously prior to sacrifice. Sacrifice was carried out under pentobarbital anesthesia by transcardiac perfusion of 5% formalin or 2.5% glutaraldehyde. Photographic records of the extent of spread of dye tracer was made. Fixed brain was retained for light microscopy, histochemistry, fluorescence microscopy, and electron microscopy. In *Group II* cold lesions were made in an identical fashion in 24 cats. One-half of these animals were treated with dexamethasone from the time of lesion production. Animals were sacrificed at 24, 48, and 72 h for wet weight/dry weight determinations of grey and white matter on the side of lesion production, and in the opposite control hemisphere. 24 additional animals were studied in *Group III.* Identical cold lesions were made, however, instead of dexamethasone, these animals received cortisone, 1.25 mg/kg per day, prednisone, 2.5 mg/kg, and prednisolone, 2.5 mg/kg/day. One-half of the animals were sacrificed 24 h after lesion production and the other half at 48 h. Identical methods for the evaluation of the degree of brain edema were employed in this group. *Group IV* consists of a small series of animals in which specific histochemical determinations were carried out. Since a sizable number of untreated animals had been processed for histochemistry, this entire group was treated with dexamethasone. One-half of the animals were given the drug 48 h prior to lesion production. The other half received it only after the lesion was made. The dose of dexamethasone was 2.0 to 2.5 mg/kg per 24 h. All animals were sacrificed at 24, 48, 72 h; or 4 or 7 days. After sacrifice, the tissue was processed for the following histochemical reactions: LDH; SDH; 6-glucose phosphorylase; glycogen; amino peptidase; and acid and alkaline phosphatase. In *Group VI,* in an effort to determine the effects of glucosteroids upon spinal cord edema, a similar cold lesion was made in the

thoracic spinal cord of 36 *cats*. One-half of these animals were treated with dexamethasone in the dose 2.5 mg/kg per 24 h. The evaluation of spinal cord edema was made by gross examination of the spinal cord, the extravasation of protein-labeled dyes, wet weight/dry weight determinations, and light, fluorescence, and electron microscopy.

Table 2. Methods of Evaluation of Effects of Steroids

1. Gross Photography
2. Spread of Dye (Planimetry)
3. Wet/Dry Weight Determinations
4. Light Microscopy
   a) Hematoxylin-Eosin
   b) Luxol-fast Blue
   c) PAS
   d) Holzer or PTAH
   e) FAN
5. Fluorescence Microscopy
6. Histochemistry
7. Electron Microscopy (Morphometrics)

Results

The basic results of our studies of the effects of glucosteroids upon experimental cerebral edema in all of the preparations, except the extensive studies on the cortical cold lesion, have previously been summarized [17]. Basically, in all groups of animals treated with large doses of steroids, the characteristic clinical course of untreated animals did not develop. For instance, untreated *rabbits* with intracranial psyllium seeds were uniformly comatose at 48 h and the majority expired from 72–96 h after their lesion production. However, in treated animals, only minor signs of irritability and reluctance to eat developed, and the survival rate was high. Few animals passed beyond the stage of lethargy. In all of these preparations, a decrease in the amount of extravasated protein-labeled dye tracer was found. All of these methods were imprecise enough and there was great variability in wet weight/dry weight determinations, making statistical validation by this method difficult. Light microscopic findings were not striking. These studies were primarily ultrastructural in type. While at the time the ultrastructural characteristics of brain edema were not well accepted, these have now been studied in detail and it serves no purpose to reiterate them here. On an ultrastructural level, there was a marked difference in the extent and degree of edema in these animals treated with dexamethasone. Astrocytic swelling was remarkably reduced and the general appearance of the grey matter near the offending lesion was close to normal. Astrocytes within the white matter were more swollen than those within the cortex but still significantly less enlarged than those seen in untreated animals. The white matter extracellular space was enlarged in all of these animals, but the degree of enlargement was significantly less than in their untreated counterparts. The degree of edema which developed was directly related to the amount of steroid administered and the timing of its administration. That is, animals pretreated with large doses of steroids had the least edema, those in which treatment was started at the time of lesion production developed more, and those in which treatment was delayed for 24 to 48 h developed the largest amount of edema. However, the eventual amount of edema was reduced in all three of these groups of treated animals. In an attempt to quantitate these ultrastructural observations, random morphometric examinations were carried out throughout the various edema preparations by the method of Hartmann [16]. These results are briefly summarized in Table 3. Basically, they indicated a 3–4 fold increase in astrocyte volume in untreated animals as compared with treated animals, and an increase in white matter extracellular space in untreated animals of up to 4 times that seen in treated animals. These differences are statistically significant and certainly seem to validate the morphological impressions [17, 18].

Table 3. Ultrastructural Morphometrics

Psyllium Seed Edema – Rabbits	
Treated	
Astrocyte Volume	10–14%
White Matter Excellular Space Volume	4–12%
Untreated	
Astrocyte Volume	33–55%
White Matter Extracellular Space Volume	37–45%

The Effects of Glucosteroids on Cold Induced Brain Edema

The extensive studies undertaken on the highly reproducible cold injury edema model provided multiple measures of the effects of glucosteroids upon brain edema. The first effect could be demonstrated by measurement of the gross area of edema seen on cut brain section as estimated by the extent of extravasation of Evan's blue albumin or sodium fluorescein labeled albumin. Mechanical planimetry was utilized to measure the area delineated by the extravasated dye in four regular sections taken at lesion midpoint (two sections) and at either extremity of the lesion (one section each). 24 h after lesion production, control animals averaged 2.44 sq. cm of dye stained white matter. Animals pretreated for 24 h before lesion production with glucosteroids averaged 1.24 sq. cm of edema, and the group in which treatment was begun at the time of lesion production averaged 1.95 sq. cm at 24 h. At 48 h comparable figures were 4.5 sq. cm for controls, 2.7 sq. cm for pretreated animals, and 3.14 sq. cm for post-treated animals. In addition to the fact that the area stained by dye was greatly reduced in treated animals, it was also apparent that a significantly smaller amount of dye had extravasated as judged by the blue coloration of the brain. However, dye which had extravasated in treated animals migrated at approximately the same rate and approximately the same distance as in control animals. The effect appeared to be on the amount of extravasated material.

Wet weight/dry weight determinations also demonstrated a significant effect of the glucosteroids. These results are summarized in Table 4. At 24 h, the increase in water per gram of original tissue weight in grey matter in animals receiving steroids was only 25 % of that seen in untreated animals. The comparable figure for increase in white matter was 50 %. At 48 h, increase in grey matter wet weight in treated animals was 44.5 % of the increase seen in untreated animals, and white matter edema was

70

found to be 72.5 % of the comparable figure in untreated animals. At 72 h, the difference between grey matter edema in treated and untreated animals was no longer present, however, there had been no further increase in white matter edema and edema remained 71 % of that seen in the untreated group. These figures are statistically significant.

Table 4. Increase in Water per gram of Original Brain Tissue

Hours after Cold Lesion		Tissue Weight Increase (gms)	
		Steroids	No Steroids
24	Grey	0.038	0.15
	White	0.335	0.67
48	Grey	0.08	0.18
	White	0.45	0.62
72	Grey	0.07	0.09
	White	0.34	0.48

The effects of cortisone, prednisone, and prednisolone were equivalent with dexamethasone as judged by these two parameters of edema [16, 17, 20, 21].

Light Microscopy

In the routine light microscopic studies employed in this investigation, no really significant differences were seen between treated and untreated groups of animals in the acute phase of edema, except for the changes seen in astrocytes. In untreated animals, an astrocytic reaction in the area of pure edema was apparent even a few hours after lesion production. The hypertrophied astrocytes were quite apparent and steadily increased so that by 3–6 months the previous area of edema could almost be outlined by the reactive glial cells. This glial reaction continued to 18 months, the longest time point sampled in this study. The effects of glucosteroid administration upon this gliosis were striking. Very little astrocytic reaction occurred early. Swollen astrocytes were obviously seen, but these were greatly reduced as compared with untreated edema. These cells had essentially disappeared by two weeks when the last vestiges of acute edema were gone. At later time points, very few reactive glial cells were seen in the previous areas of edema. The administration of steroids did not have any significant effect upon the gliosis of the lesion itself, or the maturation of this glial scar. However, the prevention of post-edema gliosis by glucosteroids in the previous edematous white matter well away from the lesion itself was striking, both in light and electron microscopy [21].

Fluorescence Microscopy

There were also significant differences seen by the use of fluorescence microscopy tracing the extravasated Evan's blue albumin or sodium fluorescein. In untreated animals there was widespread extravasation of the fluorescent tracer in the general vicinity of the lesion, similar to the pattern described by Klatzo *et al.* [10, 11, 12]. The dye first appeared diffusely as if it were extracellular in location. However, many neurons in the vicinity of, but not incorporated in, the lesion itself, fluoresced brightly and even at a very early stage, many astrocytes in the white matter beneath the lesion and in the surrounding grey were also filled with the fluorescent material. Whether or not these are viable cells is a moot point for the difference between this picture of widespread cellular fluorescence in which the entire cell was filled with the fluorescent tracer was strikingly different from that seen in steroid treated animals. In the latter group there seemed to be less extravasation and less background fluorescence from the extracellular fluorescent material. The striking difference, however, was in the cellular content of the fluorescence. Very few neurons even in the immediate vicinity of the lesion demonstrated any fluorescence and the number of fluorescent astrocytes was also markedly reduced. When fluorescent material was seen within these astrocytes and neurons, it was small in amount and globular in form, suggesting that it was being handled by some cellular mechanism in a viable cell. At later time points, differences by fluorescence studies continued to be present. In the untreated animals long chains of astrocytes appeared filled with fluorescent globules throughout the areas of edema, and shortly thereafter, huge swollen pericytes filled with fluorescent material and cellular debris were apparent. This astrocytic reaction was certainly suggestive of a phagocytic process. Such a reaction was present much earlier in treated animals, and the huge swollen pericytes disappeared much earlier as well.

Histochemistry

With the exception of one enzyme, the histochemical studies carried out on treated and untreated animal groups were not really rewarding [32]. There were no significant differences between treated and untreated animals in the enzymes studied except for the acid phosphatase reaction. Of course, differences demonstrable through the presence of increased numbers of astrocytes were present, but these were not different from those previously described by Rubinstein, and did not appear to be significant in terms of the action of the glucosteroids [31]. There were very suggestive differences in the appearance of acid phosphatase between treated and untreated animals, however. At 24 h, the amount of acid phosphatase present in areas of edema in untreated animals was definitely increased as compared with that present in the treated group. Utilizing the speed of appearance of acid phosphatase as a measure of lysosomal fragility, animals treated with glucosteroids demonstrated a definitely decreased fragility as compared with animals left untreated. Since these observations are highly qualitative, we are currently attempting to validate them by a quantitative method, but it certainly appears that glucosteroids may have a protective effect preventing the release of lysosomes in the area of edema.

Electron Microscopy

Thirty of the animals from the large series were processed for electron microscopy. These studies extended from one day through 18 months. The complete report of this temporal study of brain edema describing both the evolution and resolution of the process with and without treatment has been previously published, so only a summary is appropriate here. At 24, 48, and 72 h, the expected acute changes of brain edema were obviously present in untreated animals with the major volume abnormality being increase in white matter extracellular space and astrocytic swelling. In treated animals the amount of increase in the extracellular space of the white matter was consistently less and astrocytic swelling was even more dramatically reduced. While morphometric studies were not employed, these observations were validated by the use of large numbers of survey micrographs randomly selected through white matter at standard magnification. These micrographs were then reviewed by two independent observers and grouped according to degree of astrocytic swelling and size of extracellular space. Excellent correlation between the results of the two observers in terms of correctly grouping treated and untreated animals at the various time periods was obtained. At periods up to one week, definite evidence of accelerated resolution of the edema in treated animals was present with long chains of astrocytes appearing in the white matter and cortex. Shortly thereafter, swollen pericytes filled with cellular debris were found and their appearance in treated animals preceded their appearance in untreated animals by several weeks. As judged by electron microscopy, untreated edema was resolved in about 14 days, whereas it was largely gone within 5–7 days in treated animals. As previously stated, beyond the one month period, the major change in untreated animals was a progressive gliosis. In animals which had been treated this gliosis was markedly reduced [16, 17, 18, 19, 20, 21].

Spinal Cord Edema

The administration of glucosteroids in experimental spinal cord edema has been studied by the same basic battery of tests. A beneficial effect of the same general type has been noted by all of the parameters utilized. Wet weight/dry weight determinations reveal significant reduction in edema in animals receiving steroids at all time points from 6 to 72 h (Table 5, 6).

Table 5. Spinal Cord Edema (Treatment begun 24 h before)

Hours after Injury	Water content at lesion, % wet weight Untreated	Treated
1	64.8	64.3
2	65.4	65.0
3	67.3	65.1
6	69.6	65.6
12	77.1	70.0
24	75.1	69.0
48	72.6	68.0
72	67.5	64.0

Table 6. Spinal Cord Edema

Treatment begun	Water content at lesion, % wet weight at 12 h
24 h before	66.9
At lesion time 0	70.0
3 h after	71.9
6 h after	75.1
No treatment	77.1

Discussion

We believe that these studies, utilizing a great variety of experimental edemas un-equivocally demonstrate a beneficial effect of the glucosteroids in reducing brain edema. The failure of several investigators to corroborate our early morphological and biochemical studies may have several explanations. The type of lesion which pro-duces the edema is certainly important, and the timing of steroid administration is also a major factor. We have not demonstrated significant changes in less than 12 h, and most do not become obvious for 24 h after lesion production. The dose and admini-stration of the steroids and the type of steroids employed may also be important for variations in steroid metabolism between species do occur. An additional species factor is the size of the brain and the amount of white matter available for study. Since the edema process in man is primarily a white matter phenomenon, at least in terms of volume, larger animals with brains more closely analogous to humans are preferable for study, and the changes seen with steroids certainly are more definite in these animals [26].

Since all of the factors involved in the production of brain edema have not been clarified, it is not likely that all of the actions of glucosteroids can be classified at this time. There are many possibilities. Klatzo has shown that the basic mechanism for the development of brain edema is an increase in cerebrovascular permability, particu-larly to protein, and with the protein, water, and other ions [11]. In other models this change in vascular permeability has been shown to be secondary to direct injury to ca-pillary walls with actual mechanical disruption, and also to temporary physiological disruption of capillary endothelial junction with later reconstitution of the barrier [8, 9]. One definite fact from our studies appears to be a beneficial effect of glucoste-roids upon the so-called blood-brain barrier. There is consistently less extravasation of dye-protein tracer in animals receiving glucosteroids. This may well be effected through stabilization of the pentalaminar capillary endothelial junctions. Direct ef-fects upon sodium, potassium, and water transport across the capillary-glial inter-face have also been postulated as important in the genesis of brain edema. In other systems, glucosteroids have definite effects upon such transfers, and a analogous beneficial effect in the injured brain capillary is certainly possible [16]. The sug-gestions that the release of the histamine or histamine-like substance at the site of brain injury was responsible for the increased vascular permeability of brain edema was made thirty years ago and this postulation has recently been revived both in brain and spi-nal cord injury [13]. Glucosteroids have a well-known anticatecholamine effect and this is another possibility for their beneficial effects in brain edema. Iron is a potent peroxidizing agent and certainly iron, through the desintegration of hemoglobin, is present in most kinds of brain injuries. The role of peroxidation/oxidation in the development of brain edema has not yet been defined, but the postulation that even subtle changes in the lipoprotein structure of cell membranes induced by these chemical reactions could be responsible for brain edema is certainly attractive. Glu-costeroids have a rather nonspecific anti-oxidizing effect, and, therefore, could be ex-pected to have a beneficial effect upon this kind of peroxidizing system. Glucosteroids are generally known as nonspecific membrane stabilizers and effects upon membrane transport systems would not have to be limited to the capillary-glial complex. Widespread effects upon sodium/potassium transfers are certainly possible, and might

74

be particularly important in neuronal function. A stabilizing effect upon lysosomal membranes seems quite likely from our study and has been demonstrated in other non-neural systems. The glucosteroids have also been said to have a stabilizing effect upon intercellular cement substance. Gutterman and Shenkin have shown a decrease in post-operative water and salt retention in patients undergoing craniotomy who have been treated with glucosteroids [32]. While the exact contribution of this aspect of steroid function has not yet been studied experimentally, it certainly could retard the development of brain edema. Blood flow is also known to be decreased in edematous areas. Reduction in the amount of edema with subsequent reconstitution of more normal blood flow through the area, while not a primary effect, may certainly be important in the rapid recovery of function in many patients treated with glucosteroids and in the increased speed of resolution of edema.

In summary, our morphological and biochemical studies in the effect of glucosteroids upon brain edema cover many species of animals in many models of edema development. The results in all of the models of vasogenic brain edema appear to be qualitatively the same. A decreased extravasation of protein bound tracers, definite diminution in water content, decreased lysosomal activity, and striking decrease in post-edema gliosis are the morphological hallmarks of steroid effect upon brain edema. The exact mechanism by which these are effected is still unknown. An effect upon the pentalaminar capillary junctions and capillary permeability either directly or through catecholamine antagonism, stabilizing effects upon membranes and their transport systems, and a possible anti-oxidizing effect appear to be the most tenable theories at the present time.

References

1. Blinderman, E. E., Graf, C. J., Fitzpatrick, T.: Basic studies in cerebral edema: Its control by cortico-steroid (solu-medrol). J. Neurosurg. **19**, 319–324 (1962).
2. Brown, W. E., Long, D. M., French, L. A.: Brain edema in Rhesus monkeys harboring intracerebral tumors (in press).
3. Clasen, R. A., Cooke, P. M., Pandolfi, S. *et. al.*: Steroid-antihistamine therapy in experimental cerebral edema. Arch. Neurol. (Chic.) **13**, 584–592 (1965).
4. French, L. A., Galicich, J. H.: Use of steroid for control of cerebral edema. Clin. Neurosurg. **10**, 212–223 (1966).
5. Galicich, J. H., French, L. A.: Use of dexamethasone in the treatment of cerebral edema resulting from brain tumors and brain surgery. Amer. Practit. **12**, 169–174 (1961).
6. — — Melby, J. C.: Use of dexamethasone in treatment of cerebral edema associated with brain tumors. J. Lancet **81**, 46–53 (1961).
7. Gårde, A.: Experiences with dexamethasone treatment of intracranial pressure caused by brain tumors. Acta. neurol. scand. Suppl. **13**, 439–443 (1965).
8. Hammargren, L. L., Geise, A. W., French, L. A.: Protection against cerebral damage from intracarotid injection of hypaque in animals. J. Neurosurg. **23**, 418–424 (1965).
9. Harris, A. B.: Steroids and blood-brain barrier alterations in sodium acetrizoate injury. Arch. Neurol. (Chic.) **17**, 282–297 (1967).
10. Klatzo, I., Miquel, H., Otenasek, R.: The application of fluorescein labeled serum proteins (FLSP) to the study of vascular permeability in the brain. Acta. Neuropath. (Berl.) **2**, 144–160 (1962).
11. — Piraux, A., Laskowski, E. J.: The relationship between edema, blood-brain barrier, and tissue elements in a local brain injury. J. Neuropath. exp. Neurol. **17**, 548–564 (1958).
12. — Wisniewski, H., Smith, D. E.: Observations in penetration of serum proteins into the central nervous system. In: DeRobertis, E. D. F., Carrea, E. (Eds.) Progress in Brain Research, Vol 15, pp. 83–88. Amsterdam: Elsevier 1965.

13. KLATZO, I.: (personal communication).
14. Kotsilimbas, D. G., Meyer, L., Berson, M. *et. al.*: Corticosteroid effect on intracerebral melanomata and associated cerebral edema. Neurology (Minneap.) **17**, 223–226 (1967).
15. Lippert, R. G., Svien, H. J., Grindlay, J. H. *et al.*: The effect of cortisone on experimental edema. J. Neurosurg. **17**, 538–589 (1960).
16. Long, D. M.: An electron microscopic evaluation of cerebral edema and its response to steroid administration. Thesis: University of Minnesota 1964.
17. — Hartmann, J. F., French, L. A.: The response of experimental cerebral edema to glucosteroid administration. J. Neurosurg. **25**, 843–854 (1966).
18. — — — The response of human cerebral edema to glucosteroid administration. Neurology (Minneap.) **16**, 521–528 (1966).
19. — Maxwell, R. E., French, L. A.: The effects of glucosteroids upon cold induced brain edema. II. Ultrastructural evaluation. J. Neuropath. exp. Neurol. **30**, 680–697 (1971).
20. — — — The effects of glucosteroids upon cold induced brain edema. III. Prevention of gliosis following brain edema. (in press).
21. Maxwell, R. E., Long, D. M., French, L. A.: The effects of glucosteroids upon cold induced brain edema. I. Gross morphological and vascular permeability changes. J. Neurosurg. **334**, 477–487 (1971).
22. Pappius, H. M., Gulati, D. R.: Water and electrolyte content of cerebral tissues in experimentally induced edema. Acta. neuropath. (Berl.) **2**, 451–460 (1963).
23. — McCann, W. P.: Effects of steroids on cerebral edema in cats. Arch. Neurol. (Chic.) **20**, 207–216 (1969).
24. Plum, F., Alvord, E. C., Jr., Posner, J. B.: Effect of steroids on experimental cerebral infarction. Arch. Neurol. **9**, 571–573 (1963).
25. — Posner, J. B., Alvord, E. C.: Edema and necrosis in experimental cerebral infarction. Arch. Neurol. **9**, 563–570 (1963).
26. Prados, M., Strowger, B., Feindel, W.: Studies in cerebral edema. II. Reaction of the brain to exposure to air; physiologic changes. Arch. Neurol. **54**, 290–300 (1945).
27. Raimondi, A. J., Clasen, R. A., Beattie, E. J. *et al.*: The effect of hypothermia and steroid therapy on experimental cerebral injury. Surg. Gynec. Obstet. **108**, 333–338 (1959).
28. Rasmussen, T., Gulati, D. R.: Cortisone in the treatment of postoperative cerebral edema. J. Neurosurg. **19**, 535–544 (1962).
29. Rovit, R. L., Hagen, R.: Steroids and cerebral edema: The effects of glucosteroids on abnormal capillary permeability following cerebral injury in cats. J. Neuropath. exp. Neurol. **27**, 277–299 (1968).
30. Rubinstein, L. J., Klatzo, I., Miquel, J.: Histochemical observations on oxidative enzyme activity of glial cells in a local brain injury. J. Neuropath. exp. Neurol. **21**, 116–136 (1962).
31. Shenkin, H. A., Gutterman, P.: The analysis of body water compartments in postoperative craniotomy patients. III. The effects of dexamethasone. J. Neurosurg. **3**, 400–407 (1969).
32. Taylor, J. M., Levy, W. A., McCoy, G. *et al.*: Prevention of cerebral edema induced by triethyl-tin in rabbits by cortico-steroids. Nature **204**, 891–892 (1964).
33. — — Herzog, I. *et al.*: Prevention of cerebral edema by corticosteroids. Neurology (Minneap.) **15**, 667–674 (1968).
34. Yanagihara, T., Goldstein, N. P., Svein, H. *et al.*: Experimental cerebral edema: enzyme-histochemical study. Neurology (Minneap.) **17**, 669–679 (1967).

The Influence of Dexamethasone on Water Content, Electrolytes, Blood-Brain Barrier and Glucose Metabolism in Cold Injury Edema

H.-D. Herrmann, D. Neuenfeldt, J. Dittmann, and H. Palleske

Neurochirurgische Universitätsklinik, 6650 Homburg/Saar, W. Germany

With 5 Figures

Summary. 1. Cerebral edema in rabbits, induced by a local cold lesion, is influenced by dexamethasone. The "BBB" disturbance is reduced; an already disturbed "BBB" is restored faster, the sodium as well as the initial water content is reduced, so that the total water content is significantly lower than in the control series. This effect of dexamethasone seems to be localized not only at the capillary-tissue junction but also at the cellular membranes or intercellular junctions.

2. No influence of dexamethasone could be seen during the later course of the edema (later than 70 h), possibly due to a second "compartement" not influenced at all. *In vitro* no influence of dexamethasone on the glucose metabolism could be observed.

3. Extremely high doses of dexamethasone increase the water uptake of cortex slices *in vitro* so that the effect of dexamethasone seems to be dose-dependent.

Introduction

The mode of action of dexamethasone upon cerebral edema is still unknown and the quantitative aspect of its ability to inhibit the development and to enhance the resolution of brain edema is still controversial. To gain some more informations about these problems 3 sets of experiments were performed to examine:

1. The influence of dexamethasone on the time course of the changes in sodium and potassium in cold induced edema.

2. The influence of dexamethasone on the development and regression of the disturbance of blood-brain barrier and on the time course of the water accumulation in cold induced edema.

3. The influence of dexamethasone on swelling and glucose metabolism of incubated brain slices.

General Method of Series 1 and 2

Brain edema was induced in one hemisphere of rabbits using the method of Klatzo *et al.* [3], i. e., by epidural application of a copper cube cooled with acetone-dry ice for 30 sec. Groups of animals were killed at certain time intervals after the cold injury. The brains were removed immediately and the arachnoid and pia membranes stripped off. The water content was determined by weighing the fresh and dried samples.

77

1. Determination of Water Content and Na^+/K^+ Ratio [4]

Method. The entire injured hemisphere was analysed after removal of the necrotic area in the center of the lesion. Sodium and potassium were determined by flame photometry after preparation of the tissue according to Reulen *et al.* [7]. The electrolyte concentration was calculated on the dry weight basis, the water content was expressed as percent of total weight. Untreated controls were compared with steroid-treated animals. Dexamethasone (0.3 mg/kg body weight) was given daily starting one day prior to the injury.

Results. The control series (dashed lines) showed an increase in the water content up to 2 % and a comparable increase in the Na^+/K^+ ratio reaching a maximum about 24 h after the lesion and a slow decrease towards normal thereafter (Fig. 1). The increase of the Na^+/K^+ ratio [4, 5] was mainly due to the sodium increase, since on the dry weight basis potassium did not change significantly. Under dexamethasone medication the increase in water content as well as the increase of the Na^+/K^+ ratio was significantly lower as compared to the controls, the time course, however, almost remained the same.

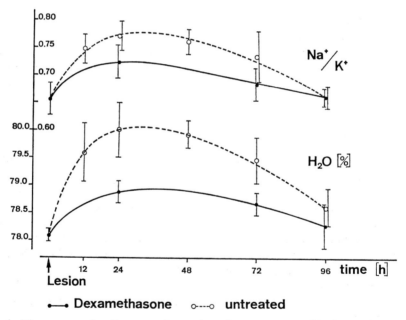

Fig. 1. Time course of sodium potassium ratio and water content of brain tissue after a cold lesion in rabbits. Untreated animals = dashed lines; dexamethasone-treated animals = drawn out lines

In these experiments the entire hemisphere, including the lamina quadrigemina, was examined. Thus, areas of severely damaged, though not necrotic tissue as well as non edematous areas distant to the lesion, including cortex, white matter and basal ganglion – with somewhat different reaction to trauma [9] – were analysed together.

In a second series of experiments we therefore only examined a small strip of tissue free of necrosis or petechial bleeding adjacent to the lesion, containing only cortical tissue.

2. Determination of the Blood-Brain Barrier [BBB] Disturbance and the Water Content in the Perifocal Edema

Method. As indicator for the BBB function ^{125}I-diiodo-fluoresceine was used. The erythrocytes of 8–10 ml blood of each rabbit were tagged with ^{51}Cr. The BBB indicator and the ^{51}Cr-erythrocytes were injected intravenously shortly after the cold lesion was applied. From each animal sacrificed at certain time intervals a small strip of brain cortex close to the lesion but free of necrosis or petechial bleeding as well as an analogous strip from the uninjured hemisphere was dissected out. Brain tissue water content and the BBB indicator concentration were measured in these strips. The concentration of the BBB indicator and of the ^{51}Cr-tagged erythrocytes was measured in 1 ml blood drawn by cardiac puncture as well as in the slices of both hemispheres. From the ^{51}Cr-erythrocytes content of the brain slices, the blood content could be estimated. From the total ^{125}I-activity of the brain slices, the calculated ^{125}I-activity of the blood, which the slices contained, was subtracted. The thus determined net BBB indicator concentration of the brain tissue was recorded as difference between injured and "healthy" hemisphere in counts per minute per gram tissue fresh weight. The edema was recorded as percentage difference of water content between injured and uninjured hemisphere. After a control series one series of animals received 0.3 mg/kg dexamethasone twice a day starting at the time of injury, in a second series this medication was started 48 h prior to the injury.

Results. a) *Controls.* The control series showed that the disturbance of the BBB reaches the maximum 21 h after the injury (Fig. 2). Thereafter a rapid and nearly complete restitution of the BBB takes place, thus limiting the water uptake so that the maximum of the water content is reached 3 h later and enabling elimination of the indicator from the tissue against a concentration gradient. Within this phase of repair a minimum of BBB disturbance (10 % of the maximum) and of the water content (55 % of the maximum) is reached 36 h after lesion production followed by a small second maximum 10 h later [2].

b) *Dexamethasone-treatment started at the time of injury.* The increase of the BBB disturbance to the maximum was not as straight as in the untreated group. The maximum was reached however, at the same time, 21 h after the injury (Fig. 2). The indicator concentration at maximum was 10 % lower than in the controls. The phase of repair was dramatically faster as compared to the controls. The minimum concentration was reached already 3 h after the time of maximal disturbance. The second maximum at 36 h could not be observed.

The water content increased at the same rate as in the controls but reached maximum value at the same time as the BBB disturbance which is 3 h earlier than in the controls. The percentage of water retained at maximum was 23 % lower than in the controls. This significantly lower water content was maintained up to 70 h after the lesion. At this time, there was no more difference between the treated and the untreated group; the water content in both groups, however, was still significantly above normal.

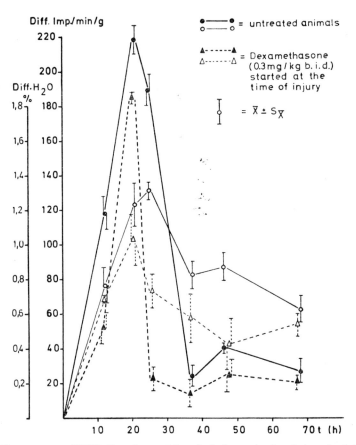

Fig. 2. Time course of BBB-disturbance (closed circles and triangles) and of the cortical water content (open circles and triangles) in untreated (drawn out lines) and in dexamethasone-treated animals (dashed lines). Treatment started at the time of injury

These results evidence a much faster restoration of the BBB disturbance and suggest a protection of the BBB against a disturbance following dexamethasone treatment. If the latter assumption is correct than a pretreatment with dexamethasone should be able to reduce BBB-disturbance to a minimum.

c) *Dexamethasone-treatment started 48 h before injury*. The BBB disturbance reached a maximum at exactly the same time as in the controls and under the condition 2b (Fig. 3 and 4). The maximum concentration of the BBB-indicator, however, was about 50 % lower than in the control group and about 35 % lower than in the group 2b. The phase of repair was not as rapid as in either of the former groups so that the 36 h concentration – a minimum concentration in the former groups – was significantly higher than the respective concentrations of the mentioned groups. About 70 h after the lesion there was no more difference between the three groups.

The tissue water content increased during the first 12 h at the same rate as in the controls and under the condition 2b (Fig. 5). The maximum of water accumulation occured at the same time as in the group 2b but was about 25 % less pronounced com-

80

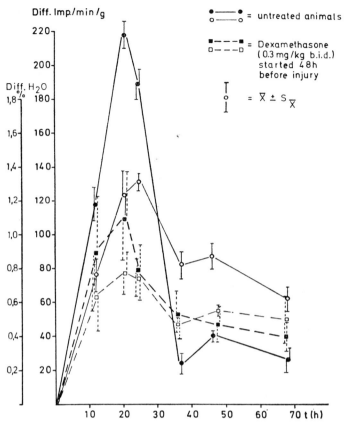

Fig. 3. Time course of BBB-disturbance (closed circles and squares) and of the cortical water content (open circles and squares) in untreated (drawn out lines) and in dexamethasone-treated animals (dashed lines). Treatment started 48 h before injury

pared to this group and about 43 % less than in the untreated group. Thereafter the water content did not differ at all from that determined in group 2b.

This series proved that dexamethasone exerts some protection against the BBB disturbance caused by a cold lesion in a cortical region adjacent to this lesion. This protecting effect, however, inhibits only the initial water uptake so that the maximum value is lower than in group 2b, while the further course remains the same.

The mechanism by which dexamethasone protects the BBB against disturbance or restores a disturbed BBB faster is unknown. *In vitro* examinations could throw some light on this problem if the glucose metabolism of the tissue is directly and mainly influenced by dexamethasone.

3. Determination of the Water Content and some Parameters of the Glucose Metabolism in Rabbit Brain Slices after in vitro Incubation according to Warburg's two-vessels method

Method. Rabbit brain cortex freed of arachnoid and pia membrane was sliced and incubated according to Warburg's two-vessels method. These slices swell during incubation. In these experiments the Q_{O_2}, $Q_{CO_2}^{O_2}$ as well as the glucose consumption and lactate and pyruvate production during incubation were determined. The "extracellular space" was estimated with inulin and the "intracellular space" by the difference between sucrose and inulin uptake with all the caution of interpretation Pappius [6] has stressed. Water content was determined by fresh and dry weight determinations of comparable samples without and after incubation.

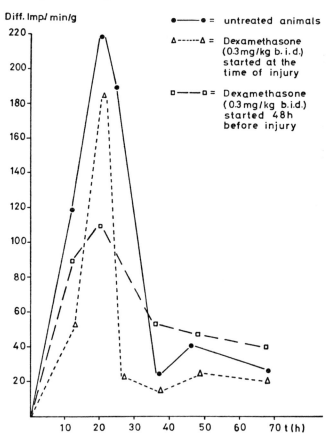

Fig. 4. Time course of the BBB-disturbance of the control series and the two dexamethasone-treated series 2b and 2c for comparison

Results. High concentrations of dexamethasone (0.25 mg/ml) added to the incubation medium increased the water uptake of the brain slices.

Lower concentrations of dexamethasone (2.5 μg/ml; 10 μg/ml; 25 μg/ml) caused in 8 out of 10 experiments a small but significant decrease of the water uptake, in 2 experiments, however, a slight increase. In the experiments with a decreased water uptake the "extracellular" as well as "intracellular space" were reduced.

The metabolic studies also disclosed differing results: in some experiments a slight augmentation, in others a small reduction of the glycolytic breakdown of glucose was observed. The respiratory metabolism of the slices was not influenced by dexamethasone.

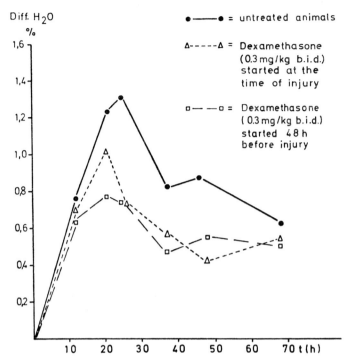

Fig. 5. Time course of the water content of the control series and of the two dexamethasone-treated series 2b and 2c for comparison

These results show that dexamethasone has no direct and unique effect on the glucose metabolism. They suggest, however, a membrane effect reducing the water uptake of the slices. (The glucose uptake was uninhibited.) Under *in vitro* conditions this effect cannot be localized at the capillary-tissue junction, it rather must be localized directly at the cell membranes and intercellular junctions.

Discussion

Many points of this paper are open for discussion, a few shall be presented:

1. The curves shown in Figure 1 do not correspond in their time course to the figures of series 2 (Fig. 5). This may be due to the different brain areas examined in these series. The untreated group of series 1 showed a maximal increase of brain water content of 2 % and a slower normalization (at 70 h a decrease of 0,5 % of maximum) compared to a maximal increase in cortical water content of 1,3 % with a decrease of 0,7 % at 70 h in series 2. It can be assumed that a greater part of more severely damaged tissue or a greater part of white matter was examined in series 1 which is known to be more edematous and to retain water longer probably due to the greater amount of proteins penetrated into these areas.

2. The reduction of the Na^+/K^+ ratio following dexamethasone-treatment in series 1 is comparable to the reduction of the BBB-disturbance in series 2c (in both series 50 % of the maximum value of the control series).

The reduction in water content, however, was more pronounced in series 1 than in series 2c. This has to be investigated in more detail. One explanation may be the different dosage of dexamethasone in these series. In series 2c each aimal received daily twice the dose as in series 1 and the medication was started 48 h before the injury whereas in series 1 it was started 24 h before. The *in vitro* experiments show a significant increase in water uptake at high dexamethasone concentration. If in series 2c dexamethasone accumulated then relatively high blood concentrations could have been attained already at the time of injury. It therefore could be possible that the concentrations used in series 1 were more effective in protecting the BBB even in unfavourable areas than the concentrations used in series 2c.

3. The time curve of the water content of the cortex samples (Fig. 5) of series 2b compared to that of the control series is lower in the maximum and shows this lower level almost parallel to the control curve up to about 70 h following the lesion. The time curve of the water content of series 2c only differs in the maximum from the curve of series 2b, the further course is exactly the same in both curves. This means that neither under condition 2b nor under 2c it is possible to reduce the edema in the later course. If one roughly extrapolates the curve formed by the maximum towards zero by connecting maximum and the first minimum by a straight line in each curve these extrapolated zeropoints all lie between 60 and 70 h which is roughly the time when the three curves join at a much higher level. This suggests that each curve presented in Figure 5 actually consists of 2 overlying curves; one that gives the initial maximum with a short time constant and another with a long time constant. It furthermore suggests that only the first or rapid curve is influenced by dexamethasone, whereas the slow curve remains unchanged. It may be conceived that the dimensions of such two compartments differ from species to species which could explain some of the discrepancies in the action of dexamethasone reported in the literature. This problem is a matter of our present investigation.

4. In spite of the obvious ability of dexamethasone to reduce the disturbance of the BBB after a cold lesion it was not possible to protect the BBB completely as shown by Figure 4. Two explanations seem possible for this: Either in our series 2c we already have overdosed dexamethasone so that – as in our *in vitro* experiments – a contrary effect, a disturbance of the BBB, takes place, or one part of the initial disturbance cannot be influenced by dexamethasone at all. This again shall be the aim of a further investigation.

5. Observing the time course of the tissue concentration of ^{125}I-diiodo-fluresceine following a cold lesion we concluded that there is a disturbance of the BBB. As the *in vitro* experiments suggest, some influence of dexamethasone is exerted on the membranes or intercellular junctions directly. If this is correct then the "BBB" which we examined should not be localized entirely at the capillary-tissue junction but at least to some extent within the tissue itself.

References

1. Herrmann, H.-D., Dittmann, J.: Examination of the metabolism of oedematous brain tissue. I. Alterations of the metabolism in the cold induced oedema of the rabbit brain measured manometrically in vitro. Acta neurochir. **22**, 167–175 (1970).

2. Herrmann, H.-D., Neuenfeldt, D.: Development and regression of a disturbance of the blood-brain-barrier and of edema in tissue surrounding a circumscribed cold lesion. Exp. Neurol. **34**, 115–120 (1972).
3. Klatzo, J., Piraux, A., Laskowski, E. J.: The relationship between edema, blood-brain-barrier and tissue elements in a local brain injury. J. Neuropath. exp. Neurol. **17**, 548–564 (1958).
4. Palleske, H., Herrmann, H.-D., Kremer, G.: Verlaufsuntersuchungen über Veränderungen des Elektrolyt- und Wassergehaltes des Gehirns im experimentellen Hirnödem und deren therapeutische Beeinflussung durch Dexamethason. Zbl. Neurochir. **31**, 31–37 (1970).
5. Pappius, H. M., Gulati, D. R.: Water and electrolyte content of cerebral tissues in experimentally induced edema. Acta neuropath. (Berl.) **2**, 451–460 (1963).
6. — Distribution of water in brain tissues swollen in vitro and in vivo. Brain Res. **15**, 135–154 (1965).
7. Reulen, H. J., Aigner, P., Brendel, W., Messmer, K.: Elektrolytveränderungen in tiefer Hypothermie. Pflügers Arch. ges. Physiol. **288**, 197–219 (1966).
8. — Medzihradsky, F., Enzenbach, R., Marguth, F., Brendel, W.: Electrolytes, Fluids and Energy Metabolism in Human Cerebral Edema. Arch. Neurol. **21**, 517–525 (1969).
9. — Steude, U., Hilber, C., Prusiner, S., Brendel, W.: Energetische Störungen des Kationentransports als Ursache des intracellulären Hirnödems. Acta neurochir. **22**, 129–166 (1970).

Multiple Therapeutic Approaches in the Treatment of Brain Edema Induced by a Standard Cold Lesion

Don M. Long, Robert E. Maxwell, Kil Soo Choi, Harry O. Cole, and Lyle A. French

Department of Neurosurgery, University of Minnesota Health Sciences Center, Minneapolis, MN 55455, USA

Summary. Brain edema was produced by a standard cortical freezing lesion. The temporal course of the evolution and resolution of this edema has been reported elsewhere in detail. The effects of many types of therapy, both standard and investigational, upon this model of brain edema have been employed. Osmotic diuretics were found to have no effect upon the edema itself, but a reduction in the bulk of normal brain was evident. Maintenance of hypotension after lesion production essentially eliminated brain edema whereas prolonged hypertension increased brain edema dramatically. Focal excision of the cold injury itself immediately after lesion production prevented the development of brain edema. A beneficial effect on brain edema by focal excision was evident up to 24 h after injury at all time points from 6 h on. The addition of glucosteroids to focal excision reduced edema even further. Treatment of animals with dibenzyline, dimethyl sulfoxide, and diphenyl-p-phenylenediamine also had a beneficial effect upon the development of edema. Combination of steroids and osmotic diuretics was not of value. Focal excision with acetazolamide was extremely effective in reducing brain edema. A combination of DMSO and dexamethasone was more effective than either drug alone. Detailed studies to elucidate the effects of hypotension or hypertension in each of these therapeutic regimens were carried out.

Introduction

The first treatment for brain edema was removal of the causative lesion and/or widespread bony decompression to allow expansion of the intracranial contents and to reduce pressure inside the skull. Before the days of angiography and pneumoencephalography, a temporal decompression for the nonspecific reduction of brain edema secondary to an unlocalizable brain tumor was a standard neurosurgical operation. While removal of an edemagenic lesion is still a cardinal feature of the treatment of many patients with brain edema, these bony decompressions are rarely necessary now. The second form of therapy available for brain edema began with Weed's classic experiments on the effects of hypotonic and hypertonic solutions upon brain bulk [11]. The clinical significance of Weed's experiments was recognized, and over the next twenty years, a large variety of osmotically active agents were tried for the reduction of brain bulk. None were remarkably successful until Javid introduced urea for this purpose [4]. In order to obviate some of the problems with urea, mannitol was subsequently employed and glycerol has also been utilized, particularly orally. All of these osmotic diuretics have approximately the same effect. By increasing

This research was supported by USPHS Grant No. NBO 7341 and the Lyle A. French Fund for Neurosurgical Research and Training.

the osmolarity of the blood, they extract water from normal brain, but unfortunately do not reduce the water content of edematous brain [8]. As Klatzo has pointed out, they also can cross the damaged blood-brain barrier responsible for the edema, increasing the osmolarity locally in the region of edema, and at a later time when the blood level has fallen, actually increase the amount of water passing into the edematous area [6]. In spite of these two drawbacks, the drugs have obvious advantages in that they act rapidly over 15 to 45 min; reduce intracranial pressure and brain bulk dramatically; and maintain this reduction for 6–8 h. They are relatively innocuous and complications of their use are few. That steroids might have an effect upon brain edema was suggested by experimental data as early as 1945 [9]. The glucosteroids were introduced by Galicich and French in 1959 for the specific treatment of brain edema complicating brain tumors, and later expanded by these authors into the treatment of vasogenic edema of many causes [1, 3]. Their clinical effectiveness is undoubted [10]. Nevertheless, the use of glucosteroids does not completely solve the edema problem. The effects of the steroids are rarely evidenced before 12 h and are rarely maximal before 24 h [7]. There appears to be degrees of edema so severe that the effects of the steroids are not satisfactory to completely relieve the mass effect. Some patients cannot be given steroids and the development of complications may occasionally force their discontinuation. Hypothermia has been used extensively in neurosurgery, and has been recommended as a treatment for brain edema. On an experimental basis, hypotension is also effective in reducing the amount of edema expected from the standard cold cortical lesion, and, conversely, hypertension tremendously increases the amount of edema present [5].

In an attempt to improve the treatment of human brain edema, we have undertaken a study comparing the use of standard therapies in combination, and we are also exploring several new avenues of edema therapy. This paper summarizes the preliminary results of some of these investigations to date.

Methods

The edema model employed is the standard cortical freezing lesion described by Klatzo. Adult male and female cats averaging from 2.5 to 4 kg in body weight have been employed. The technique, as we have modified it, is as follows. All animals are anesthetized with pentobarbital administered intraperitoneally. A midline scalp incision is made and the temporalis muscle cut away from one side of the skull. A one-half inch trephine is utilized to remove a bone button and the dura opened in a cruciate fashion exposing the suprasylvian gyrus. A metal plate measuring 2 × 5 mm, previously cooled to —50° C with a mixture of acetone and dry ice, is then applied by hand to the exposed gyrus for 30 sec. The adherence of the plate to the pia is broken by a wash of physiologic saline. The dura is replaced by a small pledget of gellfoam. The bone button is put loosely in place and the skin closed with clips.

In order to provide accurate assessment of the effect of hypothermia, hyperthermia, hypotension, and hypertension, as well as to separate direct effects of drug therapies from the effects of drugs on blood pressure alone, the following studies were carried out. An intra-arterial cannula was introduced via the femoral artery for monitoring blood pressure. Rectal and esophageal temperature probes were put in place and precordial electrocardiographic leads employed. Respiration and pulse rate were also monitored. All of this material was displayed visually, simultaneously on a Hewlett-Packard ink writing recorder either throughout the period of treatment, or in the case of animals surviving for more than 24 h, at regular intervals during the course of treatment.

Edema was estimated grossly, by spread of dye-protein tracers, and by wet/dry weight determinations in each animal [6, 8]. Multiple types of therapies have been employed in this study (Table 1).

Table 1. Methods of therapy

---

1. Osmotic diuretics
2. Hypotension
3. Steroids
   Hypotension
   Osmotic diuretics
   DMSO
4. Focal excision
   Steroids
   Hypotension
   Furosemide
   Acetazolamide
5. Drugs
   Dibenzyline
   Thorazine
   DMSO
   DPPD
   Acetazolamide
   Furosemide

---

1. *Osmotic diuretics.* In order to make satisfactory comparisons the result of the administration of osmotic diuretics in our model was studied. Eight animals were employed. One group of animals received the drug immediately after lesion production, another group 24 h after lesion production. One-half the animals were sacrificed 24 h after administration of the drug, and one-half after 180 min. All animals were given intravenous mannitol 20% in a total dose of 3 gm/kg of body weight in rapid intravenous infusion.

2. *Hypotension/hypertension.* Hypotension to the level of 30, 50, or 70 mmHg was induced by an intravenous drip of Arfonad employed as necessary to maintain the blood pressure at a constant level. In three of the animals treatment was begun immediately after lesion production. In the second group, treatment was begun only after 24 h of edema developed. Hypertension (180 mmHg) was induced in a similar manner in three animals by the use of intravenous infusions of levarterenol begun at the time of lesion production and continued for 24 h.

3. *Focal excision of lesion.* In this group of 36 animals, the edemagenic lesion was removed at varying time points after its production. The effect of this removal upon the developing edema alone and in combination with other therapies was then assessed. In all animals the method of removal was the same [2]. Each animal had been

given intravenous Evan's blue-albumin just before lesion production, and within a few minutes after standard cold lesion production. The area of injury was well demarcated by the extravasated dye. Using the operating microscope, microsurgical techniques and bipolar coagulation, the pia was opened only along the crest of the lesion gyrus, and the lesion itself carefully removed maintaining immaculate hemostasis. In one-third of the animals, the gyrus removed was replaced with blood so that bulk remained the same. Focal brain excision animals were sacrificed 24, 48, or 72 h later. In a second group of animals, edema was allowed to develop for 6, 24, 48, and 72 h before excision. These animals were then allowed to live 24 h before sacrifice.

4. *Investigational drugs.* In this group of eight animals, we have created a standard cold lesion and then treated the resultant edema with a variety of investigational drugs. These include dimethyl sulfoxide (DMSO), diphenyl-p-phenylenediamine (DPPD), and the alpha adrenergic blocking agent dibenzyline. Sacrifice in each case was at 24 h.

5. *Combination therapies.* In the area of combination therapy, we have utilized several modes of treatment which may have application in the clinical situation. These include a combination of dexamethasone and hypotension (4 animals), and excision of the lesion 24 h after its production in combination with either hypotension, furosemide, or acetazolamide (6 animals). In addition, we have used DMSO and dexamethasone in combination 24 h after lesion production, dexamethasone and focal excision have been combined in an extensive study (36 animals).

Results

The results of these multiple experiments are included in Tables 2, 3 and 4. These effects of focal excision are expressed as increment of water per gram of original tissue weight so these data can be compared with our other published material. In Tables 2 and 3 the effects of various therapies are expressed as per cent increase or decrease in original white matter wet weight. Since the actual number of animals employed is large (over 100), presentation of numerical data in tabular form would be prohibitive. These percentages are derived by individually calculating increases or decreases in white matter water as compared with original tissue weight and then averaging the group. An extensive statistical analysis of these data will soon be published.

1. *Osmotic diuretics.* The administration of mannitol starting at the time of lesion production resulted in white matter wet weight reductions of 10 % in the normal hemisphere at 3 h. The amount of edema in the lesion hemisphere was unchanged. In animals so treated with sacrifice at 24 h the wet weight figures were the same as for untreated animals. Mannitol administered 24 h after lesion production brought about a similar immediate reduction of 10 % on the normal side without significant effect upon the edema. Delay of sacrifice by 24 h eliminated the effect upon normal brain and there was no effect upon the amount of edema. As demonstrated by Pappius the reduction appeared to be in the normal rather than edematous white matter primarily [8] (Table 2).

2. *Hypertension/hypotension.* The administration of intravenous levarterenol continuously after lesion production (180 mmHg) produced a marked increase in brain wet weight and this increased edema was verified by increased extravasation of Evan's

blue albumin. At 24 h the wet weight of the edematous hemisphere had increased by 34 %. Hypotension induced by a continuous intravenous infusion of Arfonad brought about a marked decrease in brain edema. At the lowest levels no significant edema occurred. Averaging all levels (30–70 mmHg), only a 3 % increase in percent wet weight in the lesion hemisphere occurred.

Table 2. Percent wet weight, white matter

	24 h	48 h
1. Control (sham operation)	64–66%	64–66%
2. Lesion (no therapy)	80–82% (+24%)	82–84% (+28%)

Change in % wet weight by therapy, compared to normal white matter

1. Mannitol				
	Immediate	lesion	+25%	
		normal	−10%	
	24 h	lesion	+26%	
		normal	± 0%	
2. Hypertension (180 mmHg)			+34%	
3. Hypotension (30–70 mmHg)			+ 3%	
4. Dexamethasone			+10%	+12%
5. Focal excision (see Table 3)				
6. Dibenzyline			+14%	
7. DMSO				
	Immediate		+10%	
	After 24 h		—	+20%
8. DPPD			+14%	

Table 3. Combination therapy, % change in wet weight compared to normal white matter

	24 h	48 h
1. Focal excision and steroid immediate	0	0
30 min	+ 6%	+12%
24 h	+10%	+12%
2. Focal excision (24 h) + hypotension	+12%	
3. Focal excision (24 h) + furosemide	+17%	
4. Focal excision (24 h) + acetazolamide	+ 5%	
5. DMSO + dexamethasone	+10%	

3. *Steroids.* These data have been reported in detail elsewhere in this symposium. Treatment with dexamethasone (2.0–2.5 mg/kg/24 h IM) results in edema reduction of 50 % at 24 h, 45 % at 48 h, and 28.5 % at 72 h [7].

4. *Excision.* Immediate excision of the injured tissue essentially completely prevented the development of edema. No significant changes in wet weight occurred. If excision was delayed for 30 min edema development was reduced by almost 50 % at

91

24 h; at 48 h an even greater reduction occurred; at 72 h, the beneficial effects were still present though reduced. Excision of the lesion 24 h after production resulted in a reduction in edema of 32%, but surprisingly enough the effects at 48 and 72 h were very comparable to those seen with excision much earlier (Table 4).

Table 4. Effects of focal excision, white matter increment of H_2O/gram of original tissue weight

	24 h	48 h	72 h
No therapy	0.68	0.62	0.48
Immediate excision	—	—	—
Immediate excision and dexamethasone	—	—	—
Excision, $^1/_2$ h	0.39	0.26	0.37
Excision, $^1/_2$ h and dexamethasone	0.19	0.18	0.31
Excision, 24 h	0.47	0.26	0.32
Excision, 24 h and dexamethasone	0.31	0.18	0.34

5. *Experimental drugs.* The administration of dibenzyline, 5 mgm, intravenously at the time of lesion production definitely decreased edema, at 24 hours % wet weight increase was 14% (Table 2). DMSO administered at the time of lesion production resulted in +10% edema as contrasted with wet weights in untreated controls. DMSO administered 24 h after lesion production brought about a wet weight increase of 20%. The dose of DMSO was 0.5–1.5 cc intravenously. DPPD 2 cc intravenously also brought about a moderate reduction in edema formation on a comparative basis (+17%) (Table 2).

6. *Combination therapies.* The results of the various combination therapies are found in Tables 3 and 4.

a. Focal excision plus steroids. The addition of steroids to the results of immediate focal excision were not apparent since essentially no edema developed in this model with excision alone. However, as the excision was performed further and further away from the actual time of lesion production, the effect of focal excision alone became less prominent and the effects of steroids became more obvious. Excision carried out one-half hour after lesion production coupled with dexamethasone led to reduction in edema of about 70% at 24 and 48 h and about 40% at 72 h. Delaying excision to 24 h coupled with steroids reduced edema only about 50% at 24 h, but at 48 and 72 h effects were comparable to the earlier excisions. Focal excision at 24 h coupled with Arfonad-induced hypotension for 24 h after brought about only minimal reduction in brain edema (+20%).

b. Focal excision with furosemide was accompanied by minimal reduction in edema development, comparative weights were +17%.

c. Focal excision plus acetazolamide, 10 mgm/kg administered intravenously were accompanied by a marked reduction in brain edema. Comparative weights were +5% at 24 h compared with controls.

d. The combination of DMSO 0.5–1.5 cc intravenously and dexamethasone 2.5 mgm/kg IM begun 24 h after lesion production brought about a moderate reduction in edema and there seemed to be little cummulative effect of the two drugs. Comparative wet weights in these animals were 14% higher than in normal animals.

The figures reported here have been compared both in terms of the raw data and also with consideration for the effect of the various modes of therapy upon the cardio-respiratory status of these animals. In the dosage utilized, none of the drugs employed brought about hypotension to the degree induced by Arfonad, and hypertension was not a factor in any of those animals except those treated with levarterenol.

Discussion

While these studies represent survey work exploring new avenues for improving the therapy of brain edema and most of them must be elaborated to be statistically significant, and explored further in terms of drug dosage and timing of administration, there are several points which appear to be of clinical relevance. First of all, the effects of glucosteroids in the prevention and reduction of brain edema are significant both in grey matter and in white matter though the mechanisms for this effect are not entirely clarified. Excision of the edemagenic lesion is also beneficial and the addition of glucosteroids with excision during the period of time in which extravasation of protein, ions, and water is continuing, gives an increased reduction of edema as compared with steroids alone or focal excision alone [7]. The use of steroids and osmotic diuretics in combination does not appear to have a significant advantage in terms of long term effect. Though the immediate reduction in brain bulk with mannitol administered 24 h after production of the cold lesion was obvious, at 48 h or 72 h, in similar animals allowed to survive after mannitol therapy, the amount of edema present was more or less comparable to those animals treated with steroids alone.

As Klatzo has previously reported, hypertension definitely increased the amount of brain edema in relation to the degree of elevation and hypotension markedly decreased brain edema [5]. The addition of dexamethasone to the hypotensive regimen brought about a further minimal decrease in edema which was significant but not striking.

New drugs which were utilized were the alpha adrenergic blocking agents, DMSO and DPPD. All of these had an effect upon brain edema. The decrease in the development of edema with dibenzyline was not due to the hypotensive effect of dibenzyline alone. This drug is still an experimental agent, but these results appear to be promising enough to warrant further trials in this and in other models of edema. DMSO employed in several ways brought about a modest reduction in edema as did the use of DPPD, an anti-oxidant. It has been postulated that much of the disruption in brain edema may be secondary to lipid peroxidation and oxidative processes going on throughout the area of injury. It is of significance that the use of an anti-oxidant definitely does reduce the amount of brain edema developing after a standard lesion. The addition of dexamethasone to the DMSO brought about a further minimal reduction. We have not utilized steroids in combination with anti-oxidants as yet.

Focal excision combined with hypotension, acetazolamide, and furosemide all brought about additional reductions in expected development of edema. The most striking of these occurred with the use of acetazolamide. In view of the suggestion that at least the cellular swelling of brain edema may result from abnormalities of the carbonic anhydrase system, the effect of acetazolamide is extremely interesting and remains to be explored further.

These preliminary studies simply indicate a beneficial effect of several modes of therapy upon brain edema which would be expected to develop after a standard cold cortical lesion. By analogy with the human situation, several important points can be made. It appears obvious that avoidance of hypertension is extremely important and that a reduced development of vasogenic brain edema can be expected if hypertension can be eliminated. Hypotension is extremely effective in prevention brain edema in this model, however, it cannot be inferred from this information that clinical trials of controlled hypotension are warranted. There is a very critical balance between perfusion of brain tissue and arterial pressure. Without more information about this balance in the presence of brain edema and without better ways to measure tissue perfusion during this hypotension, the clinical use of hypotension as an anti-edema tool is not feasible yet. In vasogenic brain edema, removal of the abnormal area of increased cerebrovascular permeability, whether this be tumor, contused brain, abscess, or whatever, appears to be a feasible way of preventing additional edema from developing. Treatment of the edema already present with glucosteroids in addition to the focal excision provides additional benefit. There are several new avenues of therapy utilizing alpha adrenergic blocking agents, DMSO, carbonic anhydrase inhibitors, and anti-oxidizing and peroxidizing agents which appear promising. The mechanisms of action of these drugs and their eventual clinical usefulness remains to be defined.

A major factor which has not been considered in this study is the effect of these various drugs upon total water balance, electrolyte balance and excretion in these animals. Quantitative metabolic balance studies will have to be undertaken before these variables can be elucidated.

References

1. French, L. A., Galicich, J. H.: Use of steroid for control of cerebral edema. Clin. Neurosurg. **10**, 212–223 (1966).
2. — Maxwell, R. E., Long, D. M.: The effect of focal cortical excision upon traumatic spreading edema. In: Head Injuries. Proc. Internat. Symp. Edinburgh-London: Churchill Livingstone 1971.
3. Galicich, J. H., French, L. A., Melby, J. C.: Use of dexamethasone in treatment of cerebral edema associated with brain tumors. J. Lancet **81**, 46–53 (1961).
4. Javid, M.: Urea – New use for an old agent. Surg. Clin. N. Amer. **38**, 907–928 (1958).
5. Klatzo, I., Wisniewski, H., Steinwall, O., Streicher, E.: Dynamics of cold injury edema. In: Klatzo, I., Seitelberger, F. (Eds.): Brain Edema. Berlin-Heidelberg-New York: Springer 1967.
6. — Neuropathological aspects of brain edema. J. Neuropath. exp. Neurol. **26**, 1–14 (1967).
7. Maxwell R., E., Long, D. M., French, L. A.: The effects of glucosteroids on experimental cold-induced brain edema. I. Gross morphological alterations and vascular permeability changes. J. Neurosurg. **34**, 477–487 (1971).
8. Pappius, H. M.: Biochemical studies on experimental brain edema. In: Klatzo, I., Seitelberger, F. (Eds.): Brain Edema. Berlin-Heidelberg-New York: Springer 1967.
9. Prados, M., Strowger, B., Feindel, W.: Studies on cerebral edema. II. Reaction of the brain to exposure to air; physiologic changes. Arch. Neurol. Psychiat. **54**, 290–300 (1945).
10. Rasmussen, T., Gulati, D. R.: Cortisone in the treatment of postoperative cerebral edema. J. Neurosurg. **19**, 535–544 (1962).
11. Weed, L. H., McKibben, P. S.: Experimental alterations of brain bulk. Amer. J. Physiol. **48**, 531–558 (1919).

Steroid-Induced Inhibition of Growth in Glial Tumors: a Kinetic Analysis

Charles B. Wilson, Marvin Barker, Takao Hoshino, Anthony Oliver, and Robert Downie

H. C. Naffziger Laboratories for Neurosurgical Research, University of California, School of Medicine, San Francisco, CA, USA

Introduction

The ability of corticosteroids to alleviate symptoms, prolong life, and inhibit growth of tumors under both clinical and experimental conditions is well known [5, 13, 20, 29, 30]. Conversely, a complete lack of response and even enhancement of tumor growth have also been observed [18, 19, 36]. Corticosteroids have assumed a major role in the treatment of brain tumors based upon their effect in reducing related cerebral edema. The possible oncolytic properties of these drugs have received less emphasis, and most clinical reports dealing with prolonged corticosteroid therapy for intracranial tumors concern secondary, rather than primary tumors. The relief afforded is thought to be due to reduction of cerebral edema rather than a direct inhibitory effect upon the tumor. However, in cases of meningeal leukemia, clinical "cures" have been reported following the systemic administration of corticosteroids [31, 33].

Experimentally, cell lines exhibit marked variation in their response to steroids [1, 8, 9, 10, 12, 17, 19, 21, 23, 26, 27, 32, 37, 39]. Transplantable tumors of the lymphoid series show a transient inhibitory reaction to cortisone but there is no such action on tumors of an epithelial origin [2].

Laboratory data are lacking regarding the anti-tumor effects of corticosteroids when used against primary brain tumors *in vivo*. Kotsilimbas *et al.* [22], studying the effects of corticosteroids upon cerebral edema accompanying intracerebral transplants of a mouse melanoma, unexpectedly found much smaller tumors with prolonged survival in the animals receiving corticosteroids when compared to tumors in nontreated animals. He concluded that corticosteroids inhibited the growth of the melanoma. Wright *et al.* [40] reported that a subcutaneous transplant of a murine ependymoblastoma failed to grow when treated with adrenal corticoids. Inhibition of cell growth of human brain tumors by corticosteroids *in vitro* has been demonstrated by Mealey *et al.* [25].

Adrenal glucocorticoids can effect a direct or indirect inhibition of the mitotic cycle in both normal and neoplastic tissues [6, 7, 11, 15, 21, 28, 34, 35, 38], but the

This work was supported in part by the Clinical Cancer Research Center USPHS Grant # 5-PO2-CA-11067; NIH Cancer Research Center Grant # CA-11249; the American Cancer Society, California Division; NIHNDS Training Grant # 5593; and by a gift from the Phi Beta Psi Sorority.

95

mechanisms responsible for the diverse effects of steroids remain obscure. Cortisone has been shown to reduce the number and increase the size of rat liver mitochondria and these structural changes are accompanied by the uncoupling of oxidative phosphorylation and other defects in the mitochondrial respiratory pathway [16].

Baxter *et al.* [3, 4, 24] have proposed that the first step in the cellular action of steroid hormones in many tissues is an intracellular binding of the hormone by cytoplasmic receptors. Possession of such receptors dictates the sensitivity of the cell to steroids. Most investigators agree that the inhibitory effect of corticosteroids upon normal and neoplastic cells is mediated through a reduction in protein synthesis with little or no change in the rate of protein catabolism. There remains conflicting evidence as to whether the reduced protein synthesis is effected through inhibition at the level of RNA or DNA.

Methods and Results

In our laboratory, interest in the cytotoxic properties of corticosteroids was acquired after observing the effect of hydrocortisone acetate upon cell cultures of human central nervous system tumors. Cultures of oligodendrogliomas, glioblastomas and metastatic melanomas ranging in age from 25 to 1633 days were incubated in graded concentrations of hydrocortisone for 24 h. Reduced growth rates and morphological abnormalities were observed at concentrations higher than 100 micrograms/ml. Complete lysis, a lethal endpoint determined with other drugs *in vitro*, was seldom noted even in concentrations of 5,000 micrograms/ml or higher. It was also found that low concentrations of hydrocortisone, i.e., 1 microgram/ml, actually stimulated the growth of brain tumors in cell culture. Although tumor response to hydrocortisone varied, no correlation between tumor type, degree of malignancy, or age in culture and drug response could be made.

We have recently studied the effect of methylprednisolone acetate (MPA) on the *in vitro* population kinetics of a chemically-induced rat glioma carried in cell culture (Table 1). MPA (1.25 micrograms/ml) added at the time of passage to culture bottles seeded with 125,000 rat glioma cells allowed proliferation to a population of 1.2×10^6 cells four days later, while untreated cultures had attained a population of 2.3×10^6 cells. After six days of contact with MPA a population of only 1.3×10^6 cells was reached while control cultures had attained a population of 9×10^6 cells.

Table 1. Effect of methylprednisolone acetate (MPA) on the growth of rat glioma cells in culture

	Cell population	
	Untreated	MPA (1.25 μg/ml)
Day 4	2.3×10^6	1.2×10^6
Day 6	$9 \ \times 10^6$	1.3×10^6

To observe the long-term effect of MPA on the population kinetics of rat glioma cells, a number of three ounce prescription bottles were seeded with 20,000 cells. One day after seeding, the bottles were divided into three groups. One group served as an untreated control culture. The second group received 0.09 micrograms/ml of dexamethasone, while the third group received 0.34 micrograms/ml of MPA. Thereafter, every two days, bottles from each group were harvested by trypsinization and a cell count performed (Table 2).

Table 2. Effect of methylprednisolone acetate and dexamethasone on growth of rat glioma in culture

Days in culture	Cell population		
	Untreated	Dex (0.09 μg/ml)	MPA (0.34 μg/ml)
2	4×10^4	4×10^4	4×10^4
4	1.5×10^5	1.3×10^5	8×10^4
6	2.5×10^5	1.8×10^5	1.5×10^5
8	5×10^5	3×10^5	2.3×10^5
10	6.5×10^5	3×10^5	2.3×10^5
12	6×10^5	2×10^5	2.5×10^5

MPA reduced the population of cells by the fourth day. Dexamethasone showed no such inhibition until the sixth day. Inhibition became more apparent on succeeding days with the final population for the three experimental groups on the twelfth day being: Control – 600,000; MPA – 250,000; and dexamethasone – 200,000.

The mechanism responsible for the effects observed could be due to: 1. increasing cell loss (cytotoxicity); 2. increasing numbers of cells in the non-proliferating pool; or 3. lengthening of the cell cycle. Overt cell loss is possible but unlikely at the concentrations of drugs used, and indirect evidence against cell loss was the absence of cell debris in the medium of the cultures. Since the effect was delayed, an indication of some drug metabolic interaction is supported. Although no attempts have been made to determine the size of the proliferating pool, we believe that lengthening of the cell cycle is the most tenable explanation for the effect of steroids on these cultures. This would agree with the work of Kollmorgen and Griffin [21] on HeLa cells.

The use of an animal model for brain tumors appeared to offer the next step in determining the effect of steroids on brain tumors. As previously reported [14], MPA had a dramatic effect on both tumor weight and survival time of rats bearing transplanted intracerebral glial tumors. On the tenth, thirteenth and nineteenth days after tumor implantation, animals in one group received 100 mg/kg IM of MPA, and animals in a second group received 50 mg/kg.

Twenty-one days after tumor implantation all animals were killed, and the tumors were removed and weighed. Average wet weights of the tumors from the two treated groups were 36.25 mg and 34.1 mg, while those from the two control groups weighed 157.5 mg and 113 mg.

Average survival of tumor-bearing animals treated with 50 mg/kg IM of MPA on days 10, 13 and 19 was 37.4 days. Untreated control animals survived an average of 28.7 days. Water content and sodium and potassium levels of the surrounding brain tissue indicated that MPA had reduced edema as well as exhibited anti-tumor activity.

A study of *in vivo* proliferation kinetics of this animal model for brain tumors yielded the parameters analyzed on 100 mg tumors shown in Table 3. These kinetic parameters can be used to analyze the effects of MPA on tumors *in vivo*. As previously noted, untreated tumors weighed approximately 140 mg on day 21. This

Table 3. Tumor kinetics of a 100 mg rat glioma *in vivo*

Cell cycle time	20 h
G_1 phase	6–7 h
DNA synthesis	10 h
G_2 phase	2–2.5 h
Mitotic time	1–2 h
Labeling index	15–20%
Growth fraction	0.34–0.46
Doubling time	72 h
Cell loss factor	0.42

corresponds to a tumor mass of 1.4×10^8 cells. The MPA-treated tumors weighed approximately 35 mg, a tumor mass of 3.5×10^7 cells. The difference in survival of treated and control animals was eight days. Since the observed doubling time of the tumor was 72 h, it is apparent that the treated tumors have lost the equivalent two doubling times. Thus it appears that in the *in vivo* system, MPA again acts by affecting the cell cycle rather than by a direct cytotoxic effect. Whether this effect is a lengthening of the cell cycle or whether cells move into the non-proliferating pool is a question under present investigation.

Conclusions

Although cell culture and an experimental rat glioma model are far removed from human brain tumors, the evidence that steroids do inhibit tumor growth in these situations should promote further investigation. The lack of evidence for an anti-tumor response in brain tumor patients treated with steroids is not discouraging for several reasons. First, one steroid, dexamethasone, has been used almost exclusively. Secondly, daily maintenance dosages of steroids given to control brain edema might not be the optimal schedule. Intermittent short-term massive doses, limited by toxicity, would be one possibility for future study. Thirdly, as the proliferation kinetics of human brain tumors become defined, scheduling of steroid therapy, as well as combination therapy with other effective agents, would be feasible. Finally, there remains the possibility that some or all human brain tumors are not sensitive to steroids due to lack of cytoplasmic receptors or rapid metabolic adaptation of the neoplastic cell population.

References

1. Arpels, C., Babcock, V. I., Southram, C. M.: Effect of steroids on human cell cultures; sustaining effect of hydrocortisone. Proc. Soc. exp. Biol. **115**, 102–106 (1963).
2. Baserga, R., Schbik, P.: The action of cortisone on transplanted and induced tumors in mice. Cancer Res. **14**, 12–16 (1954).

3. Baxter, J. P., Tomkins, G. M.: Glucocorticoid Hormone Receptors Advances in the Biosciences. Raspe, G. (Ed.). New York: Pergamon Press 1970.
4. — — Specific cytoplasmic glucocorticoid hormone receptors in hepatoma tissue culture cells. Proc. nat. Acad. Sci. 68, 932–937 (1971).
5. Blinderman, E. E., Graff, C. J., Fitzpatrick, T.: Basic studies in cerebral edema: Its control by a corticosteroid (Solu-Medrol). J. Neurosurg. 19, 319–324 (1962).
6. Bruce, W. R., Meeker, B. E., Valeriote, F. A.: Comparison of the sensitivity of normal hematopoietic and transplanted lymphoma colony-forming cells to chemotherapeutic agents administered *in vivo*. J. Nat. Cancer Inst. 37, 233 (1966).
7. Bullough, W. S., Laurence, E. B.: The role of glucocorticoid hormones in the control of epidermal mitosis. Cell Tiss. Kinet. 1, 5 (1968).
8. Burton, A. F., Storr, J. M., Dunn, W. L.: Cytolytic action of corticosteroids on thymus and lymphoma cells *in vitro*. Canad. J. Biochem. 45, 289–297 (1967).
9. Connor, J. D., Marti, A.: Reversal of contact inhibition in primary ammion cultures by hydrocortisone. Proc. Soc. exp. Biol. 123, 730–735 (1966).
10. Dell'Orco, R. T., Melnykovych, C.: Lipid composition of heteroploid cells in culture: Effects of prednisolone. J. cell. Physiol. 76, 101–106 (1970).
11. Foley, G. E., Lazarus, H.: The response *in vitro* of continuous cultures of human lymphoblasts (CCRF-CEM cells) to chemotherapeutic agents. Biochem. Pharmacol. 16, 659 (1967).
12. Gabourel, J. E., Arnow, L.: Growth inhibitory effects of hydrocortisone on mouse lymphoma ML-388 *in vitro*. J. Pharmacol. exp. Ther. 136, 213–221 (1962).
13. Grenell, R. G., McCawley, E. L.: Central nervous system resistance. II. The effect of adrenal cortical substances on the central nervous system. J. Neurosurg. 4, 508–518 (1947).
14. Gurcay, O., Wilson, C., Barker, M., Eliason, J.: Corticosteroid effect on transplantable rat glioma. Arch. Neurol. 24, 266 (1971).
15. Hydes, T. A., Davis, J. G.: The effects of corticortisol and chloranzanil on the mitotic rate in mouse liver and skin. Europ. J. Cancer 2, 227–230 (1966).
16. Kimberg, D. V., Loud, A. V., Wiener, J.: Cortisone-induced alterations in mitochondrial function and structure. J. Cell Biol. 37, 63–79 (1968).
17. Kline, I., Leighton, J., Belkin, M., Orr, H. C.: Some observations on the response of four established cell strains to hydrocortisone in tissue culture. Cancer Res. 17, 780–784 (1957).
18. Kodama, M.: Effect of hydrocortisone on Ehrlich ascites tumor. Cancer Res. 22, 1212–1219 (1962).
19. — Kodama, T.: Effect of steroid hormones on the *in vivo* incorporation of glycine-2-^{14}C into solid Ehrlich tumor, kidney and liver. Cancer Res. 30, 228–235 (1970).
20. Kofman, S., Garvin, J. S., Nagamani, D., Taylor, S. G.: Treatment of cerebral metastasis from breast carcinoma with prednisolone. J. Amer. med. Ass. 163; 1473–1476 (1957).
21. Kollmorgen, G. M., Griffin, M. J.: The effect of hydrocortisone on HeLa cell growth. Cell Tiss. Kinet. 2, 111–112 (1969).
22. Kotsilimbas, D. G., Meyer, L., Berson, M., Taylor, J. M., Scheinberg, L. C.: Corticosteroid effect on intracerebral melanomata and associated edema. Some unexpected findings. Neurology 17, 223–226 (1967).
23. Kupiecki, F. P.: Cell culture studies with unique cytotoxic steroids. Cancer Res. 25, 417–420 (1965).
24. Levinson, B. B., Baxter, J. D., Rousseau, G. G.: Cellular site of Glucocorticoid receptor complex formation. Science 175, 189–190 (1972).
25. Mealey, J., Ehen, T. T., Schanz, G. P.: The effects of dexamethasone and methylprednisolone on cell cultures of human glioblastoma. J. Neurosurg. 34, 324 (1971).
26. Melnykovych, H. G., Swayze, M. A., Bishop, C. F.: Effects of cultural condition on alkaline phosphatase and cell culture survival in the presence of prednisolone. Exp. Cell Res. 47, 167–176 (1967).
27. Omura, E. F., Schwartz, M. S., Jahiel, R. I. *et al.*: Effect of hydrocortisone on growth and detachment of human heteroploid cells in maintenance media. Proc. Soc. exp. Biol. 125, 447–451 (1967).

28. Pearson, O. H., Li, M. C., Maclean, J. P. *et al.*: The use of hydrocortisone in cancer. Ann. N. Y. Acad. Sci. **61**, 393 (1955).
29. Prados, M., Stowger, B., Feindel, W. H.: Studies on cerebral edema: I. Reaction of the brain to air exposure; pathologic changes. Arch. Neurol. Psychiat. **54**, 163–174 (1945).
30. Rasmussen, T., Gulati, D. R.: Cortisone in the treatment of postoperative cerebral edema. J. Neurosurg. **19**, 535–544 (1962).
31. Ruderman, N. B., Hall, T. C.: Use of glucocorticoids in the palliative treatment of metastatic brain tumors. Cancer **18**, 298–306 (1965).
32. Schafer, I. A., McManus, T. J., Sullivan, J. C. *et al.*: Inhibition by hydrocortisone of iododeoxyuridine incorporation into the DNA of cultured mammalian cells. Exp. Cell Res. **44**, 108–118 (1966).
33. Shaw, R. K., Moore, E. W., Freireich, E. J., Thomas, L. B.: Meningeal Leukemia. Neurology (Minneap.) **10**, 823–833 (1960).
34. Simpson-Herren, L., Lloyd, H. H.: Kinetic parameters and growth curves for experimental tumors systems. Cancer Chemother. Rep. **54**, 143–174 (1970).
35. Stock, C. C., Karnofsky, D. A., Sugiura, K.: Studies on steroids for inhibition of normal and abnormal growth in experimental animals. In: White, A. (Ed.): Symposium on Steroids in Experimental and Clinical Practice. Philadelphia: Blakiston Co. 1951.
36. Toolan, H. W.: Growth of human tumors in cortisone-treated laboratory animals: The possibility of obtaining permanently transplantable human tumors. Cancer Res. **13**, 389–394 (1953).
37. Weinger, E., Marmary, Y.: The *in vitro* effect of hydrocortisone on cultures of peritoneal monocytes. Lab. Invest. **21**, 525–511 (1969).
38. Wellings, S. R., Moon, H. D.: Morphologic and functional effects of hydrocortisone in tissue culture. Lab. Invest. **10**, 539–547 (1961).
39. Wellington, J. S., Moon, H. D.: Effect of hydrocortisone on human cells in tissue culture. Proc. Soc. exp. Biol. **107**, 556–559 (1961).
40. Wright, R. L., Shaumba, B., Xeller, J.: The effect of glucocorticosteroids on growth and metabolism of experimental glial tumors. J. Neurosurg. **30**, 140–145 (1969).

Effects of Steroids on Edema Associated with Injury of the Spinal Cord

Marcial G. Lewin, Hanna M. Pappius, and Robert R. Hansebout

Department of Neurology and Neurosurgery and the Donner Laboratory for Experimental Neurochemistry, The Montreal Neurological Institute, McGill University, Montreal, Canada

With 4 Figures

Summary. Standardized spinal cord injury was produced in cats by impact. Some were untreated and others treated with dexamethasone before and up to 24 h after injury.

The neurological condition of the cats was rated throughout the experimental period. Water and electrolyte content determinations and histological observations were made of injured spinal cord tissue.

Edema as demonstrated by increasing water content of the injured tissues begins a day after injury and thence increases significantly to a maximum three to six days after the trauma when segments adjacent to the lesion are involved. Edema has begun to recede on the ninth day.

Cats treated with dexamethasone before or up to 24 h after cord injury have significantly better recovery and less histological abnormality in the spinal cord than untreated cats, but the course of post-traumatic edema is similar. The beneficial effects of dexamethasone on functional recovery of animals with potentially reversible cord lesions does not seem to be mediated by its effects on edema alone.

Introduction

Spinal cord injury can cause immediate complete sensori-motor paralysis due to irreversible cord destruction. Some patients may retain minimal function early after injury but in some cases this can disappear permanently during the next few hours. The effects of spinal cord trauma can therefore be immediate or delayed. Animal studies confirm that severe cord trauma may induce delayed [6] and progressive [3, 12, 27] pathological changes of an auto-destructive nature [7].

Various derangements such as mechanical deformation [11], vascular factors [7], hypoxia [15] and ischemia [10] have been linked in the pathogenesis of progressive cord injury but edema has often been invoked as a main or potentiating factor [7, 9, 14, 24]. Freeman and Wright [9] hypothesized that following cord injury the pia might serve as a limiting membrane. As edema became superimposed on hemorrhage, the increasing pressure could be transmitted to adjacent segments decreasing capillary circulation and finally causing anoxia which might induce permanent damage. Scarff said that edema of the cord could itself cause neurological dysfunction and that minutes following injury the cord could swell to double its size to fill the dural sac [24]. It has been suggested that in the face of internal pressure and its unyielding coverings the edematous cord might undergo "ischemic" transection [1].

101

The arrest of this delayed response to cord trauma would be of great clinical interest and accordingly investigators have proposed various treatments. Allen improved the clinical course in dogs and later humans with cord injuries by longitudinal myelotomy for the relief of pressure [3]. Although the beneficial effects of myelotomy were confirmed by others [9, 17] Scarff discouraged myelotomy as a form of treatment of cord injury since the procedure itself could cause irreversible damage and might lead to cord rupture [24]. Instead he recommended the use of intravenous 50 % glucose in water to decrease edema [24]. Later intravenous urea was also shown to be beneficial [14]. Local hypothermia has also proven encouraging for treatment of the injured cord. Since these forms of treatment are directed against the hypothesized spinal cord edema, and steroids are known to decrease cerebral edema [22], it is logical to investigate the effects of steroids in treating spinal cord injury.

Edema has usually been gauged by histological or electron microscopic means, but few actual chemical determinations have been undertaken to verify its presence. The following study was designed to characterize traumatic spinal cord edema and to evaluate the possible ameliorative effects of steroid administration on the injured spinal cord.

Materials and Methods

Eighty-two mature cats of either sex were selected randomly and anesthetized using intraperitoneal pentobarbital (Nembutal). Under sterile conditions an incision was made in the thoraco-lumbar region to expose the spinous processes and laminae. Following the removal of the T-13 and L-1 spines a burr hole was made in the neural arch of T-13 using the Smith-Peterson automatic drill. The epidural fat was gently removed. Impact injury was delivered to the dura and underlying cord at T-13. The wound was then closed. The cats were then given intraperitoneal 5 % dextrose and saline until they were eating. Incontinent cats had their bladders expressed manually.

The apparatus for induction of impact injury is essentially Allen's method [4] as modified by Albin *et al.* [1], with the exception that the saddle was made of "lucite". The impounder measured 0.6 cm in diameter by 1.2 cm long. The vented Teflon tube was 30 cm long. A 10 gm weight was used to strike the impounder resting on the dura to produce impact injury. The results of the pilot study indicated that the optimum force to cause injury in this investigation would be obtained by dropping the 10 gm weight a distance of 15 cm (150 gram-centimeter force equals 150 GCF).

The operative day (day of lesion) was designated "day 0" while the day after the lesion was "day 1" and so forth.

The animals were divided into various groups as follows:

Group	Number of cats
I Normal control cats – without injury	8
II Cats with 150 GCF spinal cord injury	74 (total)
Breakdown	
A. Untreated group	33
B. Group treated with intramuscular steroid	41 (74)
Breakdown	
1. 48 h pretreated subgroup	17
2. 5 h post-treated subgroup	12
3. 24 h post-treated subgroup	12 (41)

Normal control cats were neither operated upon nor given steroids. The rest of the animals sustained a cord lesion and were randomly divided into an untreated and a treated group. The treated cats were given 0.25 mg of dexamethasone per kg per day divided into two intraperitoneal doses until death. Subgroup B1 had treatment initiated 48 h before injury while subgroups B2 and B3 were given the steroid respectively 5 and 24 h after the cord injury.

Post-operative clinical examinations were done daily to evaluate voluntary motor movements, muscle tone, reflexes, righting response, sensation and bladder functions. The evaluation of voluntary movements was based on Tarlov's rating system [26] which is as follows:

Rating	Condition
1	Complete paraplegia
2	Minimal voluntary movements
3	Animal able to stand but not run
4	Animal able to run with some spasticity and incoordination
5	Normal

The normal control cats were killed to obtain fresh cord tissue for baseline determinations of percentage dry weight and electrolyte content. The untreated cats were allocated to random lots and killed on days 1, 2, 3, 6 and 9 following clinical observation. One-half of the cats in each treated subgroup were killed on day 3 while the remaining one-half were killed on day 6. The cats were fully anesthetized and killed by exsanguination. Following laminectomy the dura and cord were sectioned transversely at the junction of the T-10 and T-11 cord segments and again at the junction of the L-1 and L-2 cord segments. The intervening tissue ws removed *en bloc* and placed in a humidity chamber to prevent drying. The meninges were removed and the gross pathological features recorded. Each cord specimen was divided into 10 consecutive blocks (5 mm long) of cord tissue numbered in order from cephalad to caudad. Each block was analyzed for percentage dry weight (water content) by weighing before and after drying overnight at 100 degrees Celsius [21]. The dried samples were digested with nitric acid and the sodium and potassium concentrations were determined [20]. All 10 blocks were analyzed to obtain sequential data of the lesion and adjacent cord.

Histological evaluations were performed on the spinal cords of 13 cats by taking 3.5 mm long cross sections of the cord at the center of the lesion and at levels 2.5 cm above and below this point. The remaining tissue was processed as above. After fixation in formalin, the specimens were imbedded in paraffin, and sectioned and stained using hemotoxylin and eosin or according to the Bodian or Heidenhain methods.

Results and Discussion

Water and Electrolytes

Percentage water content and sodium and potassium concentrations were the same in all blocks of normal cord tissue. The normal average percentage dry weight is about 34.5 mg %. The average normal sodium and potassium concentrations are respectively about 55 and 86 mEg per kilogram of wet weight.

103

The course of traumatically induced spinal cord edema could be plotted using the data obtained by processing the cord speciments of untreated cats for water and electrolyte content. This is seen in Figure 1. Edema is indicated by a fall in the percentage dry weight (increase in water content), a rise in tissue sodium concentration and a fall in the potassium concentration. The average water and electrolyte content of the consecutive blocks of cord tissue are shown for days 1, 3 and 9 after the lesion. Observations for days 2 and 6 are not illustrated for sake of brevity. Block 1 is rostal and 10 caudal while blocks 6 and 7 include the impact area located anatomically in the T-13 cord segment.

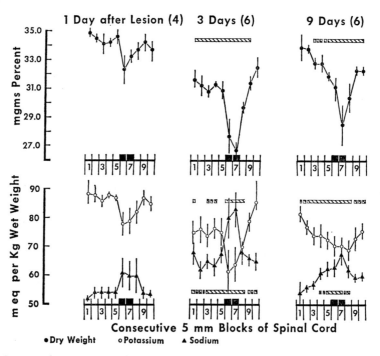

Fig. 1. Percent dry weights (●) and sodium (▲) and potassium (○) concentrations in adjacent spinal cord blocks: 1,3 and 9 days after impact. Number of animals in brackets. ■ = segment of injury; ▨ = $p < 0.01$; ▨ ▨ ▨ = $p < 0.05$

Significant alterations in water and electrolyte content are seen throughout most of the observation periods. On day 1 minimal abnormalities are noted in the water and electrolyte content of blocks 6 and 7 at the site of impact indicating a trend towards edema. On day 3 there is a significant decrease in the % dry weight and potassium concentration and a rise in sodium concentration. The blocks nearest the lesion show the greatest abnormality in values. At this stage edema is therefore present in segments adjacent to the lesion, as well as the lesion itself. On day 9 edema has begun to regress and is reflected by alterations in the water and electrolyte content of all blocks toward the normal baseline values both at the lesion and in adjacent segments. The potassium concentration values seem further from normal baseline values than the sodium concentration at this stage. This is discussed elsewhere [13]. Significant water and electrolyte abnormalities were also found in cord tissue obtained on days 2 and 6. The abnormalities were better developed on day 2 than day 1 but not as striking as on day 3. Results obtained on day 6 gave similar results to those seen on day 3.

Comments. By definition, edema is increased fluid content of the tissues. As measured above, progressive edematous changes are induced in spinal cord tissues by trauma. Edema begins at the site of injury on the day after injury; its presence becomes significant on day 2 and remains so through to day 9. It becomes maximal between 3 and 6 days after injury and also involves segments adjacent to the injury. Regressive changes are seen on day 9, but the water and electrolyte abnormality has not completely abated.

Histological changes have been described which are referred to as edema. This edema can involve the grey matter [12] but is said to manifest itself by enlargement of the periaxonal spaces [5], swelling of axons [17], and the appearance of vacuolated spaces [8] in the white matter. The ultrastructural abnormalities of spinal cord edema are thickening of the capillary wall, swelling of the astrocytic vascular feet and enlargement of the extracellular spaces, especially in the white matter [23].

Edema defined histologically becomes maximal between 2 and 3 days after injury and resolves about 7 days after the injury [17, 24]. Thus, edema determined histologically seems to follow the time course of the edema described in this study. However, the abnormal water contents shown in this study were decreased but still present on the ninth day. Detection of significant edema by chemical means is possible on the second day after injury. Histologically it has been described as beginning fifteen [5] to thirty [3] minutes after trauma, and may become well developed in the white matter by four [3, 12, 27] to eight [2, 6] hours after trauma. These differences in the time course raise the possibility that the histological abnormality and edema detected by chemical means may not be equivalent. However, they may be the same with the histological variant representing a more restricted local edema, which later becomes chemically measurable as it increases.

The cord has been observed to swell within minutes after injury [24] even to double its normal size. Such swelling is often equated with edema [1]. Again, this observation is not consistent with our finding that the maximal increase in water content of the injured tissues occurs after 3 days. It may be that the early swelling often observed following cord injury reflects an expanding central hematoma, some true edema and possibly other phenomena such as vessel dilatation.

The Effect of Dexamethasone on Post-Traumatic Spinal Cord Edema

Water and electrolyte content in the three treated groups of cats was determined on cord tissue obtained on the third and sixth day after injury. There was no apparent difference in the course of edema in the three subgroups so their results were pooled.

The percentage of dry weight and sodium and potassium concentration in cord tissue from treated cats are compared with results obtained by analysis of comparable tissues in normal and cord-injured but untreated cats 3 and 6 days after trauma (Fig. 2). On day 3 when the edema is well-developed the dry weights of injured cord its-sues are somewhat higher (water content less) in cats treated with dexamethasone than in untreated cats, but there is really little difference. This trend continues until day 6.

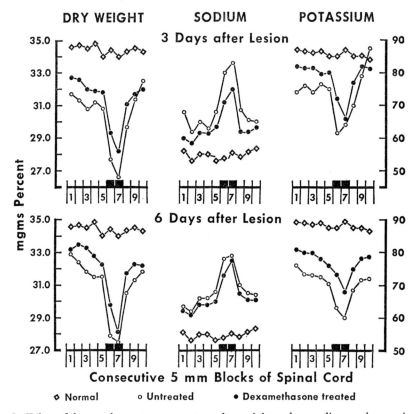

DRY WEIGHT **SODIUM** **POTASSIUM**

Fig. 2. Effect of dexamethasone on percentage dry weight and on sodium and potassium of injured spinal cord. Sodium and potassium are expressed as meq/kg wet weight

There is also a consistent trend for sodium and potassium concentration in cords of treated animals to lie closer to normal baseline levels. However, none of these differences in % dry weight or sodium and potassium concentration are statistically significant except for the difference in potassium concentration between treated and untreated cats on day 6. The possible meaning of this observation is discussed elsewhere [13].

Comment. The administration of dexamethasone by intramuscular injection shows a consistent but minimal tendency to reduce posttraumatic spinal cord edema. This is in agreement with the ultrastructural studies of Richardson and Nakamura who noted better structural preservation of traumatized spinal cord tissues in cats treated with steroids over untreated control animals. In treated animals there was increased electron density of cytoplasm and the basement membranes were reduced in thickness compared with untreated animals. However despite steroid treatment, the astrocytic feet and mitochondria remained swollen. Also the extracellular space in the white matter was reduced, but still larger than normal [23].

106

Neurological Studies

Marked neurological deficit occurred after the lesion was made. The impact injury itself caused an immediate mass extension reflex of the hind limbs and spinal column. The cats had flaccid hindlimbs devoid of sensation on awakening and were incontinent of urine. The day following injury (day 1) spastic paraplegia in extension developed. Sequential return of motor power included first proximal, then distal hindlimb movements, and later the ability to stand. The cats then began to walk and run and finally became normal. Sensation and bladder control returned coincident with the ability to walk. Various degrees of the above course were noted in individual cats.

There was considerable variation in the individual Tarlov ratings. Cats in the untreated group and steroid-treated subgroups were tabulated according to whether they had minimal movements or less (Tarlov 1 and 2), were able to stand (Tarlov 3) or could run with incoordination or normally (Tarlov 4 and 5).

Table 1. Effects of dexamethasone on Tarlov ratings of cats with spinal cord injury

	Tarlov rating	Untreated			Pre-treated (48 h)			Post-treated (5 h)			Post-treated (24 h)		
		No.	%		No.	%		No.	%		No.	%	
3 days after injury	4–5	3	12.5	} 37.5	5	31	} 68.5	5	41.5	} 83	1	8	} 66
	3	6	25		6	37.5		5	41.5		7	58	
	1–2	15	62.5		5	31.5		2	17		4	34	
Total		24	100 %		16	100 %		12	100 %		12	100 %	
6.days after injury	4–5	3	16	} 32	4	40	} 80	4	67	} 83.5	2	33	} 83
	3	3	16		4	40		1	16.5		3	50	
	1–2	13	68		2	20		1	16.5		1	17	
Total		19	100 %		10	100 %		6	100 %		6	100 %	

Dramatic clinical differences were seen in comparing steroid-treated and untreated cats (Table 1). All subgroups on steroid therapy consistently had better functional recovery than the untreated group. Less than $1/3$ of cats in any treated subgroup had severe paraparesis on day 3 (Tarlov 1 and 2) while $2/3$ of untreated cats were in this category. Over $2/3$ of the cats in any treated subgroups were able to stand or run (Tarlov 3 to 5) but less than $1/3$ of untreated cats had comparable function. On day 6 little change had occurred in the untreated cats whereas in each treated subgroup over 80 % of cats could then stand or run. Improvement in the 24 h post-treated subgroup was less dramatic than the other treated subgroups, but superior to the untreated group.

The average Tarlov ratings of untreated cats are compared with those treated in Figure 3. The treated cats were assigned to one "pooled" treated group regardless as to when treatment began. Cats in which treatment began 24 h after trauma were added to the untreated group on day 1. The number of cats decreased on succeeding days as they were killed for post-mortem studies. The individual Tarlov ratings of cats in each group were averaged to one decimal place and plotted. On day 1 the average

Tarlov ratings for untreated and treated cats were respectively 2 and 2.5. The rate of improvement of treated cats was faster than untreated cats as indicated by comparing the steepness of the recovery curves of averaged Tarlov ratings. On day 6 untreated cats averaged Tarlov 2.3 whereas the average for the treated group was more than a full rating higher at 3.4. Remarkably treated cats averaged a higher Tarlov rating on day 1 than the average Tarlov rating for untreated cats on day 6. These clinical differences are statistically significant. It is particularly noteworthy that once improvement in function began in any animal or group it continued regardless of the day of onset.

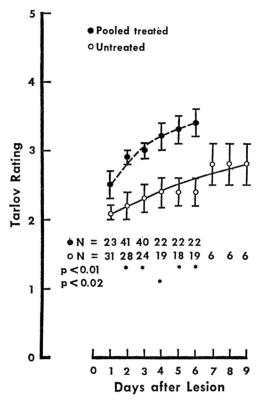

Fig. 3. Effect of dexamethasone on Tarlov ratings of cats with spinal cord injury. Averages ± S.E.

Comment. Cats with spinal cord injuries treated with steroids improve more rapidly and attain a higher functional recovery over the experimental period than untreated cats. These differences are statistically significant. Such clinical improvement is in agreement with that noted by Ducker and Hamit who observed dogs with spinal cord injuries which were treated by daily injections of intramuscular steroids [7]. Progressive improvement in individual cats or groups is therefore present while significant edema (increased water content) progresses in the injured spinal cords. Steroid administration significantly improves functional recovery in injured animals while it does not significantly alter the course of edema.

Steroids may affect structural abnormalities favorably. However, Ducker *et al.* [8] noted the progression of the pathological abnormalities while clinical improvement occurred in monkeys after cord injury. Thus additional actions of steroids must be considered.

Osterholm and Mathews say that after cord injury, norepinephrine accumulates in cord tissues to provide a neural (electrical depressive) response causing immediate weakness and a vasospastic response which might cause permanent dysfunction due to hemorrhagic auto-destruction of the cord tissues [18]. They claim steroids significantly reduce norepinephrine concentration in the traumatized tissues and may protect the wounded spinal cord [19].

The time interval following cord trauma in which any treatment can still be effective is important clinically. There is evidence that local cooling is of no avail if started later than 8 h after trauma [2], however, hyperbaric oxygen administration for the treatment of such an injury is equally effective whether started immediately or 4 h after injury [16]. The current study suggests that intramuscular steroid therapy can still be beneficial even when started within 24 h after trauma. The investigators above [1, 16] have used a greater force to induce cord trauma than the current study. Direct comparison may not be applicable unless the extent of cord damage could be compared in all studies. However, it may be that with non-disruptive cord injury even administration of steroids several hours following trauma may possibly arrest the progressive pathological changes.

Pathological Changes

In the current study cats which underwent a sham operation without induced cord trauma had normal cords at autopsy and in subsequent histological studies. There were gross changes in the cords of all cats undergoing impact injury whether treated or untreated. In untreated cats the cord was increased in girth at the site of impact and was often tight against the dura. The only difference seen in the treated cats was that the area of increased girth was more confined to the zone near the lesions. On sections early after trauma a central hematoma was seen which later became a syrinx.

In order to increase objectivity the histological sections were examined without prior knowledge as to whether the animal had been treated or not. Various parameters studied were graded (Fig. 4) and later correlation was attempted between these histological findings and functional recovery.

Considerable variation in the severity of the pathological abnormalities between individual animals was seen whether treated or not. However, using the objectively recorded histological parameters a computerized lesion was reconstructed for six studied treated and seven studied untreated cats (Fig. 4). The damage noted was not confined to the zone of impact but involved the cord in diminishing degree above and below the injury.

Comments. This experimental model reduplicates the classical pathological findings in animals [2, 3, 4, 12] and humans [24, 25] after cord injury.

Steroid treatment in this study has enhanced the preservation of the cord structures, especially the white matter, as studied histologically (Fig. 4). This relative preservation of the functional integrity of the white matter may explain the better clinical improvement noted in the treated cats compared with the untreated cats.

109

Steroids have also been noted to exert a protective effect on the white matter by others [19].

Parameters	Area of Cavitation	Area of Demyelination	Neuronal Integrity	Loss Large Axons (approx.)	Swelling Large Axons (approx.)	Loss Small Axons
Untreated N=6	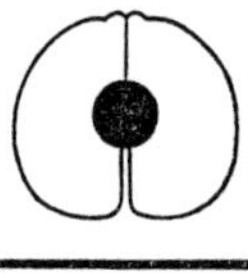	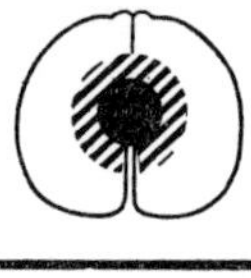	Marked cell loss eosinophilia & loss of detail	1/2	1/2	Moderate
Treated N=7	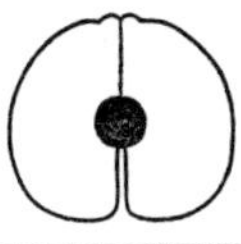	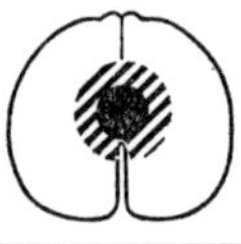	Many present Chromatolysis & some loss of detail	1/3	1/3	Light

Fig. 4. Effects of dexamethasone on histological characteristics of traumatized spinal cord

The mechanism of such a protective effect of steroids on the white matter is incompletely understood and theoretical. Since the post-treated cats fare about as well as those pretreated, it is unlikely that steroids make the white matter more resistant to the initial trauma. Alterations in the grey matter precede those in the white matter [12] at a time when the animal is clinically the worst [8]. Therefore, consideration must be given to the possibility that the white matter is influenced secondarily by occurences in the grey matter.

After severe cord trauma the lesions are found initially behind the central canal [17]. This site of involvement has often been explained on the basis of mathematical [17] and structural considerations [8]. There is then a delay in the pathological sequence followed by progression to central hemorrhagic necrosis [6] with involvement of the white matter by necrosis at a later stage [12]. The above mechanisms do not account for the delay in progression of the pathological sequence which may be related to other abnormalities of the grey matter. Recent evidence indicates that the grey matter is richer in concentration of the vasoconstrictor norepinephrine than the white matter [20]. It has been postulated that after trauma this may be released into the cord tissues to temporarily halt conductive functions in the white matter. The norepinephrine then may cause vasospasm with resultant autodestructive hemorrhagic necrosis and permanent loss of cord function [18]. Such a theory may account for the delayed consequence observed pathologically. Steroids are said to reduce the effects of the abberent metabolism of norepinephrine and to protect the cord [19].

In view of the possibility of toxic factors influencing cord function after injury and causing delayed damage, it is interesting to reflect on the past. Allen in 1911 [4] after a study of impact injury theorized the following: "either there is a destruction of axis cylinders directly consequent to the impact, or else owing to the impact there is an edematous and hemorrhagic outpouring into the cord tissue, which by its pressure and chemical activity inhibits temporarily all conduction function or destroys permanently the spinal cord." Allen showed improvement by relief of the pressure phenomenon by longitudinal myelotomy in dogs in 1914 [3]. Possibly the advent of steroid therapy will lend a new dimension to the treatment of this deleterious "chemical activity" which could destroy the cord.

Acknowledgements. This work was supported in part by M.R.C. Canada Grant MA 3988.

References

1. Albin, M. S., White, R. J., Locke, G. S., Massopust, L. C., Kretchmer, H. E.: Localized spinal cord hypothermia. Anesth. Analg. Curr. Res. **46**, 8–16 (1967).
2. — — Yashon, D., Harris, L. S.: Effects of localized cooling on spinal cord trauma. J. Trauma **9**, 1000–1008 (1969).
3. Allen, A. R.: Remarks on the histopathological changes in the spinal cord due to impact. An experimental study. J. nerv. ment. Dis. **41**, 141–147 (1914).
4. — Surgery of experimental lesion of spinal cord equivalent to crush injury of fracture dislocation of spinal column. J. Amer. med. Ass. **57**, 878–880 (1911).
5. Dohrmann, G. J., Wagner, F. C., Bucy, P.: Transitory traumatic paraplegia: electron microscopy of early alterations in myelinated nerve fibers. J. Neurosurg. **36**, 407–415 (1972).
6. Ducker, T. B., Assenmacher, D. R.: Microvascular response to experimental spinal cord trauma. Surg. Forum **20**, 428–430 (1969).
7. — Hamit, H. F.: Experimental treatments of acute spinal cord injury. J. Neurosurg. **30**, 693–697 (1969).
8. — Kindt, G. W., Kempe, L. G.: Pathological findings in acute experimental spinal cord trauma. J. Neurosurg. **35**, 700–708 (1971).
9. Freeman, L. W., Wright, T. W.: Experimental observations of concussion and contusion of the spinal cord. Ann. Surg. **137**, 433–443 (1953).
10. Fried, L. C., Goodkin, R.: Microangiographic observations of the experimentally traumatized spinal cord. J. Neurosurg. **35**, 709–714 (1971).
11. Gelfan, S., Tarlov, I. M.: Physiology of spinal cord, nerve root and peripheral nerve compression. Amer. J. Physiol. **185**, 217–229 (1956).
12. Goodkin, R., Campbell, J. B.: Sequential pathologic changes in spinal cord injury: a preliminary report. Surg. Forum **20**, 430–432 (1969).
13. Hansebout, R. R., Lewin, M. G., Pappius, H. M.: Evidence regarding the action of steroids in injured spinal cord. In: Steroids and Brain Edema. Berlin–Heidelberg–New York: Springer 1972.
14. Joyner, J., Freeman, L. W.: Urea and spinal cord trauma. Neurology (Minneap.) **13**, 69–72 (1963).
15. Kelly, D. L., Lassiter, K. R., Calogero, J. A., Alexander, E.: Effects of local hypothermia and tissue oxygen studies in experimental paraplegia. J. Neurosurg. **33**, 554–563 (1970).
16. — — Vongsvivut, A., Smith, J. M.: Effects of hyperbaric oxygenation and tissue oxygen studies in experimental paraplegia. J. Neurosurg. **36**, 425–429 (1972).
17. McVeigh, J. F.: Experimental cord crushes with especial reference to the mechanical factors involved and subsequent changes in the areas of the cord affected. Arch. Surg. **7**, 573–600 (1923).
18. Osterholm, J. L., Mathews, G. J.: Altered norepinephrine metabolism following experimental spinal cord injury. Part 1: Relationship to hemorrhagic necrosis and post-wounding neurological deficits. J. Neurosurg. **36**, 386–394 (1972).
19. — — Effect of hypothermia and steroids upon spinal injury norepinephrine metabolism. Presented at the meeting of the American Association of Neurological Surgeons, Boston 1972.
20. Pappius, H. M., Dayes, L. A.: Hypertonic urea: its effect on the distribution of electrolytes in normal and edematous brain tissues. Arch. Neurol. **13**, 395–402 (1965).
21. — Gulati, D. R.: Water and electrolyte content of cerebral tissues in experimentally induced edema. Acta neuropath. (Berl.) **2**, 451–460 (1963).

22. Rasmussen, T., Gulati, D. R.: Cortisone in the treatment of post-operative cerebral edema. J. Neurosurg. **19**, 535–544 (1962).
23. Richardson, H. D., Nakamura, S.: An electron microscopic study of spinal cord edema and the effect of treatment with steroids, mannitol, and hypothermia. Presented at the meeting of the American Association of Neurological Surgeons, Boston 1972.
24. Scarff, J. E.: Injuries of the vertebral column and spinal cord. In: Broch, S. (Ed.): Injuries of the Brain and Spinal Cord and Their Coverings. 4th Edition. Berlin-Heidelberg: Springer 1960.
25. Schneider, R. C., Cherry, G., Pantek, H.: The syndrome of acute central cervical spinal cord injury with special reference to the mechanisms involved in hyperextension injuries of cervical spine. J. Neurosurg. **11**, 546–577 (1954).
26. Tarlov, I. M.: Spinal Cord Compression: Mechanism of Paralysis and Treatment. Springfield, Ill.: Charles C. Thomas 1957.
27. Wagner, F. C., Dohrmann, G. J., Bucy, P.: Histopathology of transitory traumatic paraplegia in the monkey. J. Neurosurg. **35**, 272–276 (1971).

Effect of Dexamethasone on Triethyl Tin Induced Brain Edema and the Early Edema in Cerebral Ischemia

Barry A. Siegel, Rebecca K. Studer, and E. James Potchen

The Edward Mallinckrodt Institute of Radiology, Washington University, School of Medicine, St. Louis, MO 63110, USA

Summary. The effects of dexamethasone were investigated in experimental brain edema induced by triethyl tin intoxication and cerebral microembolism. Large doses of steroid (1.25 mg/kg/day) significantly reduced brain water and sodium in triethyl tin poisoned rats. However, in experimental microembolism, steroids had no effect on mortality, severity of edema, brain electrolyte changes, or cerebral isotope spaces.

Introduction

The use of steroids in the treatment of cerebral edema was initiated by the recognition, in 1945, that adrenal cortical extract prevented swelling of the cat brain after exposure to air [28]. Subsequently, their utility has been demonstrated in edema of several origins [19].

We have recently become interested in potential methods for brain edema detection with radionuclides [27] and our interest soon expanded to evaluation of steroid therapy in selected experimental models. In the present discussion, we shall describe our results in edema due to triethyl tin intoxication and cerebral microembolism and summarize the contributions of other investigators.

Triethyl Tin Edema

The toxicity of alkyl metal compounds has been known for almost 100 years [11, 49, 54], but these compounds subsequently received little attention until the mid-1950's when their use as fungicides was proposed [50] and the report of 110 fatalities in France following the use of a preparation containing diethyl tin dii odide [32]. The studies by Stoner and his coworkers [40] provided a general description of the consequences of acute and chronic administration of a series of tetra-, di-, and monoalkyl tin compounds in rats, rabbits, guinea pigs, and fowl. Triethyl tin sulfate was found to be highly toxic with intraperitoneal doses of 10 mg/kg in rats, causing initial stupor and weakness from which the animals apparently recovered before passing through stages of hemiplegia, paraplegia, generalized weakness, and death within 3 days. Rabbits responded similarly to even smaller doses. Chronic administration of 20 p.p.m. of triethyl tin hydroxide in the diet caused progressive weight loss and paralysis which

This project was supported in part by NIH Research Grant RO1HE-12237, Training Grant TO1-GM0747, and the United States Atomic Energy Commission Grant AT(11-1)-1653 under which this document becomes AEC No. CO-1653-131.

113

progressed from a weakness of the hindlimbs to total immobility and death in 3–4 weeks.

Following these initial studies more detailed investigations were undertaken to study the histopathology of the cerebral lesion, the biochemical effects of triethyl tin compounds on the brain tissue, both *in vivo* and *in vitro*, and the changes in compartments, water, and electrolyte movement in affected tissues.

Light microscopy [18] on the brains of chronically poisoned rats showed an interstitial edema of the white matter without obvious damage to the neurons. The lesion was found to be reversible with return to a normal histological appearance after removal of the toxic material from the diet. The cerebral hemispheres of mice on a diet containing triethyl tin sulfate exhibited glial swelling and endothelial swelling in the terminal stages when examined by both light and electron microscopy [48]. However, these findings were not confirmed by others [2] in studies of rabbits given intraperitoneal triethyl tin sulfate in a dose of 1 mg/kg/day. With light microscopy, there appeared to be a diffuse sponginess of myelinated areas with no evidence of phagocytosis or inflammatory processes. The neuron and glial elements appeared to be essentially normal, except for mild, focal swelling of the glial elements. Improved techniques allowed the white matter to be examined by electron microscopy without artifact. The myelin sheaths of the spinal cord and white matter of the cerebellum were split along the intraperiod line forming a series of fluid filled clefts and vacuoles. Similar clefts were seen scattered diffusely in the cortex, but were not as large or as plentiful. The structure of the brain vasculature appeared to be normal. Lee and Bakay [16] recorded similar observations in the brains of rats fed triethyl tin hydroxide but did not find splitting of the myelin in the cortex of the cerebrum. Recovery was seen in approximately 45 days after return to a normal diet. Bakay [4] also observed some grey matter changes in the form of vacuolar degeneration in neuronal cytoplasm of the basal ganglia and other highly myelinated areas.

More recently, Torack and coworkers [47] have provided a detailed description of the acute development of edema after intraperitoneal injections of 2, 7, 8, or 9 mg/kg in rats. The changes in 24 h resembled those previously described, but at 12 h post-injection there was a transient focal dilation of axons which was inversely related to the presence of myelin clefts. Astrocytic swelling in the neuropil was observed from 12–24 h, while in the white matter it was seen only at 12 h. Swollen cells were most often observed at doses of 9 mg/kg, and by 18 and 24 h post-injection, the cells appeared to have shrunk. The oligodendrocytes and the cerebral vessels appeared normal at all times.

These morphological studies have been accompanied and supplemented by chemical determinations of several brain constituents and isotopic studies of functional brain compartments and ion kinetics. Early studies by Magee *et al.* [18] demonstrated increased brain water and sodium content in intoxicated animals while potassium, lipids, nucleic acids, phospholipids, and cholesterol remained normal. The results of phosphorous-32-uptake studies were inconclusive.

The brain extracellular space in triethyl tin induced cerebral edema has been assessed histologically [2, 47, 48], by thiocyanate distribution [41], and by estimation of the ^{35}S-sulfate space [15, 47], and the ^{14}C-sucrose space [29, 47]. All these results indicate that the extracellular space is not enlarged, although some controversy exists with respect to the interpretation of these data [47].

114

A constant observation is elevation of the brain water, sodium, and chloride content while potassium content remains normal when expressed per unit of dry weight of brain. The water and electrolyte changes are most pronounced in white matter and are of a much lesser magnitude in the grey matter [2, 4, 29]. Analysis of radioactive sodium kinetics has given divergent results. Katzman et al. [15] found ^{24}Na exchange to be delayed in edematous white matter and decided the most probable explanations were: 1) a reduced sodium extrusion due to inhibition of the sodium pump or 2) a "sink" action of the myelin clefts, i. e. an accumulation of a non- or slowly exchanging sodium pool in the edema fluid sequestered in these clefts. On the other hand, Reed et al. [29] analyzed ^{22}Na and ^{36}Cl uptake curves of cortex in rats fed triethyl tin acetate and felt they indicated an increase in the permeability of glial cell membranes to sodium and chloride and not a decrease in the sodium efflux.

Brain equilibration of ^{42}K is normal, as might be expected from the observed tissue electrolyte values and results of ^{32}P uptake were again too variable to yield reliable information [4]. The permeability of the blood -brain barrier in triethyl tin induced edema has been tested by dye injection techniques [4, 18] and the distribution of ^{131}I-albumin [4, 15]. These studies have shown the barrier to be intact. Similarly, uptake of ^{14}C-glycine did not differ from that in normal animals in contrast to the elevation of such uptake in cold injury edema [4]. However, the studies of Kalsbeck and Cummings [14] have demonstrated increased albumin and alkaline phosphatase in the edema fluid suggesting origin from the plasma. More recently, Joo et al. [12] have presented evidence for abnormal penetration of Evans blue and thorotrast.

Many studies have been done in vivo and in vitro to elucidate the biochemical mechanisms underlying triethyl tin induction of cerebral edema, but the results of such studies are difficult to integrate with other phenomena studied. Aldridge and Cremer [1] found triethyl tin to be a potent inhibitor of in vitro oxygen uptake by brain brei. There was little effect on glycolytic enzymes but apparently a marked inhibition of Krebs cycle enzymes was observed. Brain tissue slices from rats treated in vivo with triethyl tin showed approximately 50 % inhibition of oxygen uptake in vitro [7]. This observation was expanded and confirmed by the work of Moore and Brody [21]. They found that in vitro respiration of brain slices, but not liver slices, from rats given triethyl tin in vivo was inhibited while both tissues showed similar responses when treated with triethyl tin in vitro. This might be explained by the intracellular distribution of triethyl tin in vivo; in the brain, 40 % of intracellular content is associated with the mitochondria, while only 14 % is bound to mitochondria in the liver [31]. On the basis of their findings, Moore and Brody concluded that decrease in respiration and uncoupling of oxidative phosphorylation could lead to a decrease in the brain energy reserves, thus causing the toxic effects commonly seen.

In vitro exposure of brain cortex slices to triethyl tin causes a decrease in tissue potassium content of 73 % when glucose is the substrate or by 18 % when pyruvate is the substrate [8]. This would indicate that the primary effect at least in vitro is one of altered metabolism and not altered cellular permeability. Later studies [9] showed that the metabolic effects of in vivo triethyl tin poisoning were a decrease in the oxidation of pyruvate formed from glucose while glycolysis was not inhibited.

Torack [47, 48] has observed the inhibition of a peculiar membrane bound, magnesium-activated, glutaraldehyde-resistant adenosine triphosphatase in the white matter of triethyl tin intoxicated rats. While the impaired utilization of adenosine triphosphate appears to be a specific inhibitory effect, there remains some question as to the reliability of the histochemical technique used.

Several means of therapy have been found to reduce the edema of triethyl tin intoxication. The administration of glycerol [20], hypertonic urea [17], mannitol [52], escin [51], and silymarin [53] serve to lessen the ultrastructural or chemical alterations in the poisoned animals. Taylor and her coworkers [43, 44] have reported on the use of corticosteroids to alleviate the abnormalities of triethyl tin induced edema. Rabbits given 0.75 mg/kg dexamethasone concurrently with 1 mg/kg/day triethyl tin sulfate showed a marked clinical improvement compared to those given triethyl tin alone. Water and sodium content were reduced and structural changes in the edematous white matter were improved. Although fluid accumulation in the myelin sheaths was still seen in animals treated with dexamethasone, it was of a focal rather than a diffuse nature.

We have studied the effects of dexamethasone on the development of triethyl tin bromide edema induced by the intraperitoneal injection of 1.25 mg/kg/day for a period of 7 days [42]. Dexamethasone was administered intramuscularly in doses of 0.25 mg/kg or 1.25 mg/kg daily in both normal animals and those receiving triethyl tin. 5 min prior to sacrifice, ^{59}Fe-red cells, ^{131}I-albumin, and ^{99m}Tc-pertechnetate were injected intravenously. The cerebral distribution of technetium was normal, confirming previous impressions of the state of the blood-brain barrier. The sum of the red cell and albumin spaces was used to estimate the cerebral blood content (Table 1) which was significantly reduced from normal in animals receiving triethyl tin alone. The administration of the larger dose of dexamethasone with triethyl tin resulted in a significant improvement of the blood volume. The lower dose of dexamethasone was ineffective. Brain water content of animals receiving triethyl tin alone was increased,

Table 1. Effect of dexamethasone on triethyl tin induced brain edema

	Control	Steroid only 1.25 mg/kg/day	triethyl tin	Triethyl tin plus steroid 0.25 mg/kg/day	Triethyl tin plus steroid 1.25 mg/kg/day
Brain water gm/gm dry wt.	3.52 ± .04[b]	3.39 ± .06[a b]	3.73 ± .09[a]	3.78 ± .16[a]	3.61 ± .09[a b]
Brain Na meq/kg dry wt.	279 ± 12[b]	268 ± 13[b]	338 ± 25[a]	312 ± 28[a]	302 ± 33[b]
Brain K meq/kg dry wt.	465 ± 35	433 ± 28	442 ± 33	460 ± 38	460 ± 33
Brain blood volume ml/100 gm wet wt.	2.83 ± .18[b]	3.34 ± .50[b]	2.15 ± .10[a]	2.30 ± .40	2.66 ± .30[b]

Results expressed as mean ± standard deviation (n = 5 — 8).
[a] Statistical significance at p < .05 compared to control.
[b] Statistical significance at p < .05 compared to triethyl tin.

as was that of animals in both steroid treatment groups. However, those animals receiving the larger dose of steroid plus triethyl tin exhibited a brain water content which was significantly lower than those receiving triethyl tin alone. Administration of this dose of dexamethasone decreases brain water content in normal animals as well. A similar decrease in brain water content has been reported by Timiras *et al.* [45] after treatment of normal animals for nine days with hydrocortisone, but Taylor and her coworkers [44] did not find such changes after 6 days of dexamethasone treatment at a lower dose (0.75 mg/kg/day) than used in our studies. The brain sodium content showed the same pattern as the water, i.e. the higher dose of dexamethasone caused a significant reduction of accumulation. Brain potassium values were essentially normal in all groups studied.

Thus, administration of dexamethasone decreased cerebral edema in rats poisoned with triethyl tin bromide. Since the brain water and sodium content of steroid-treated control animals was also reduced, this may be simply a nonspecific dehydrating effect. As suggested by Taylor *et al.* [43], the effects of dexamethasone could also be related to alterations in the pharmacology of the triethyl tin compounds. Possible explanations would include 1) prevention of cerebral uptake of triethyl tin, 2) enhancement of its urinary excretion, or 3) interference with its local absorption from the injection site. We are currently investigating these potential indirect effects of steroid therapy.

Cerebral Ischemia

Brain edema frequently accompanies ischemic brain injury. Pathologic studies have shown that edema is a significant contributing factor to the fatal outcome in patients dying within the first week of acute cerebral infarction [22, 36]. Plum has shown that brain swelling contributed to clinical deterioration or death in 21 % of 106 patients with acute hemispheric infarcts [25].

The use of corticosteroids in the treatment of stroke remains a controversial issue. Early uncontrolled studies suggested that such therapy might be useful [30, 34]. Controlled studies have yielded discrepant results. Dyken and White [10] found a slightly higher mortality (statistically insignificant) in patients treated with cortisone. Subsequently, Rubinstein [33] reported favorably on the use of steroids. Most recently, Patten *et al.* [24] have conducted a double blind study of the effects of dexamethasone and concluded that there was significant improvement in the treated group.

Few experimental studies of steroid effectiveness in ischemic brain injury have been performed. Plum *et al.* [26] evaluated a single 0.55 mg/kg dose of dexamethasone in rats subjected to hypoxia alone or hypoxia plus unilateral carotid ligation. Steroid treatment resulted in greater mortality and, in surviving animals, did not benefit clinical status, severity of edema, brain electrolyte shifts, or abnormal vascular permeability to trypan blue. Cantu and Ames [5] found no beneficial effect of methyl-prednisolone given 45 min to 2 h prior to aortic ligation. This model results in cerebrovascular obstruction after restoration of aortic flow which is believed to be due to edema with both endothelial and astrocytic swelling [3, 6]. However, the results of both these groups may be criticized because the observations did not extent beyond 24 h [23].

Recently, Kahn and coworkers [13] have studied a model of experimental infarction produced by unilateral carotid ligation in the gerbil. Treated animals received the human equivalent of a 40 mg daily dose of dexamethasone in divided doses beginning 1 h after ligation and every 8 h thereafter. Infarction developed in 57 % of the treated animals compared to 40 % of saline-treated controls. Similarly, mortality was higher in the steroid group (47 % versus 37 %). Dexamethasone had no beneficial effect on either the length of survival or the degree of infarction determined pathologically.

We have recently described a model of ischemic brain injury in the rat produced by the intracarotid injection of 80 micron carbonized microspheres [37]. Cerebral edema is a constant accompaniment of microembolism and is present by 4 h after sphere injection. The brain ^{59}Fe-red cell and ^{131}I-albumin spaces are initially decreased as a reflection of diminished cerebral blood volume due to increased intracranial pressure and vascular compression. The ^{99m}Tc-pertechnetate space is significantly elevated by 8–16 h after embolization, and by 16–14 h the ^{131}I-albumin space increases above normal values. These changes are believed to result from abnormal permeability of the blood-brain barrier as a consequence of vascular injury. Other workers have also found evidence of increased capillary permeability to macromolecules under similar circumstances [35, 39, 55].

Table 2. Effect of dexamethasone on edema of cerebral microembolism

| | Time after embolization (h) | | | |
	4	24	48	72
Water (gm/gm dry wt.)				
Control	3.55 ± .07	3.69 ± .05	3.69 ± .06	3.69 ± .06
Steroid only	3.58 ± .11	3.55 ± .04ᵃ	3.59 ± .09ᵃ	3.66 ± .11
Microembolism	4.09 ± .22ᵃ	4.26 ± .26ᵃ	4.31 ± .26ᵃ	4.21 ± .22ᵃ
Microembolism + steroid	4.09 ± .16ᵃ	4.20 ± .44ᵃ	4.77 ± .17ᵃ	4.38 ± .62ᵃ
Sodium (meq/kg dry wt.)				
Control	197 ± 12	198 ± 9	217 ± 13	217 ± 13
Steroid only	207 ± 12	205 ± 17	217 ± 11	243 ± 9ᵃ
Microembolism	276 ± 40ᵃ	282 ± 40ᵃ	338 ± 43ᵃ	342 ± 57ᵃ
Microembolism + steroid	314 ± 55ᵃ	274 ± 53ᵃ	417 ± 19ᵃ ᵇ	412 ± 103ᵃ
Potassium (meq/kg dry wt.)				
Control	378 ± 13	425 ± 16	428 ± 14	428 ± 14
Steroid only	388 ± 8	410 ± 16	422 ± 21	439 ± 7ᵃ
Microembolism	361 ± 19ᵃ	378 ± 31ᵃ	387 ± 9ᵃ	392 ± 19ᵃ
Microembolism + steroid	329 ± 16ᵃ ᵇ	374 ± 24ᵃ	354 ± 32ᵃ	363 ± 55ᵃ

Determinations are results for both hemispheres in control and steroid only groups; for right hemisphere only in microembolism and microembolism + steroid groups.
Results expressed as mean ± standard deviation.
ᵃ Statistical significance compared to control group at $p < .05$.
ᵇ Statistical significance compared to microembolism group at $p < .05$.

Subsequently, we have tested the effects of dexamethasone (0.25 mg/kg at the time of embolization and every 8 h thereafter for up to 72 h) in this model [38]. Steroid therapy had no significant effect on mortality which ranged from 14 % to 73 % and increased progressively with time in both treated and untreated groups. The results of brain water and electrolyte determinations are shown in Table 2. Brain water and sodium values were increased and those for potassium decreased in both treated and untreated animals at all times studied. Steroids had no significant ameliorative effect. Similarly, steroid treatment did not significantly alter the changes in cerebral spaces of ^{59}Fe-red cells, ^{131}I-albumin, or ^{99m}Tc-pertechnetate.

In summary, the available experimental evidence fails to demonstrate a beneficial effect of steroid therapy on the edema of ischemic brain injury. This is contrasted with the good results of some authors in clinical instances of cerebral infarction. At the present time, the role of steroids in the treatment of stroke remains controversial and larger clinical series will probably be necessary to resolve the question.

References

1. Aldridge, W. N., Cremer, J. E.: The biochemistry of organo-tin compounds. Diethyltin dichloride and triethyltin sulphate. Biochem. J. **61**, 406–418 (1955).
2. Aleu, F. P., Katzman, R., Terry, R. D.: Fine structure and electrolyte analyses of cerebral edema induced by alkyl tin intoxication. J. Neuropath. exp. Neurol. **22**, 403–413 (1963).
3. Ames, A., III, Wright, R. L., Kowada, M. et al.: Cerebral ischemia. II. The no-reflow phenomenon. Amer. J. Path. **52**, 437–453 (1968).
4. Bakay, L.: Morphological and chemical studies in cerebral edema: Triethyltin induced edema. J. neurol. Sci. **2**, 52–67 (1965).
5. Cantu, R. C., Ames, A., III.: Experimental prevention of cerebral vasculature obstruction produced by ischemia. J. Neurosurg. **30**, 50–54 (1969).
6. Chiang, J., Kowada, M., Ames, A., III, et al.: Cerebral ischemia. III. Vascular changes. Amer. J. Path. **52**, 455–476 (1968).
7. Cremer, J. E.: The metabolism in vitro of tissue slices from rats given triethyltin compounds. Biochem. J. **67**, 87–96 (1957).
8. — Studies on brain cortex slices. The influence of various inhibitors on the retention of potassium ions and amino acids with glucose or pyrurate as substrate. Biochem. J. **104**, 223–228 (1967).
9. — Selective inhibition of glucose oxidation by triethyltin in rat brain in vivo. Biochem. J. **119**, 95–102 (1970).
10. Dyken, M., White, P. T.: Evaluation of cortisone in the treatment of cerebral infarction. J. Amer. med. Ass. **162**, 1531–1534 (1956).
11. Harnack, E.: Über die Wirkungen des Bleis auf den thierischen Organismus. Naunyn-Schmiedeberg's Arch. exp. Path. Pharmak. **9**, 152–225 (1878).
12. Joo, V. F., Zoltan, Ö. T., Csillik, B. et al.: Untersuchungen über das durch Triethylzinn-sulfat verursachte Hirnoedem bei der Ratte. 5. Mitteilung: Die Wirkung von Triaethyl-zinnsulfat auf die Permeabilität der Blut-Hirn-Schranke. Arzneimittel-Forsch. **19**, 296–297 (1969).
13. Kahn, K., Pranzarone, G. F., Newman, T.: Dexamethasone treatment of experimental cerebral infarction (Abstract). Neurology **22**, 406–407 (1972).
14. Kalsbeck, J. E., Cummings, J. N.: Experimental edema in the rat and cat brain. J. Neuropath. exp. Neurol. **22**, 237–247 (1963).
15. Katzman, R., Aleu, F., Wilson, C.: Further observations on triethyltin edema. Arch. Neurol. (Chic.) **9**, 88–97 (1963).
16. Lee, J. C., Bakay, L.: Ultrastructural changes in the edematous central nervous system. 1. Triethyltin edema. Arch. Neurol. (Chic.) **13**, 48–57 (1965).
17. Levy, A., Taylor, J. M., Herzog, I. et al.: The effect of hypertonic urea on cerebral edema in the rabbit induced by triethyl tin sulfate. Arch. Neurol. (Chic.) **13**, 58–64 (1965).
18. Magee, P. N., Stoner, H. B., Barnes, J. M.: The experimental production of oedema in the central nervous system of the rat by triethyl tin compounds. J. Path. Bact. **73**, 107–124 (1957).
19. Maha, G. E.: Adrenal corticosteroid therapy of cerebral edema. Penn. Med. **73**, 50–55 (1970).

20. Mandell, S., Taylor, J. M., Kotsilimbas, D. G. *et al.*: The effect of glycerol on cerebral edema induced by tri-ethyltin sulphate in rabbits. J. Neurosurg. **24**, 984–986 (1966).
21. Moore, K. E., Brody, T. M.: The effect of triethyltin on oxidative phosphorylation and mitochondrial adenosine triphosphatase activation. Biochem. Pharmacol. **6**, 125–133 (1961).
22. Ng. L. K. Y., Nimmannitya, J.: Massive cerebral infarction with brain swelling. A clinicopathological study. Stroke **1**, 158–163 (1970).
23. Pappius, H. M., McCann, W. P.: Effects of steroids on cerebral edema in cats. Arch. Neurol. (Chic.) **20**, 207–216 (1969).
24. Patten, B. M., Mendell, J., Bruun, B. *et al.*: Double-blind study of the effects of dexamethasone on acute stroke. Neurology **22**, 377–383 (1972).
25. Plum, F.: Brain swelling and edema in cerebral vascular disease. Proc. Ass. Res. nerv. ment. Dis. **41**, 318–348 (1964).
26. — Alvord, E. C., Jr., Posner, J. B.: Effect of steroids on experimental cerebral infarction. Arch. Neurol. (Chic.) **9**, 571–573 (1963).
27. Potchen, E. J., Adatepe, M. H., Studer, R. *et al.*: Radioisotopic assessment of cerebral edema. Arch. Neurol. (Chic.) **24**, 287–290 (1971).
28. Prados, M., Strowger, B., Feindel, W.: Studies on cerebral edema. II. Reaction of the brain to exposure to air: Physiologic changes. Arch. Neurol. Psychiat. (Chic.) **54**, 290–300 (1945).
29. Reed, D. J., Woodbury, D. M., Holtzer, R. L.: Brain edema, electrolytes and extracellular space. Arch. Neurol. (Chic.) **10**, 604–616 (1964).
30. Roberts, H. J.: Supportive adrenocortical steroid therapy in acute and subacute cerebrovascular accidents with particular reference to brain stem involvement. J. Amer. Geriat. Soc. **6**, 686–702 (1952).
31. Rose, M. S., Aldridge, W. N.: The interaction of triethyltin with components of animal tissues. Biochem. J. **106**, 821–828 (1968).
32. Rouzaud, M., Lutier, J.: Oedeme subaigu cerebro-meninge du a une intoxication d'actualite. Presse méd. **62**, 1075 (1954).
33. Rubinstein, M. K.: The influence of adrenocortical steroids on severe cerebrovascular accidents. J. nerv. ment. Dis. **141**, 291–299 (1965).
34. Russek, H. I., Russek, A. S. Zohman, B. L.: Cortisone in immediate therapy of apoplectic stroke. J. Amer. med. Ass. **159**, 102–105 (1955).
35. Russell, R. W. R.: A study of the microcirculation in experimental cerebral embolism. Angiologica **3**, 240–258 (1966).
36. Shaw, C. M., Alvord, E. C., Jr., Berry, R. G.: Swelling of the brain following ischemic infarction with arterial occlusion. Arch. Neurol. (Chic.) **1**, 161–177 (1959).
37. Siegel, B. A., Meidinger, R., Elliott, A. J. *et al.*: Experimental cerebral microembolism: Multiple tracer assessment of brain edema. Arch. Neurol. (Chic.) **26**, 73–77 (1972).
38. — Studer, R. K., Potchen, E. J.: Steroid therapy of brain edema: Ineffectiveness in experimental cerebral microembolism. Arch. Neurol. (Chic.) **27**, 209–212 (1972).
39. Steegman, A. T., de la Fuente, J.: Experimental cerebral embolism: II. Microembolism of the rabbit brain with seran polymer resin. J. Neuropath. exp. Neurol. **18**, 537–558 (1959).
40. Stoner, H. B., Barnes, J. M., Duff, J. I.: Studies on the toxicity of alkyl tin compounds. Brit. J. Pharmacol. **10**, 16–25 (1955).
41. Streicher, E.: The thiocyanate space of rat brain in experimental cerebral edema. J. Neuropath. exp. Neurol. **21**, 437–441 (1962).
42. Studer, R., Potchen, E. J.: Effects of dexamethasone on triethyl tin induced brain edema in rats. (Abstract) Clin. Res. **19**, 356 (1971).
43. Taylor, J. M., Levy, W. A., Herzog, I. *et al.*: Prevention of experimental cerebral edema by corticosteroids. Neurology **15**, 667–674 (1965).
44. — — McCoy, G. *et al.*: Prevention of cerebral edema induced by triethyltin in rabbits by cortico-steroids. Nature **204**, 891–892 (1964).
45. Timiras, P. S., Woodbury, D. M., Goodman, L. S.: Effect of adrenalectomy, hydrocortisone acetate and desoxycorticosterone acetate on brain excitability and electrolyte distribution in mice. J. Pharmacol. exp. Ther. **112**, 80–93 (1954).

46. Torack, R. M.: The relationship between adenosinetriphosphatase activity and triethyltin toxicity in the production of cerebral edema of the rat. Amer. J. Path. **46**, 245–261 (1965).
47. — Gordon, J., Prokop, J.: Pathobiology of acute triethyltin intoxication. Int. Rev. Neurobiol. **12**, 45–86 (1970).
48. — Terry, R. D., Zimmerman, H. M.: The fine structure of cerebral fluid accumulation. II. Swelling produced by triethyl tin poisoning and its comparison with that in the human brain. Amer. J. Path. **36**, 273–287 (1960).
49. Ungar, E., Bödlander, G.: Über die toxischen Wirkungen des Zinns, mit besonderer Berücksichtigung der durch den Gebrauch verzinnter Conservenbüchsen der Gesundheit drohenden Gefahren. Z. Hyg. Infek.-Kr. **2**, 241–296 (1887).
50. Van der Kerk, G. J. M., Luijten, J. G. A.: Organotin compounds. III. Biocidal properties of organotin compounds. J. appl. Chem. **4**, 314–319 (1954).
51. Varkonyi, V. T., Csillik, B., Zoltan, Ö. T. *et al.*: Untersuchungen über das durch Triaethylzinnsulfat verursachte Hirnödem bei der Ratte. 4. Mitteilung: Elektronenoptische Untersuchungen. Arzneimittel-Forsch. **19**, 293–295 (1969).
52. — Maurer, M., Zoltan, Ö. T. *et al.*: Untersuchungen über das durch Triaethylzinnsulfat verursachte Hirnödem bei der Ratte. 9. Mitteilung: Die Wirkung von Mannit auf das elektronenoptische Bild der experimentell durch Triaethylzinnsulfat hervorgerufenen Vergiftung bei der Ratte. Arzneimittel-Forsch. **21**, 147–148 (1971).
53. — — — *et al.*: Untersuchungen über das durch Triaethylzinnsulfat (TZS) verursachte Hirnödem bei der Ratte. 10. Mitteilung: Die Wirkung von Silymarin auf das elektronenoptische Bild der experimentell durch Triaethylzinnsulfat hervorgerufenen Vergiftung bei der Ratte. Arzneimittel-Forsch. **21**, 148–149 (1971).
54. White, T. P.: Über die Wirkungen des Zinns auf den thierischen Organismus. Naunyn-Schmiedeberg's Arch. exp. Path. Pharmakol. **13**, 53–69 (1880–1881).
55. Zülch, K. J.: Neuropathological aspects and histological criteria of brain edema and brain swelling. In: Klatzo, I., Seitelberger, F. (Eds.): Brain Edema, pp. 95–116. Berlin-Heidelberg-New York: Springer 1967.

Effects of Ischemia on Water and Electrolyte Content of Cerebral Tissues

S. Shibata,, J. W. Norris, C. P. Hodge, and H. M. Pappius

Montreal Neurological Institute, McGill University, Montreal, Canada

As part of a long range study of various aspects of cerebral edema, we investigated the effect of ischemia on the distribution of water, sodium and potassium in brain tissues *in vivo*.

The method we chose for producing ischemia was the clipping of the middle cerebral artery (MCA) in the dog. The clip was placed as closely as possible to the origin of the artery and the area affected by the clip was clearly delineated in the exposed cerebral cortex by fluorescein angiography through the lingual artery as described by Feindel *et al.* [4]. Fluorescein angiography was carried out before and at intervals after the clipping of the artery in acute experiments. In experiments of 24 h duration or longer angiography was carried out only at the end of the experiment to avoid large exposure of the cortex necessary for this procedure. The area of non-filling, as delineated by fluorescein angiography through the lingual artery, persisted as long as the clip was in place, in our experiments up to 48 h.

In 75 % of our animals 48 h after clipping the MCA, focal areas of infarction developed in the area of caudate nucleus, the internal capsule and, occasionally, in the overlaying temporal-parietal cortex. Edema could be demonstrated chemically in the surrounding and underlying white matter. However, analysis of large uninfarcted cortical areas, apparently ischemic on the basis of fluorescein angiography, failed to show any effect of the clipping on water and electrolyte distribution [5].

We, therefore, investigated the collateral blood supply to the area normally supplied by the clipped artery. In animals in which the MCA was clipped from 1–48 h earlier, the area showing as non-filling on angiography via the lingual artery showed complete, though delayed filling when the fluorescein was injected via the femoral artery. This was verified by carbon perfusion through the heart just before the animal was killed. In all these animals although the proper placement of the clip was seen at autopsy, the carbon was uniformly distributed throughout the brain including the area supplied by the clipped artery. Thus it was clear that the affected cortical area had considerable collateral blood supply, obviously sufficient to maintain normal distribution of water and electrolytes.

To induce a more drastic impairment of the blood supply, the collateral circulation had to be compromised and after some preliminary trials the following model was developed: MCA was clipped as before. 1 h later systemic blood pressure (BP) was lowered to 50 mmHg by bleeding. Following 1 h of hemorrhagic hypotension,

BP was returned to normal by reinfusion of the citrated blood. This produced an area of ischemia in the territory normally supplied by the clipped artery which could be easily demarcated by fluorescein angiography through the femoral artery and by carbon perfusion.

Femoral injection of fluorecein during the period of hypotension resulted in patchy, much delayed filling of the cortical vessels in the area of the clipped MCA. When the blood pressure was returned to normal, fluorescein appeared in this area with much delay (50–60 sec instead of the normal 18 sec) and the appearance of the fluorescence was grossly abnormal and blurred as if it were not restricted to blood vessels. It persisted at 130 sec when the last pictures were taken, in contrast to normal conditions when the passage of the bolus of the dye through the cortical vessels was complete within a few seconds.

Complete ischemia of the affected cortex was clearly demonstrated with carbon perfusion. The perfusion could not be carried out successfully during the period of hypotension since the animals went into shock. However, within 30 min of elevation of the blood pressure, perfusion with carbon clearly delineated the area of the clipped artery as non-filling. This was demonstrated 1 h, 5 h and 24 h after restoration of BP.

Table 1. The percentage dry weight and potassium and sodium content of cerebral tissues, at intervals of time after restoration of blood pressure, in dogs in which the right middle cerebral artery was clipped and which then were subjected to hypotension for 60 min

Time after restoration of blood pressure	0	30 min	1 h	5 h	24 h	Control tissue[a]
Number of animals	3	4	3	3	3	16
Cerebral cortex						
Dry weight mg%	21.1	17.5	17.0	15.0	13.4	20.8 ± 1.2
Sodium meq/kg	63	78	90	109	136	58 ± 5
Potassium meq/kg	108	82	73	45	25	108 ± 5
White matter						
Dry weight mg%	31.8	30.1	30.6	29.2	26.0	33.3 ± 1.7
Sodium meq/kg	50	56	46	59	72	51 ± 4
Potassium meq/kg	83	87	90	72	58	89 ± 5

Averages ± S.D.

[a] Averages of values in unaffected hemisphere of all experimental animals.

The affected area was clearly visible on the outside of the brain and extended throughout the area normally supplied by the MCA. Thus, although the whole brain was subjected to hemorrhagic hypotension only in the territory of the clipped artery, an irreversible, total ischemia developed. This is an example of no-reflow phenomenon described by Ames, Chiang, Cantu and their coworkers [1, 2, 3] Discussion of the possible mechanisms involved is outside the scope of my presentation. We were interested in the consequences of this phenomenon.

Necrotic changes were demonstrated by conventional histological techniques (H & E) in the affected area within 5 h of restoration of BP. Within 24 h massive necrosis was grossly evident.

Chemical findings are summarized in Table 1. Normal dry weight and sodium and potassium were found at the end of 60 min of systemic hypotension. The cortex showed progressive changes starting immediately after restoration of BP. These consisted of a fall in percentage dry weight and in potassium content, and a rise in the sodium content, the latter approaching plasma levels within 24 h. The decrease in potassium represents a net loss from the normal level of 511 meq/100 mg dry weight at the end of the hypotensive period to 300 meq after 5 h and 187 meq after 24 h of restoration of BP.

In view of the histological changes and the gross appearance of the brain, we consider that these chemical changes represent cell death rather than tissue swelling. They are the result of massive necrosis.

In contrast, the findings in subcortical white matter are compatible with the gradual development of vasogenic edema. The decrease in the percentage dry weight was slower and more moderate, while the edematous changes in sodium and potassium were barely measurable 5 h after the hypotensive period. At 24 h, the changes in the white matter were of the order of magnitude seen in association with a cold lesion.

On the basis of these studies, we conclude that in the dog collateral circulation is sufficient to maintain normal water and electrolyte distribution in most cortical areas usually supplied by the clipped MCA. Irreversible impairment of circulation, achieved in our model when a period of hemorrhagic hypotension is superimposed on clipping the MCA results in irreversible interference with electrolyte distribution in the cortex where the resultant changes are brought about by massive necrosis and should not be considered as indicating presence of edema or swelling. In white matter, underlying the necrotic areas, edema develops gradually and is of the vasogenic type.

Further experiments will be needed to determine whether ischemia, more pronounced than that produced by clipping of the supplying artery but not as complete as obtained in our model, would induce reversible edematous changes in the cortex.

We have not studied the effect of steroids in our preparation. It would be of great interest to determine whether the extent of necrosis resulting from complete ischemia can be affected by steroid therapy.

References

1. Ames, A., III., Wright, R. L., Kowada, M., Thurston, J. M., Majno, G.: Cerebral ischemia. II. The no-reflow phenomenon. Amer. J. Pathol. 52, 437–453 (1968).
2. Cantu, R. C., Ames, A., III., Dixon, J., DiGiacinto, G.: Reversibility of experimental cerebrovascular obstruction induced by complete ischemia. J. Neurosurg. 31, 429–431 (1969).
3. Chiang, J., Kowada, M., Ames, A., III., Wright, L., Majno, G.: Cerebral ischemia. III. Vascular changes. Amer. J. Pathol. 52, 455–476 (1968).
4. Feindel, W., Yamamoto, Y. L., Hodge, C. P.: Intracarotid fluorescein angiography: a new method for examination of the epicerebral circulation in man. Can. med. Assoc. J. 96, 1–7 (1967).
5. Norris, J. W., Hodge, C. P., Pappius, H. M.: J. Neuropath. exp. Neurol. 30, 140 (1971).

Effect of Dexamethasone on the Early Edema Following Occlusion of the Middle Cerebral Artery in Cats

Daniel Bartko *, Hans J. Reulen, Herrmann Koch, and Kurt Schürmann

Department of Neurosurgery, University of Mainz, W. Germany, and Department of Neurology, Comenius University, Bratislava, Czechoslovakia

With 6 Figures

Summary. Occlusion of the middle cerebral artery (MCA) in cats results in a drop in blood flow in the territory normally supplied by the MCA, demonstrable by the measurement of rCBF with ^{85}Krypton or by angiography. As a consequence of tissue hypoxia a rise in lactate, in lactate/pyruvate ratio and a breakdown of CrP, ATP and the energy charge potential is found in the ischemic area. At the borderline zone a slight hyperemia, followed by a secondary depression in blood flow, was recorded, accompanied by comparable alterations in energy-rich phosphates and in L/P ratio. A significant increase in water content of the grey and white matter occured already after 30 or 120 min, respectively. The accumulation of edema fluid takes place in the absence of protein extravasation.

A group of cats were pre-treated with dexamethasone (0.3 mg/kg/day; intraperitoneally), starting 72 h before the occlusion. In dexamethasone-treated animals the accumulation of fluid in the ischemic as well as in the bordering zone was diminished 2 h after the occlusion as compared to untreated animals. rCBF changes were now less pronounced and the energetic situation was better preserved.

Introduction

Advances in methodology for measuring regional cerebral blood flow (rCBF) in patients and animals have stimulated the interest in pathophysiology of occlusive cerebrovascular disease. Most clinical and experimental studies, however, are concerned with the late phases of infarction. Recent studies have shown that the early phase following occlusion of a major cerebral vessel is of crucial importance for the development as well as the extent of the infarction [2, 3, 21, 22]. Since the blood flow of the occluded territory is at the mercy of collateral channels, alterations in arterial blood pressure [19, 21], in arterial pCO_2 [22], and the spreading of early edema [3] may determine the final extent of infarction and irreversible tissue damage. Therefore the therapy of the early stage, if possible, is of major importance [14].

The development of brain edema is a well recognized complication of cerebral infarction [4, 11, 18]. Shaw *et al.* showed, that swelling of infarcted brain tissue, as manifested by the shift of the midline, develops during the first tree to five days and subsides thereafter gradually. Deaths occuring during the first week are usually related to brain edema [11, 18]. Brain edema, therefore, is an important pathogenic factor of cerebral infarction.

* This investigation was supported by a Research Grant from the Deutsche Forschungsgemeinschaft. Dr. Bartko is recipient of a Fellowship of the Humboldt Foundation.

127

The present study is part of an ongoing study on the early alterations following occlusion of MCA. It was designed to examine whether dexamethasone – which has been shown to be biologically active in cat [13] – exerts an effect on the early edema induced by focal cerebral ischemia.

Methods

In this study 48 cats with body weights between 2.2 and 3.8 kg were used. Cats were anaesthetized with sodium pentobarbital (40 mg/kg intraperitoneally). The femoral artery and vein were unilaterally catheterized. Arterial blood pressure was continuously monitored with a pressure transducer. All animals were tracheotomized and had both lingual arteries cannulated for tracer injections. Following relaxation (0.2 mg Imbretil/30 min) all animals were mechanically normoventilated with a Starling pump. The acid-base status in the blood (and in the CSF) was intermittently controlled by the Astrup microequipment. Rectal temperature was measured and kept between 36° and 37.5° C. Arterial pO_2 was maintained between 100–140 mmHg and $paCO_2$ between 28–31 mmHg.

In order to produce an experimental infarction, MCA was exposed by a temporal approach using a microsurgical technique. After a small incision of the dura the vessel was permanently occluded at its origin by a silver clip. Care was taken to avoid damage to the brain. The dura was then closed. Thereafter Evans blue (2 % solution, 1 ml/kg b.w.) was injected intravenously. Regional cerebral blood flow (rCBF) was measured before as well as 30, 60, 120, 240 min and 24 h after the MCA occlusion, using the ^{85}Kr-clearance method [9]. A bilateral craniotomy was performed involving a large part of the cranial vault, the dura remaining intact. rCBF was measured over the following areas: a) the center of the occluded area; b) a borderline area (periphery); c) the contralateral "healthy" hemisphere, which served as control. In a few animals, MCA occlusion was controlled by angiography.

9 animals were pretreated with dexamethasone (0.15 mg/kg, twice daily, intraperitoneally) starting 72 h before the occlusion of the MCA was performed. rCBF in this group was measured 120 min following the clipping.

At the beginning and at the end of the experiment a CSF sample (obtained by puncture of the cisterna magna) was taken for the measurement of pH, lactate and pyruvate. Following the rCBF measurements the brain was instantaneously frozen *in vivo* with liquid nitrogen poured directly on the dura. Corresponding to the areas, in which rCBF has been measured, the brain was divided into slices using a precooled saw. These areas of cortex as well as subjacent white matter were separated from the slices, using small chisels cooled in liquid nitrogen. Tissue and CSF samples were stored in liquid nitrogen.

The water content of the samples was determined by drying to a constant weight at 105° C. The dried material was ground, extracted with 20 parts of 0.75 nitric acid for 4–6 days and centrifuged. Sodium and potassium were determined in the supernatant by flame photometry.

The tissue concentrations of CrP, ATP, ADP, AMP, lactate and pyruvate were determined enzymatically by methods previously described [16].

Results

Clipping of MCA resulted in an immediate and marked drop in rCBF in the territory usually supplied by the occluded vessel (Fig. 1). A slight and progressive further decrease was found at 60, 120 and 240 min following MCA occlusion. At the periphery mean rCBF was not significantly altered after 30 and 60 min. However, a significant diminution in blood flow was found in this area after 120 and 240 min. The question arises whether the regional diminution of tissue perfusion leads to a cellular hypoxia. A sensitive way of judging tissue hypoxia is the measurement of the energy state or the oxidation/reduction state of the tissue. Figure 2 represent the dynamics of the rCBF alterations in relation to the changes in lactate/pyruvate ratio of the respective areas. The lactate/pyruvate ratio (L/P ratio) is often used to express the oxidation/reduction state of the cytoplasmic NADH/NAD$^+$ system, as for instance in hypoxia. At 30 and 60 min following MCA occlusion, about 50 % of the borderline regions showed a slight hyperemia. At 120 and 240 min, however, the flow rate of these areas shifted towards lower values, thus resulting in the decrease in mean blood flow mentioned above (Fig. 2). The lactate/pyruvate ratio rose respectively with a) progressing drop in local flow rate and b) with progressing time delay after the occlusion. The threshold for this rise is a decrease in flow rate of about 20 % of the original value. It is interesting to note, that simultaneously in CSF a rise of lactate, of L/P ratio and a decrease of pH takes place [2].

Concomitantly with the increase of lactate and of L/P ratio in the affected tissue a decrease of the energy-rich phosphate compounds, such as CrP and ATP, has been found to occur (Fig. 6). Consequently AMP and ADP were found to have increased [2]. Since cellular lactate and CrP concentrations may be influenced by changes in intracellular pH, even if hypoxia is absent [20], the energy charge potential (ECP) of the adenine nucleotide pool [1] was calculated in order to evaluate the presence of an unbalance between the rate of utilization and the rate of production of energy-rich compounds.

$$ECP = \frac{ATP + 0.5\,ADP}{ATP + ADP + AMP}$$

A definite decrease of ECP was found in the ischemic area already 30 min after occlusion, thus indicating underoxygenation of the occluded territory. A similar decrease of ECP was found in the periphery at 240 min.

Brain edema can be assessed by the demonstration of an increased water (and sodium) content of the affected hemisphere or tissue area as compared to the control hemisphere or the control area, respectively. A difference in the water content between the control area and the ischemic area was measurable already 30 min following occlusion and continued to increase during the following 4 h (Fig. 3). This difference could be detected in the borderline areas only after 120 min. Figure 3 demonstrates that white matter participates more in edema than the cortex. In order to obtain information concerning the composition of the edema fluid, the changes of sodium and potassium content of the tissue are summarized in Table 1. These values represent data found 120 min following the clipping of MCA. The increase in water content of cortex and white matter was accompanied by an increase in sodium content and a marked loss of potassium.

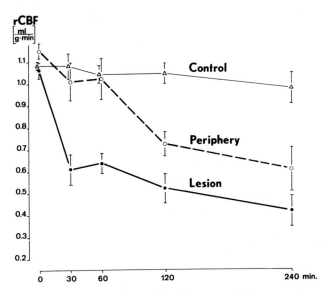

Fig. 1. Changes in rCBF after occlusion of MCA in cats. Values at time zero have been measured immediately before MCA was clipped

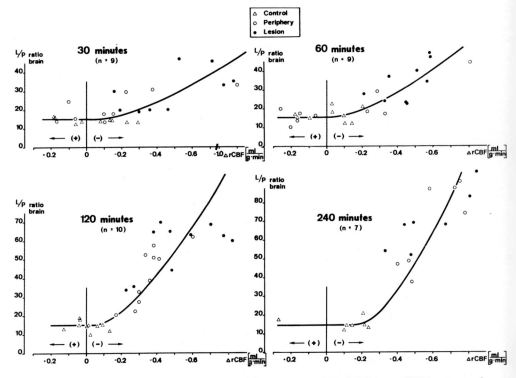

Fig. 2. Changes in lactate/pyruvate ratio in relation to the rCBF changes. △ rCBF is expressed as the change in flow rate at a definite time compared to the respective value measured in the same tissue area before the occlusion of MCA

130

Table 1. Water, sodium and potassium content of cortex and white matter in untreated and steroid-pretreated cats following occlusion of MCA

	Control area			Periphery			Ischemic area		
	untreated	steroid	P	untreated	steroid	P	untreated	steroid	P
Cortex									
Water	79.9 ± 0.2 (10)	79.4 ± 0.2 (9)	0	80.5 ± 0.1 (10)	79.6 ± 0.3 (9)	p < .005	81.9 ± 0.3 (10)	79.9 ± 0.3 (9)	p < .001
Sodium	273.0 ± 3.2 (10)	273.5 ± 6.1 (9)	0	304.3 ± 3.3 (10)	285.8 ± 9.2 (9)	p < .05	342.5 ± 5.0 (10)	307.9 ± 10.3 (9)	p < .01
Potassium	506.3 ± 4.6 (10)	523.9 ± 8.3 (9)	0	464.5 ± 7.0 (10)	500.9 ± 7.4 (9)	p < .001	418.2 ± 5.7 (10)	487.7 ± 8.4 (9)	p < .001
White Matter									
Water	70.9 ± 0.1 (4)	70.1 ± 0.4 (9)	0	71.8 ± 0.2 (4)	70.8 ± 0.5 (9)	0	72.9 ± 0.2 (4)	70.9 ± 0.5 (9)	p < .01
Sodium	182.9 ± 1.4 (4)	183.4 ± 3.3 (9)	0	204.1 ± 2.0 (4)	189.7 ± 4.9 (9)	0	221.6 ± 1.3 (4)	197.1 ± 3.8 (9)	p < .001
Potassium	303.6 ± 5.8 (4)	312.2 ± 8.5 (9)	0	279.0 ± 11.2 (4)	305.1 ± 10.2 (9)	0	263.8 ± 3.3 (4)	302.0 ± 9.0 (9)	p < .01

$\bar{x} \pm S\bar{x}$ are given. Water content is expressed as percentage of wet weight of tissue; sodium and potassium are expressed as meq/kg dry weight of tissue. P = statistically different from untreated. Total number of samples indicated in parentheses.

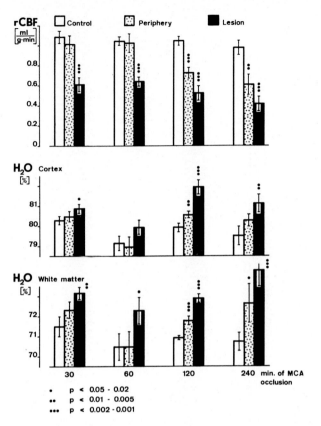

Fig. 3. Changes in the water content of cortex and white matter after occlusion of MCA in cats

Occlusion of MCA for 4 h did not result in extravasation of Evans blue, neither in the ischemic area nor in the periphery. Only one animal showed blue staining of the temporal lobe after 120 min. However, this was probably due to surgical trauma.

The effect of dexamethasone upon the early ischemic cerebral edema and the accompanying alterations is demonstrated in Figures 4–6. Pre-treatment with dexamethasone reduced significantly the accumulation of water and sodium in the ischemic cortex and white matter and prevented it almost completely in the periphery (Fig. 4 and Table 1). Table 1 also shows that the potassium loss, seen in untreated animals, was markedly reduced in dexamethasone-treated animals.

rCBF was significantly elevated in pre-treated animals, especially in the occluded area (Fig. 5). In agreement with the improvement of tissue perfusion, the increase of lactate, of L/P ratio as well as the hypoxic breakdown of CrP, ATP and of ECP were less pronounced following dexamethasone-treatment (Fig. 6).

Mean arterial blood pressure of the various groups (30, 60, 120, 240 min after MCA occlusion) amounted between 120 ± 3.8 and 136 ± 4 mmHg at the time of rCBF measurement. Mean arterial pCO_2 amounted between 29.55 ± 0.47 and 30.39 ± 0.57 mmHg.

132

Discussion

The present study provides evidence that dexamethasone exerts a beneficial effect on the early experimental ischemic cerebral edema, which develops as a consequence of the occlusion of middle cerebral artery in cats. This agrees well with recent findings of Harrison *et al.* in cerebral infarction in the gerbil. Dexamethasone, given immediately after unilateral ligation of the right common carotid artery, reduced significantly the mortality as well as the brain edema which develops in the ipsilateral hemisphere [8]. Our results are in contrast to the findings of Plum and Posner [16] who could not detect any effect of steroids on cerebral edema associated with anoxic-ischemic encephalopathy in the rat. The negative results of Plum and Posner may be related to the fact that edema following anoxic-ischemia develops as a consequence of tissue necrosis. Additionally, the anoxic-ischemic model in the rat is a different situation from the focal ischemia (occlusion of MCA) under normoxic, normocapnic and normotensive conditions in the cat.

It must be stressed that extravasation of Evans blue could not be detected neither in the ischemic areas nor in the periphery within 4 h, a finding which is in line with

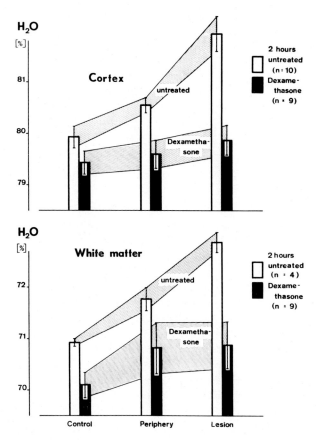

Fig. 4. Water content in cortex and white matter of untreated and of dexamethasone-treated cats 2 h after MCA occlusion

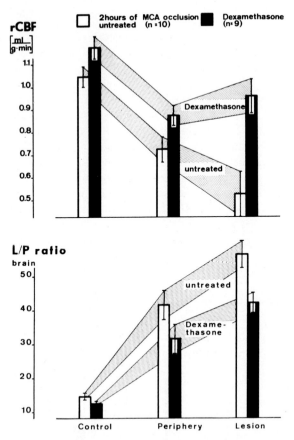

Fig. 5. rCBF and brain lactate/pyruvate ratio of untreated and of dexamethasone-treated cats
2 h after MCA occlusion

previous observations. Olsson, Crowell and Klatzo [12] only exceptionally found a
staining of brain tissue following MCA occlusion (in the rhesus monkey) within
14–24 h. The failure of Evans blue extravasation indicates the absence of protein
extravasation. Obviously, the vascular endothelium must play a crucial role in the
process, since the endothelial lining usually acts as a barrier to proteins [10]. According to electron microscopic observations, separation of inter-endothelial tight junctions or necrosis of the endothelial cells could not be noticed before 12 h after MCA
clipping [6]. The early ultrastructural changes were a swelling of glia cells in the cortex and a combination of the latter plus extracellular and intra-myelinic edema in the
white matter.

Our findings indicate that the early brain edema following occlusion of MCA is
not formed as a vasogenic type of edema with accumulation of a protein-rich fluid, but
is rather caused by a shift of water and electrolytes from the blood into the brain in
the absence of protein extravasation [3]. This is confirmed by recent observations of
Olsson, Crowell and Klatzo [12]. The mechanism underlying the formation of this
early edema is unknown. It is tempting to speculate – also with regard to the steroid

effect – that a disturbance of the permeability of the endothelial wall and/or the cellular membrane of glia cells may be involved [16].

The potassium content of the brain tissue is expressed on the basis of the dry weight of the tissue. This corrects for dilutional changes due to the accumulation of the edema fluid. The potassium content of both grey and white matter of the ischemic as well as of the borderline area was significantly diminished 120 min after occlusion of MCA. Decrease of tissue potassium has also been reported in spinal cord edema [7], as well as in edema following global cerebral ischemia, dinitrophenol, ouabain or temperature reduction [16] and seems to represent a cellular loss of this ion. Dexamethasone prevents potassium loss in the tissue following MCA occlusion as well as after spinal cord injury [7]. The latter is accompanied by an improved functional state. This would imply that dexamethasone preserves the chemical and/or the structural integrity of cellular elements as previously suggested [7, 13].

Following the occlusion of MCA the territory normally supplied by the occluded artery must reach its persisting blood supply from the borderline areas through opened collateral channels [2, 21, 22]. Autoregulation of cerebral blood flow of these

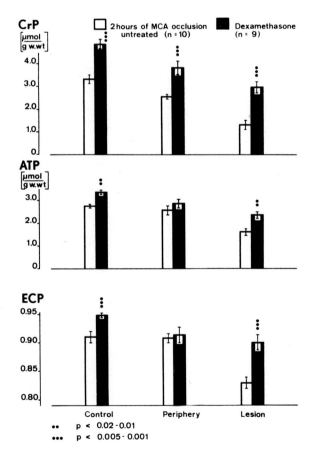

Fig. 6. CrP, ATP and ECP in brain tissue of untreated and of dexamethasone-treated cats 2 h after MCA occlusion

brain areas is impaired during the early stages of infarction. Consequently any changes in blood pressure will be reflected in the perfusion of the occluded territory [21]. The collateral blood supply, therefore, is of particular importance. The spreading of the edema from the center to the periphery, which is occuring in untreated animals 120 min after MCA occlusion, may be the reason for the reduction in flow in this areas as well as the further flow decrease in the ischemic area. It is known that local tissue perfusion in edematous areas is dependent on the local tissue pressure [17]. Edema, therefore, seems to be an important factor in the development and final extent of cerebral infarction and may produce secondary changes in the microcirculation. If dexamethasone prevents the early formation of edema at the borderline zone (and probably also in the center of the occluded territory) the blood flow can be maintained at a higher level. As a consequence the hypoxic changes, seen in the untreated animals, are clearly less pronounced in pre-treated cats. It may be assumed, that with the prevention or diminution of edema the development and extent of infarction may be reduced.

References

1. Atkinson, D. E.: The energy charge of the adenylate pool as a regulatory parameter. Interaction with feedback modifiers. Biochemistry **7**, 4030–4034 (1968).
2. Bartko, D., Reulen, H. J., Koch, H., Schürmann, K.: The time course of hemodynamic and metabolic alterations in brain following a regional brain ischemia. In preparation.
3. — — — Development of early brain edema following occlusion of middle cerebral artery in cats. In preparation.
4. Berry, R. G., Alpers, B. J.: Occlusion of the carotid circulation. Pathological considerations. Neurology **7**, 223 (1957).
5. Blinderman, E.: Effect of dexamethasone on mitochondria in anoxic brain. Arch. Neurol. **12**, 278–283 (1965).
6. Garcia, J. H., Cox, J. W., Hudgins, W. R.: Ultrastructure of the microvasculature in experimental brain infarction. Acta neuropath. (Berl.) **18**, 273–285 (1971).
7. Hansebout, R. R., Lewin, M. G., Pappius, H. M.: Evidence regarding the action of steroids in injured spinal cord. In: Reulen, H. J., Schürmann, K. (Eds.): Steroids and Brain Edema. Berlin-Heidelberg-New York: Springer 1972.
8. Harrison, M.: Discussion to this Symposium.
9. Ingvar, D. H., Lassen, N. A.: Regional blood flow of the cerebral cortex determined by Krypton 85. Acta physiol. scand. **54**, 325–338 (1962).
10. Klatzo, I.: Pathophysiological aspects of brain edema. In: Reulen, H. J., Schürmann, K. (Eds.): Steroids and Brain Edema. Berlin-Heidelberg-New York: Springer 1972.
11. Ng, L. K. Y., Nimmannitya, J.: Massive cerebral infarction with severe brain swelling: A clinicopathological study. Stroke **1**, 158–163 (1970).
12. Olsson, Y., Crowell, R. M., Klatzo, J.: The blood-brain barrier to protein tracers in focal cerebral ischemia and infarction caused by occlusion of the middle cerebral artery. Acta neuropath. (Berl.) **18**, 89–102 (1971).
13. Pappius, H. M., McCann, W. P.: Effects of steroids on cerebral edema in cats. Arch. Neurol. **20**, 207–216 (1969).
14. Patten, B. M., Mandell, J., Bruun, B., Curtin, W., Carter, S.: Double blind study of the effect of dexamethasone on acute stroke. In: Steroids and Brain Edema. Berlin-Heidelberg-New York: Springer 1972.
15. Plum, F., Alvord, E. C., Posner, J. B.: Effect of steroids on experimental cerebral infarction. Arch. Neurol. **9**, 571–573 (1963).
16. Reulen, H. J., Steude, U., Brendel, H., Hilber, C., Prusiner, S.: Energetische Störung des Kationentransportes als Ursache des intracellulären Hirnödems. Acta neurochir. (Wien) **22**, 129–166 (1970).

17. Reulen, H, J., Hadjidimos, A., Schürmann, K.: The effect of dexamethasone and diuretics on water and electrolyte content and on rCBF in perifocal brain edema in man. In: Steroids and Brain Edema. Berlin-Heidelberg-New York: Springer 1972.
18. Shaw, Ch. M., Alvord, E. C., Berry, R. G.: Swelling of the brain following ischemic infarction with arterial occlusion. Arch. Neurol. 1, 161–177 (1959).
19. Shibata, S., Norris, J. W., Hodge, C. P., Pappius, H. M.: Effects of ischemia on water and electrolyte content of cerebral tissues. In: Steroids and Brain Edema. Berlin-Heidelberg-New York: Springer 1972.
20. Siesjö, B. K., Messeter, K.: Factors determining intracellular pH. In: Siesjö, B. K., Sørensen, S. C. (Eds.): Ion Homeostasis of the Brain, pp. 244–263. Copenhagen: Munksgaard 1972.
21. Waltz, A. G.: Effect of blood pressure on blood flow in ischemic and in non-ischemic cerebral cortex. Neurology (Minneap.) 18, 613–621 (1968).
22. Yamaguchi, T., Regli, F., Waltz, A. G.: Effects of hyperventilation with and without carbon dioxide on experimental cerebral ischemia and infarction. Brain 95, 123–132 (1972).

Discussion to Chapter II see page 269

Chapter III

Mechanisms of Action of Steroids on Brain Edema

Physiology and Pathophysiology of Protein Permeability in the Central Nervous System

CHARLES F. BARLOW

Department of Neurology, Harvard Medical School and the Children's Hospital, Medical Center, Boston, MA 02115, USA

With 2 Figures

Summary. This presentation offers a brief resume discussion of the normal restriction to the entry of circulating protein into the CNS, including a discussion of the slow equilibration of radioisotope labeled albumin (1–3 days) and globulin (2–4 days) in CSF. Pathologic levels of CSF albumin are due to increased rate of entry, while pathologic levels of CSF globulin in some conditions such as subacute sclerosing leucoencephalitis can be shown to be in part derived from a nonlabeled source, presumably within the CNS or meninges.

Experiments are described in which a transient pathologic influx of protein was associated with experimental pentylenetetrazol convulsion in cats. This change was especially prominent in thalamus, and after a one hour seizure, significant increase in tissue water was also apparent. Abnormal albumin permeability was reduced, and no increase in tissue water occurred if the animal was pretreated with dexamethasone. If systemic blood pressure was maintained or elevated by norepinephrine during the convulsion, the albumin entry was increased significantly over that induced by seizures alone. Methantheline (Banthine) treatment was effective in significantly reducing the combined effect of norepinephrine enhanced convulsion permeability to values distinctly lower than those seen in convulsions alone.

Metabolic transformation of iodinated albumin into free iodine and small iodinated fragments is described in brain as one aspect of the clearance of protein from this tissue. This finding may also provide a partial explanation of increased water content due to the osmotic forces developed.

Under normal circumstances, plasma protein and substances bound to circulating proteins have very restricted access to the central nervous system (CNS), except in certain specialized areas such as choroid plexus, the area postrema and the supraoptic nucleus, etc., where there is little or no restriction to protein entry. The question as to whether there is slow entry of minute quantities of circulating albumin and globulin into the extracellular fluid of brain parenchyma generally as there is into cerebrospinal fluid (CSF) has not been directly answered. However, there is inferential evidence [11] that there may be parenchymal entry and movement of protein along with other solutes through extracellular channels in brain. This unsettled question is of interest and possible importance with reference to the pathogenesis of immunologic

Supported in part by NICHD Grant No. 1 PO1 HD 06276-01, Mental Retardation and Human Development, and NINDS Grant No. 5 PO1 NS 09704-02, Developmental Neurology, Children's Hospital Medical Center.

139

disease in the CNS and also brings up the interesting question of how "exogenous" protein is degraded and removed by the CNS. This latter issue is of special relevance to the problem of brain edema when it is recognized that in the "vasogenic" [13] varieties of edema very significant quantities of plasma protein leak into brain parenchyma.

The CSF is an extracellular solute compartment of brain which clearly contains plasma derived protein, but the level and to some extent, the relative composition of this protein differs greatly from plasma. Perhaps a review of studies from our laboratory [3, 4] on the dynamics of albumin and globulin exchange in CSF of children will serve to illustrate this point. These experiments were the result of the collaborative efforts of a number of colleagues, including R. W. P. Cutler, R. K. Deuel, G. V. Watters, J. P. Hammerstad, and E. Merler. The essential findings I shall present agree in substance with experimental work in animals [7, 10, 11], and studies in adult humans [6, 8, 9]. The experimental method involved the administration of Iodine[125] serum albumin intravenously in a dose of 5–10 μc/kg, and making serial determinations of the specific activity of albumin in serum and CSF. These measurements were plotted as the "relative specific activity"

$$\left(\frac{\text{Sp. activity CSF albumin}}{\text{Sp. activity plasma albumin}} \times 100 \right)$$

against time. The data were derived from 17 children from 3–18 years, with CSF albumin values varying from 12–1,845 mgm/100 c.c. Full equilibration of plasma and CSF albumin occurred between 24 and 72 h followed by a decline which was parallel in the two compartments. From this it was possible to say that all CSF albumin was plasma derived at both normal and grossly elevated levels. It was also possible to calculate fractional daily turnover. The average turnover value for CSF albumin in the normal range was 17.3 mgm/100 ml/day (Range 7.1–24.3 mgm/100 ml/day). Furthermore, the fractional movement of albumin out was a direct function of the level of CSF albumin and remained at about 50 % of the total per 24 h, including the patient with almost 2 gm albumin/100 ml in CSF. This observation provided indirect evidence that the abnormal levels of CSF albumin are the result of abnormal rates of movement in.

Experiments of basically similar design using intravenous injection of I[125] gamma globulin (IgG) in three patients with normal relative amounts of CSF IgG also revealed a dynamic equilibrium which was achieved after the somewhat longer interval of 2–4 days. Similar studies of three patients with subacute sclerosing panencephalitis (SSPE) who had abnormal relative levels of CSF gamma globulin led to quite different results [4]. Equilibrium between the serum and CSF was not achieved, although maximum levels of I[125] IgG in CSF were reached in 2–4 days as in the control patients. CSF globulin specific activity was approximately 15 and 28 % of the specific activity of serum globulin and this relationship was found to hold in both ventricular and lumbar fluids in the two cases where both compartments were studied. These observations indicate that a quantitatively important fraction of CSF globulin in SSPE is derived from an unlabeled pool within brain. Similar findings have been described in adult patients with multiple sclerosis [9].

Now, I should like to turn to a more complex aspect of the problem of abnormal protein permeability in the CNS, an aspect of the problem which is closely linked

140

with issues of brain edema. Destructive lesions of brain, such as tumor, infarction, inflammation, etc., cause sustained gross alteration of protein permeability in brain, well demonstrated by various techniques such as radioisotope brain scans in man and by various studies in more controlled experiments in animals. Varying degrees of brain edema usually accompany the protein influx but it is not known in what way abnormal protein entry may contribute to the pathogenesis of edema, if at all. It is clear, however, that there is not an obligatory relationship between increase in brain volume and abnormal protein entry. For example, in the specialized circumstance of experimental tri-ethyl tin edema, gross increase in white matter volume is not accompanied by protein entry. Ultrastructural studies provide the answer by demonstrating that the volumetric change is induced by prominent distortion and splitting of myelin lamellae. However, even in the "vasogenic edema" of various parenchymal destructive insults, there is often wide disparity between the development of edema and the phenomenon of protein entry.

Lesser interest has centered on the more subtle problem of transient alteration of protein permeability which occurs in CO_2 intoxication [2], and experimental convulsions. Recently, we have been interested in the regional permeability changes which are associated with experimental convulsions. We have found distinctive regional patterns of enhanced S^{35} sulfate exchange after 5 min in response to the convulsant agents pentylenetetrazol, strychnine, deoxypyridoxine, and methionine sulfoximine [14]. We then turned to the issue of convulsion induced albumin permeability [15], and I should like to report these observations in somewhat greater detail.

The basic experimental method involved the intravenous administration of I^{125} or I^{131} albumin (100 – 300 μc/kg) to curarized adult cats. Electroencephalogram, electrocardiogram, arterial, venous and CSF pressures were recorded during the experimental procedure. Convulsions were produced by intravenous injection of pentylenetetrazol, 30 mgm/kg, repeated as necessary to maintain EEG evidence of seizure activity. Various experimental procedures were then carried out, such as varying the duration of seizure, administration of drugs such as trimethadione to interrupt the seizure, infusion of norepinephrine to maintain blood pressure, and treatment with dexamethasone and methantheline bromide. Animals were killed at the end of the experiment with a lethal dose of pentobarbital (50 mgm/kg). A midline thoracotomy was performed, a cardiac blood sample drawn, and an aortic cannula was inserted, followed by saline perfusion of the head and upper trunk to clear the brain of blood. A cisternal CSF sample was drawn, the brain rapidly removed and deep frozen at $-20°$ C. Coronal sections were made and gross autoradiograms were prepared. Quantitation of radioactivity of dissected anatomical regional brain samples, etc., was accomplished by standard radioassay techniques and expressed as an arbitrary plasma ratio

$$\left(\frac{\text{cpm/mgm dry tissue}}{\text{cpm/ml plasma}} \right).$$

The separative techniques of 8 % trichloracetic acid precipitation, centrifugation, and gel filtration were employed in studies relating to the purity of labeled preparations and metabolism of iodine-protein complex.

Well known and expected changes in physiologic function occurred with electroencephalographic evidence of seizure in the curarized animals. At the outset arterial, venous, and CSF pressure rose abruptly. With seizures longer than 30 min, arterial

141

blood pressure fell to levels appreciably below preseizure levels. Arterial hypotension was compensated by administration of norepinephrine in another series of experiments.

Nonconvulsed control animals had similar minute quantities of albumin in all brain regions whether killed 15 or 70 min after radioiodinated protein injection. After a 5 min seizure, cerebral cortex, thalamus and spinal cord had significant (p < 0.05) increased albumin entry and by 60 min seizure duration, all brain regions were significantly abnormal (Fig. 1). By far the most permeable region was the thalamus. The time course of abnormal permeability was also of interest. Maximum relative increased entry occurred in most regions by 30 min, but thalamus and CSF continued a precipitous advance in the 5, 15, 30, and 60 min periods, at which time thalamus showed a 24-fold increase over controls. Autoradiograms qualitatively expressed a progressive increase in radiodensity, especially in thalamus, at first punctate and presumably in relation to blood vessels with coalescence as the process proceeds in time

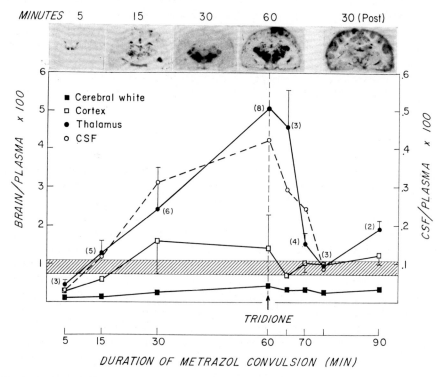

Fig. 1. Brain and CSF – plasma ratios from saline perfused samples at varying times after the onset of pentylenetetrazol induced convulsions in the cat showing increase in cerebral cortex, thalamus and CSF with time. The vertical interrupted line indicates the point of trimethadione administration which stopped the seizure, following which the radioisotope was rapidly cleared from brain and CSF. The cross hatched horizontal bar illustrates the brain-plasma ratio of unperfused brain, indicating the order of magnitude of the increased protein entry in the perfused samples. Autoradiograms of coronal brain slices depict the increasing density, its regional intensity in thalamus and the early punctate pattern with eventual coalescence. From Seventh Conference Cerebral Vascular Diseases, James F. Toole, John Moosy and Richard Janeway, editors, 1971.) (Reprinted by permission of Grune and Stratton)

142

(Fig. 1). Tissues such as muscle, nerve, liver and kidney in convulsed animals were not different from controls at all time periods.

Table 1. Albumin uptake with 60 min convulsions

	Control	Metrazol	Metrazol Norepinephrine	Metrazol Norepinephrine Methanthelene
Thalamus	0.20 ± 0.07	4.85 ± 1.34	8.70 ± 2.59	1.98 ± 0.30
Cortex	0.27 ± 0.05	1.48 ± 0.33	1.05 ± 0.33	1.55 ± 0.37
White	0.06 ± 0.02	0.31 ± 0.04	0.57 ± 0.25	0.30 ± 0.09

Norepinephrine infusion was used in order to combat the hypotensive effect of sustained convulsions (Table 1). It had the interesting result of almost doubling the albumin entry in thalamus as compared with untreated convulsed animals, while norepinephrine alone showed only a modest increase in several areas. Simultaneous administration of methantheline (Banthine), a cholinergic antagonist, reduced thalamic levels to 1.93 ± .30, as compared with 8.70 ± 2.59 in the 60 min norepinephrine convulsed series, and 4.85 ± 1.34 in animals which were convulsed 60 min without additional treatment of any kind (Table 1). It is of interest that systemic blood pressure in the convulsed animals treated with norepinephrine and methantheline attained levels generally higher than convulsed animals receiving norepinephrine alone. Therefore, the methantheline effect on permeability was in the opposite direction to the observed change in blood pressure.

Studies of regional blood flow after a 5 min seizure revealed the expected general increase, which was relatively similar in cortex and thalamus, while the greater increase in blood volume occurred in cortex.

A series of animals were sacrificed at varying times after the seizure was interrupted by intravenous trimethadione. By 15 min, the residual radioisotope was largely cleared from brain and CSF (Fig. 1). If a 60 min seizure was first interrupted and then iodinated albumin administered, it was found that permeability had been restored to normal by 15 min.

One must deal with the question of the degree of metabolic transformation of the iodinated albumin, particularly when considering the issue of the rapid loss of the material from brain. Overall, approximately 25% of the material in brain and CSF was in small molecular weight compounds, including free iodine, at the end of the 60 min seizure, as compared with about 1% in plasma. Gel filtration fractionation of the nonprotein bound iodine revealed free iodine, and two to three additional small molecular peaks in brain tissues (Fig. 2). It is clear that a significant aspect of the removal of iodinated albumin involves brain protease action, but direct extrusion of the iodine-albumin complex is probably also important.

Another set of studies [5] disclosed that seizures of 60 min duration were associated with a small increase in tissue water of thalamus. (Dry weight 23.6 ± 0.8 control, versus 20.5 ± 0.6, p = 0.05). This change was completely inhibited by pretreatment with dexamethasone (0.23 mgm/kg/24 h × 3), as well as with simultaneous treatment (0.3 mgm/kg I.V. at onset of seizure) (Table 2). In addition, the thalamic uptake of iodinated albumin was decreased from 4.85 ± 1.34 to 1.63 (pretreated) and 1.96 (simultaneous treatment).

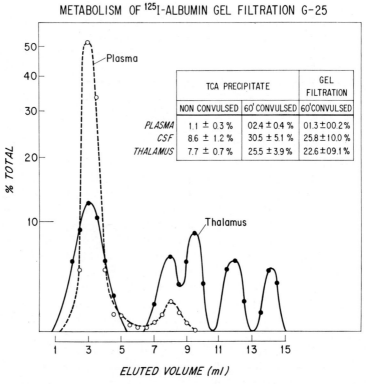

METABOLISM OF ^{125}I-ALBUMIN GEL FILTRATION G-25

	TCA PRECIPITATE		GEL FILTRATION
	NON CONVULSED	60' CONVULSED	60'CONVULSED
PLASMA	1.1 ± 0.3 %	02.4 ± 0.4 %	01.3 ± 00.2%
CSF	8.6 ± 1.2%	30.5 ± 5.1 %	25.8 ± 10.0 %
THALAMUS	7.7 ± 0.7%	25.5 ± 3.9%	22.6 ± 09.1%

Fig. 2. Gel filtration of I^{125} albumin in plasma (open circle and interrupted line) showing two peaks, the larger reflecting albumin in the early eluted volume, and a smaller fraction representing free iodine. The thalamus (solid circle and solid line) after a 60 min convulsion induced albumin entry shows a number of small molecular weight iodinated fractions in addition to iodinated albumin and free iodine. Insert box shows the quantitative percentage of compounds other than albumin and compares the results of gel filtration with trichloracetic acid precipitation

Table 2. Dexamethasone treatment

	Tissue water content		
	Dry weight nn-oconvulsed	Dry weight 60 min convulsed	Dry weight 60 min convulsed + dexamethasone
Thalamus	23.6 ± 0.8	20.5 ± 0.6	23.7 ± 0.6
	Albumin uptake (tissue/plasma × 100)		
Thalamus	0.20 ± 0.07	4.85 ± 1.34	1.63 (pre Rx) 1.96 (simultaneous Rx)

These studies have raised a number of provocative, and as yet unanswered questions, and have established a series of observations. Pentylenetetrazol seizures were associated with abnormal albumin permeability, especially in thalamus. This was detectable after a 15 min seizure and was progressive in thalamus to 60 min. At the latter time, there was also detectable increase in water content of this tissue. During the seizure, albumin permeability was greatly increased by administration of norepinephrine and was decreased by methantheline and dexamethasone. Abnormal albumin entry returned rapidly to normal after the seizure was arrested. Also, the albumin which had entered was rapidly removed from brain after the seizure was interrupted and by 30 min, radioactivity levels of brain were almost normal.

We have tentatively concluded that it is likely that the pathologic leak of protein was the result of increased vascular permeability. The ultrastructural possibilities include opening the intercellular tight junctions or activation of pinocytotic transport. Both mechanisms have been seen in more destructive insults to the vascular barrier, but the rapidly reversible disorders such as convulsion induced permeability have not been studied. Parenthetically, the possibility also exists that pinocytosis may be responsible for protein movement out as well, and may be part of the rapid process of removal of protein after it has entered, along with the process of metabolic breakdown and the possibility of flow into CSF and removal with the bulk outward movement of this fluid.

The process of metabolic breakdown of protein into smaller, osmotically more active fragments also raises the question as to whether this may account for the increased water content of thalamus which was found after a prolonged seizure, implicating protein entry more directly in the process of edema formation.

Finally, one must consider the interesting effect of substances such as norepinephrine, methantheline and dexamethasone on the abnormal permeability process. The norepinephrine effect in increasing protein entry is perhaps best explained on the basis of its observed effect of maintaining and raising blood pressure, a well known aggravating factor in the process of edema [16]. However, in the animals whose seizure-norepinephrine enhanced permeability effect was counteracted by methantheline, the blood pressure was maintained at higher levels than the seizure-norepinephrine group, yet permeability was greatly reduced. This raises the question of the relationship of a cholinergic mechanism in vascular permeability in these animals. Also, the relative preventive effect of dexamethasone is of interest in terms of its clear beneficial effect in certain varieties of human cerebral edema, although its mechanism of action is obscure.

The pathologic problem in neurology to which these experiments most directly relate is the interesting occasional child in whom a series of hemiconvulsions would seem to lead to hemispheral edema and subsequent hemiplegia [1, 12]. Therapeutic trial with dexamethasone or methantheline in an effort to prevent this process may be worth contemplating.

References

1. Aicardi, J., Ansell, J., Chevrie, J. J.: Acute hemiplegia in infancy and childhood. Develop. Med. Child Neurol. **11**, 162–173 (1969).
2. Cutler, R. W. P., Barlow, C. F.: The effect of hypercapnia on brain permeability to protein. Arch. Neurol. **14**, 54–63 (1966).

3. Cutler, R. W. P., Deuel, R. K., Barlow, C. F.: Albumin exchange between plasma and cerebrospinal fluid. Arch. Neurol. **17**, 261–270 (1967).
4. — Watters, G. V., Hammerstad, J. P., Merler, E.: Origin of cerebrospinal fluid gamma globulin in subacute sclerosing leukoencephalitis. Arch. Neurol **17**, 620–628 (1967).
5. Eisenberg, H. M., Barlow, C. F., Lorenzo, A. V.: Effect of dexamethasone on altered brain vascular permeability. Arch. Neurol. **23**, 18–22 (1970).
6. Fieschi, C., Agnoli, A.: Fractional exchange rate of albumin from cerebrospinal fluid to plasma in man. Minerva nucl. **8**, 344–347 (1964).
7. Fishman, R. A.: Exchange of albumin between plasma and cerebrospinal fluid. Amer. J. Physiol. **175**, 96–98 (1958).
8. Frick, E., Scheid-Seydel, L.: Untersuchungen mit I[131] markiertem Albumin über Austauschvorgänge zwischen Plasma und Liquor Cerebrospinalis. Klin. Wschr. **36**, 66–69 (1958).
9. — — Untersuchungen mit [131] markiertem Gamma Globulin zur Frage der Abstammung der Liquoreiweißkörper. Klin. Wsch. **36**, 857–863 (1958).
10. Hochwald, G. W., Wallenstein, M. C.: Exchange of γ-globulin between blood, cerebrospinal fluid and brain in the cat. Exp. Neurol. **19**, 115–126 (1967).
11. — — Exchange of albumin between blood, cerebrospinal fluid and brain in the cat. Amer. J. Physiol. **212**, 1199–1204 (1967).
12. Isler, W.: Akute Hemiplegien und Hemisyndrome im Kindesalter. Stuttgart: Thieme 1969.
13. Klatzo, I.: Neuropathological aspects of brain edema. J. Neuropath. exp. Neurol. **26**, 1–14 (1967).
14. Lorenzo, A. V.: Mechanisms of drug penetration in the brain. In: Black, P. (Ed.): Drugs and the Brain, pp. 41–59. John Hopkins Press 1969.
15. — Shirahige, I., Barlow, C. F.: Temporary alteration of cerebrovascular permeability to plasma protein during drug induced seizures. Amer. J. Physiol. **223**, 268–277 (1972).
16. Schutta, H. S., Kassell, N. F., Langfitt, T. W.: Brain swelling produced by injury and aggravated by arterial hypertension. Brain **91**, 281–294 (1968).

Studies on the Mechanisms of Action of Steroids in Traumatized Brain

H. P. Tutt and Hanna M. Pappius

Montreal Neurological Institute, McGill University, Montreal, Canada

Summary. Preliminary results of a study of distribution of sodium-24 between the brain and the blood in cats show that

1. The relative specific activity (RSA) of sodium-24 in cerebral cortex is increased in both the control and the experimental (traumatized) hemisphere 24 h after a freezing lesion, as compared with cerebral cortex from normal animals. The effect is not seen in the white matter. This finding does not contradict the hypothesis that active transport of solute by astrocytes may be involved in the resolution of cerebral edema. It does suggest, however, that astrocytes of cerebral cortex, as opposed to those in the white matter, would play the major role in such a mechanism.

2. Furosemide diminishes the relative specific activity of sodium-24 in cerebral cortex in both the intact and the traumatized brain to the same extent. Thus, it does not abolish the increase in RSA of sodium seen as a consequence of injury.

3. Acetazolamide had no effect on sodium distribution in traumatized brain indicating that carbonic anhydrase is not involved in the sodium fluxes studied under our experimental conditions.

4. While the results available at present are not definitive, dexamethasone appears to have little, if any, generalized effect on the electrolyte metabolism of traumatized brain.

The experiments which will be discussed under the heading of "Studies on Mechanisms of Action of Steroids" represent a preliminary attempt to investigate processes which may be involved in the resolution of cerebral edema. It is within this framework that the effects of steroids on the exchange of sodium-24 between cerebral tissues and blood were studied.

Let us summarize briefly the hypothesis which was the starting point of this work.

It is not clear why there is a preferential accumulation of fluid in white matter in vasogenic cerebral edema. Presumably, the specific cytoarchitecture of the cerebral cortex offers sufficient mechanical resistance to the influx of extravasated fluid while the parallel arrangement of myelinated fibers in the white matter would offer less resistance and allow expansion of the extracellular spaces [2, 5]. This interpretation is in keeping with a variety of experimental findings, particularly those of Klatzo and his collaborators which suggest that the mechanism of formation of cerebral edema induced by injury involves seepage of fluid from damaged blood vessels under the hydrostatic pressure of systemic circulation [7]. Venous obstruction, interfering with normal draining channels from the affected area must also be considered as a mechanical factor contributing to the accumulation of the extravasated fluid. In such a formulation no breakdown of active metabolic processes within the brain tissue elements needs to be invoked to explain the formation of cerebral edema.

The fluid which accumulates in brain under the influence of the hydrostatic pressure in the blood vessels must be somehow removed from the enlarged extracellular spaces since we know that when the lesion heals and the blood-brain barrier is repaired edema does, in fact, dissipate with time [15]. It is well established that in mammalian tissues water movement against an apparent concentration gradient is always seconary to active transport of solutes such as sodium or sugar [14]. These processes are energy-requiring and mediated by cellular elements.

As a working hypothesis, it is proposed that astrocytes may be involved in the resolution of cerebral edema in a manner not unlike that of cells in the gastrointestinal tract or in kidney tubules where active transport of solutes results in transfer of fluid against an apparent concentration gradient.

Why astrocytes? Their involvement in maintenance of normal water and electrolyte distribution in the brain as a whole has been under consideration for a long time [3]. Recently, a possible role of perivascular astrocytes in normal, physiological active transport processes at the blood-brain interface has been postulated [13]. Astrocytes are the only cell type demonstrably involved in cerebral edema [5]. Electron microscopic studies have shown swollen astrocytes in both the white matter where the bulk of the fluid accumulates and in the cerebral cortex, where only minimal changes in total water content can be demonstrated. Histochemically the activity of enzymes involved in energy metabolism was shown to increase in these cells within 12 h after trauma [18] and their pinocytotic activity is increased at the same time [8, 9]. Since under these conditions swelling of the astrocytes is obviously associated with increased metabolic activity, it is unlikely that it represents a breakdown in mechanisms for normal maintenance of water and electrolytes; to us, on the contrary, it suggests stimulation of such mechanisms.

It is difficult to design an experiment for testing this hypothesis as regards the role of astrocytes. However, demonstration of an increased rate of exchange of a suitable solute in association with edema could be considered as evidence for the involvement of active transport processes in the resolution of cerebral edema.

Sodium appeared the obvious solute to study, especially since a generalized increase in sodium-24 exchange between brain and blood was reported in rats with focal inflammatory edema some years ago [6], a finding surprisingly ignored and not followed up since.

Our experimental procedure was briefly as follows: Cats were injected intravenously with a loading dose of sodium-24 in isotonic saline and the level of the radioactivity in the blood so established was maintained for 60 min by continuous infusion of a dilute solution of the isotope. Blood samples were taken at 15 min intervals for counting and the average of the four counts was taken for subsequent calculation as the count of the blood; the counts in the individual samples were usually within 5% of this average. Exactly 60 min after the first injection of the isotope, the animal was killed by exsanguination and the brain was rapidly removed and placed in a humid chamber. Duplicate samples of cerebral cortex and single samples of white matter, each weighing approximately 500 mgms, were dissected from each hemisphere and their radioactivity measured in a well scintillation counter. The results for both the blood and the cerebral tissues were calculated as specific activity (count per minute per milli-

148

equivalent of sodium), their total sodium content having also been determined. The distribution of sodium-24 between the tissues and the blood was then expressed as the relative specific activity (RSA), or ratio of the specific activity (SA) of the tissue to specific activity of the blood.

The experimental groups consisted of animals without any lesion and animals with a standard freezing lesion (5 × 10 mm, —50° C, 45 sec) [16] on the right, or experimental, hemisphere. In both groups, some animals received no treatment, some were treated with dexamethasone (0.25 mgms/kg/day), others with furosemide (3 mgms/kg/day after an initial dose of 5 mgms/kg), and still others with acetazolamide (50 mgms/kg/day). Dexamethasone was given starting 48 h before the lesion was made; the other drugs were begun immediately following the lesion, or 24 h before the animals were killed if no lesion was made.

Dexamethasone and furosemide were used as both have been shown to diminish total cerebral edema which develops in response to our standard freezing lesion (see chapter II). Although neither of these drugs affected the water and electrolyte content of edematous tissues, we felt that this did not necessarily rule out a mechanism of action of these compounds involving electrolyte metabolism. If electrolyte transport is primarily affected, the secondary shifts of water would be rapid and the ratio of electrolytes to water could remain relatively constant, although the total edema might be significantly diminished by the over-all process. Acetazolamide was also included in this series of experiments because of its well known inhibitory action on carbonic anhydrase [12], an enzyme found in high concentrations in astrocytes [4] and known to be involved in certain sodium transport mechanisms [1].

The presentation of the tissue sodium-24 results in terms of specific activity corrects for changes due solely to variations in the total sodium content of the edematous tissues. The relative specific activity of white matter was essentially within the same range under all experimental conditions studied. This indicates that sodium exchange in white matter was not affected either by trauma or by the drugs used, even though changes in total sodium were occurring. For this reason, the data on white matter will not be considered further at this time.

The differences in the distribution of sodium-24 between the cerebral cortex and the blood under the experimental conditions studied are summarized in Table 1. It must be stressed that the data represents the relative specific activity (RSA) of cerebral cortex tissue (SA of tissue/SA of blood) at one specific time interval only, namely after 60 min of equilibration with the isotope. Consequently, no information can be derived from these results concerning the kinetics of the sodium exchange.

24 h after a freezing lesion, the RSA of cerebral cortex was significantly increased in both the control and the experimental (traumatized) hemisphere as compared to tissue from normal animals. This is in agreement with the previously quoted report of Katzman et al. [6]. It implies that there was a generalized effect on the rate of the exchange of sodium in the traumatized brain, apparently not directly related to the breakdown of the blood-brain barrier or the presence of edema both of which were restricted to the hemisphere in which the lesion was made. It is unlikely that the increase in the control hemisphere was due to the diffusion of the isotope from the injured hemisphere, especially since the effect was not demonstrable in the subcortical white matter of either hemisphere. An increase in the relative specific activity of sodium-24 measured at one time interval, in this case 60 min, gives no indication as to

whether the rate of efflux of sodium from the brain was diminished or the rate of influx was stimulated. The latter would appear more likely at a time when the total sodium content of one hemisphere was increasing.

Table 1. Distribution of sodium-24 between cerebral cortex and blood in cats

| | SA tissue/SA serum | | |
| | No lesion | 24 h after freezing lesion | |
		Control hemisphere	Experimental hemisphere
Untreated	0.235 ± 0.040 (16)	0.267 ± 0.032^a (8)	0.295 ± 0.022^b (8)
Dexamethasone, 0.25 mg/kg/day, 72 h	0.239 ± 0.048 (4)	0.236 ± 0.036^d (8)	0.278 ± 0.042^b (8)
Furosemide, 3 mg/kg/day, 24 h	0.185 ± 0.024^a (6)	$0.216 \pm 0.030^{e\ c}$ (8)	$0.252 \pm 0.028^{a\ c}$ (8)
Acetazolamide, 50 mg/kg/day, 24 h	0.219 (2)	0.279 ± 0.026^a (5)	0.298 ± 0.022^a (5)

Averages $\pm$ S.D. Number of hemispheres in brackets.
Period of equilibration with ^{24}Na: 60 min.
[a] $p < 0.01$, [b] $p < 0.02$ for difference from normal or corresponding "no lesion".
[e] $p < 0.01$, [d] $p < 0.05$ for difference from corresponding untreated.

Preliminary experiments indicate that at 48 h after the lesion the ratio of distribution of sodium-24 approaches normal values in both hemispheres. This could be due to the return to normal of the flux component initially affected or to a compensatory change in the reverse flux. Further studies will have to determine the kinetics of these exchanges and provide answers to the questions raised by the studies reported here.

The effects of acetazolamide can be dismissed very quickly – no difference was observed between the untreated animals and those given acetazolamide. Thus, carbonic anhydrase would not appear to be involved in the exchanges of sodium under these experimental conditions.

The action of furosemide as a renal diuretic is thought to involve inhibition of reabsorption of sodium in the renal tubule. Our experiments showed that furosemide significantly decreased the relative specific activity of sodium in cerebral cortex, both in the normal and in the traumatized brain. It is noteworthy that furosemide had no effect on this ratio in white matter. The results in cerebral cortex imply that either sodium influx into the brain had diminished or sodium efflux was stimulated. Unfortunately, the present data give no indication which of the two processes has been affected. As suggested earlier, an effect on electrolyte metabolism or flux need not necessarily manifest itself by a change in the electrolyte or water content of the tissue. This is borne out by the fact that neither of these parameters were affected by furosemide whether in intact or in traumatized cerebral tissue (see data presented in chapter II). Further, a diminution by furosemide of the relative specific activity of sodium in cerebral cortex in intact as well as in traumatized brain makes it uncertain as to what role, if any, this effect plays in decreasing total cerebral edema in furosemide-treated animals. The increase in the sodium distribution ratio, seen in traumatized as compared to normal brain, was not prevented by furosemide.

In contrast to furosemide, dexamethasone had no effect on the distribution of sodium-24 in intact brain and in the experimental hemisphere. The effect in the control hemisphere was borderline ($p < 0.05$ for difference from untreated). There was somewhat greater experimental variation between animals in the dexamethasone-treated group than in the other groups and more experiments will have to be done to establish unequivocally whether there is a difference in the RSA of sodium-24 of the cerebral cortex in the control hemisphere between the untreated and dexamethasone-treated animals. We are inclined to conclude, however, that the mechanism of action of steroids in traumatized cerebral tissues is not mediated by their effects on electrolyte metabolism.

References

1. Becker, B.: Carbonic anhydrase and the formation of aqueous humor. Amer. J. Ophthal. **47**, 342–361 (1959).
2. Clasen, R. A., Cooke, P. M., Pandolfi, S., Carnecki, G.: The effects of focal freezing on the central nervous system. Pres.-St. Luke Hosp. Med. Bull. **2**, 36–46 (1963).
3. De Robertis, E., Gershenfeld, H. M.: Submicroscopic morphology and function of glial cells. Int. Rev. Neurobiol. **3**, 1–65 (1961).
4. Giacobini, E.: Metabolic relations between glia and neurons studied in single cells. In: Cohen, M. M., Snider, R. S. (Eds.): Morphological and Biochemical Correlates in Neuronal Activity, pp. 15–38. Harper and Row 1964.
5. Hirano, A.: The Fine Structure of Brain in Edema. In: Bourne, G. H. (Ed.): The Structure and Function of Nervous Tissue, Vol. II. New York: Academic Press 1969.
6. Katzman, R., Gonatas, N., Levine, S.: Electrolytes and fluids in experimental focal leukoencephalopathy. Arch. Neurol. **10**, 58–65 (1964).
7. Klatzo, I.: Presidential address – Neuropathological aspects of brain edema. J. Neuropath. exp. Neurol. **26**, 1–14 (1967).
8. — Miquel, J.: Observations on pinocytosis in nervous tissue. J. Neuropath. exp. Neurol. **19**, 475–487 (1960).
9. — — Otenasek, R.: The application of fluorescein-labelled serum proteins (FLSP) to the study of vascular permeability in the brain. Acta neuropath. (Berl.) **2**, 144–160 (1962).
10. Lee, J. C., Bakay, L.: Ultrastructural changes in the edematous central nervous system. II. Cold-induced edema. Arch. Neurol. **14**, 36–49 (1966).
11. Long, D. M., Hartmann, J. F., French, L. A.: Ultrastructure of human cerebral edema. J. Neuropath. exp. Neurol. **25**, 373–395 (1966).
12. Maren, T. H.: Carbonic anhydrase: chemistry, physiology and inhibition. Physiol. Rev. **47**, 595–781 (1967).
13. Pappenheimer, J. R.: On the location of the blood-brain barrier. In: Proceedings of the Wates Symposium on the Blood-Brain Barrier, pp. 66–74 (privately circulated). Oxford 1970.
14. Pappius, H. M.: Water transport at cell membranes. Canad. J. Biochem. **42**, 945–953 (1964).
15. — Gulati, D. R.: Water and electrolyte content of cerebral tissues in experimentally induced edema. Acta neuropath. (Berl.) **2**, 451–460 (1963).
16. — McCann, W. P.: Effects of steroids on cerebral edema in cats. Arch. Neurol. **20**, 207–216 (1969).
17. Raimondi, A. J., Evans, J. P., Mullan, S.: Studies of cerebral edema: III. Alterations in the white matter; an electron microscopic study using ferritin as a labelling compound. Acta neuropath. (Berl.) **2**, 177–197 (1962).
18. Rubinstein, L., Klatzo, I., Miquel, J.: Histochemical observations on oxidative enzyme activity of glial cells in a local brain injury. J. Neuropath. exp. Neurol. **21**, 116–136 (1962).

Evidence Regarding the Action of Steroids in Injured Spinal Cord

Robert R. Hansebout, Marcial G. Lewin, and Hanna M. Pappius

Montreal Neurological Institute, McGill University, Montreal, Canada

With 2 Figures

Summary. 1. Dexamethasone (0.25 mg/kg/day) prevents the loss of potassium from the injured spinal cord which occurs in untreated animals between the third and sixth day and persists on the ninth day.

2. The level of potassium in the spinal cord on the sixth day after injury correlates with the functional state of the animal at the same time.

3. These results indicate that in spinal cord injury, as in cerebral trauma, the beneficial effects of dexamethasone do not appear to be mediated through their action on edema. In both instances, functional integrity appears better preserved in dexamethasone-treated animals while effects on edema are not particularly impressive.

In the studies on impact injury of the spinal cord discussed by Dr. Hansebout earlier (see chapter II), two findings made us look more closely at the net content of potassium in the cord. First of all, 9 days after injury when the edematous changes in the cord were regressing and both the percentage dry weight and the sodium content appeared to be returning towards the normal levels, the same trend was not as obvious with respect to potassium concentration. Secondly, while dexamethasone appeared to have only minimal effects on the edematous changes in the injured spinal cord, on the sixth day after injury significantly higher levels of potassium were noted in the cord of the dexamethasone-treated animals.

The experimental design of these studies was described in detail elsewhere in this book [2]. The point to stress with respect to the data to be presented here is that the potassium values obtained for each of the 10 blocks of the injured cord which were subjected to analysis were recalculated on the basis of dry weight of tissue. This corrects for the dilutional changes in potassium associated with the accumulation of low-potassium edema fluid and the data represent the net content of potassium of the spinal cord.

When the potassium content of the spinal cord was expressed per kg of dry weight of tissue it was clearly seen that the potassium level was maintained for the first two days after the injury, then it started to decrease so that 6 and 9 days following injury there was a significant loss of potassium from the cord. This applied not only to the blocks which were injured and might be expected to lose potassium from the area of necrosis, but was observed to the same extent throughout the whole section of the cord subjected to analysis. The decrease in potassium content was not directly related to edema which was receding by the ninth day. The fall did occur, however, between the third and sixth day, at which time edema was at its maximum.

The values for the 10 blocks were averaged for each cat and then the averages for each experimental group of animals were plotted with their standard deviations against time after lesion (Fig. 1). It will be seen that, as mentioned earlier, two days after the cord was injured there was no change in its potassium content. Thereafter the potassium level decreased and became statistically highly significantly different from normal on the sixth and ninth day.

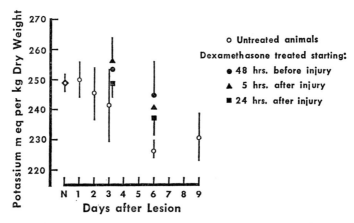

Fig. 1. Effect of dexamethasone on net changes in potassium content of spinal cord of animals with impact injury to the cord. Each point represents an average of four to eight animals. Vertical bars represent standard deviation

Dexamethasone treatment prevented this loss of potassium, the effect being statistically significantly different from the untreated group on the third day in both the pre-treated group and in the animals treated within 5 h after injury. On the sixth day in all the three treated groups potassium content was significantly different from the corresponding untreated group.

These results indicate that dexamethasone has a significant effect on the potassium content of the injured spinal cord, preventing a loss of this ion which occurs with time after injury in the untreated animals. This effect is unlikely to be mediated by the effect of dexamethasone on edema, as edema was only minimally affected in the treated animals [2].

At the same time, data presented by Dr. Hansebout showed that the functional state of the animals with impact injury was also significantly affected by dexamethasone treatment [2].

For this reason, the potassium content of the spinal cord of the individual cats 6 days after impact injury, regardless of the treatment they received, were plotted against their final Tarlov ratings in Figure 2. The correlation between these two parameters was found to be statistically highly significant (N = 41; r = 0.57; p < 0.001).

Our findings are compatible with the hypothesis that steroid treatment maintains the integrity of the cellular elements in traumatized and/or edematous brain and cord [1, 3, 4, 5]. This would be reflected in the maintenance of a relatively normal potassium content of the cord, on the one hand, and a better functional state of the animal, on the other. Because of the importance of potassium in normal functioning of nervous tissues, it is tempting to postulate that the improved functional state with

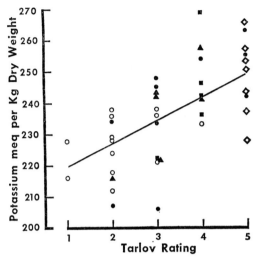

Fig. 2. Correlation between potassium content of the spinal cord and Tarlov rating of cats 6 days after impact cord injury. Data for 8 normal cats also included. Each point represents the results with a single animal. Regression line was calculated by the method of least squares

steroid treatment is directly correlated with the effects of dexamethasone on the potassium content of the injured cord. The results presented, however, do not warrant such a far-reaching conclusion at this time. Both effects may be secondary to a common underlying cause – the preservation of structural integrity of cellular elements by dexamethasone by mechanisms unknown at present.

References

1. Ducker, T. B., Hamit, H. F.: Experimental treatments of acute spinal cord injury. J. Neurosurg. 30, 693–697 (1969).
2. Lewin, M. G., Pappius, H. M., Hansebout, R. R.: Effect of steroids on edema associated with injury of spinal cord. In: Steroids and Brain Edema, pp. 101–112. Berlin-Heidelberg-New York: Springer 1972.
3. Long, D. M., Hartmann, J. F., French, L. A.: The response of experimental cerebral edema to glucosteroid administration. J. Neurosurg. 24, 843–854 (1966).
4. Pappius, H. M., McCann, W. P.: Effect of steroids on cerebral edema in cats. Arch. Neurol. 20, 207–216 (1969).
5. Richardson, H. D., Nakamura, S.: An electron microscopic study of spinal cord edema and the effect of treatment with steroids, mannitol and hypothermia. Proceedings of the American Association of Neurological Surgeons, Paper 39, 1971.

The Role of Necrosis and Inflammation in the Response of Cerebral Edema to Steroids

Raymond A. Clasen, Walid A. Hindo, Sylvia Pandolfi, and Iris Laing

University of Illinois, College of Medicine, Presbyterian St. Luke's Hospital, Chicago, IL 60612, USA

With 2 Figures

Summary. The effect of steroids on the edema associated with lesions induced by focal cerebral freezing in monkeys was assessed. The animals were sacrificed 48 h after injury. In one group treatment was begun 48 h prior to injury and in a second group treatment was begun after injury but the lesion size was reduced. The degree of edema was assessed through measurements of changes in the concentrations of tissue water, sodium, chloride, potassium, and iron and by the increase in weight of the damaged hemisphere. In addition to this the uptake of serum albumin and Evans blue was also measured. No indication of any effect on edema in either group was found.

The degree of edema in the brains of patients with unilateral metastatic tumors was assessed through measurements of hemispheric weights. It was found that those patients having a favorable neurological clinical response to steroids at the time of death had less edema than those who did not. Histologic changes in the brains of such patients were analyzed. It was found that lesions from those patients who were not responding to steroids at the time of death showed significantly more inflammation than those who were responding.

An attempt is made to define the relative roles of necrosis and inflammation in the response of cerebral edema to steroid management. It is concluded that the presence or absence of cellular inflammation is the determining factor in this response.

Introduction

Our previous attempt to demonstrate an effect of steroids on the edema associated with cerebral cryogenic injury in the monkey proved unsuccessful [8]. Subsequent workers, on the other hand, were able to demonstrate a suppression of this edema in other animals [13, 23, 29, 30, 31], as well as cerebral edema associated with other experimental models [11, 12, 13, 14, 18, 36, 37]. Negative results, however, have also appeared [3, 15, 20]. Our paper was subjected to justified criticisms with respect to dosage and type of steroid, species response to the drug and, most importantly, the time interval between initiation of therapy and sacrifice. The following experiments were undertaken in an attempt to answer these criticisms. The results remain negative. It was felt that an explanation of these results could lead to an understanding of the basic mechanisms through which steroids suppress cerebral edema. An answer to this question was sought both through an analysis of the existing literature on experimental cerebral edema and through a study of human metastatic brain tumors.

This work was supported by a grant from the National Institute of Neurological Diseases and Stroke (NS-03677) and The Otho S. A. Sprague Memorial Institute.

157

Material and Methods

1. Experimental

Focal areas of hemorrhagic necrosis were produced in the brains of anesthetized monkeys (Macaca rhesus) by the application of a freezing instrument to the exposed intact skull. Only enough of the skull was exposed to accommodate the instrument. Lesions were produced both by our standard method using liquid nitrogen as the refrigerant [10] and by substituting solid carbon dioxide in isopentane (modified method). In the latter case acetone was placed in the inner tube of the instrument. Using the standard method, an exposure of 3–5 min was required to produce a lesion. With the modified method, 15–45 min was required. After the lesion was produced the incision was sutured and the animal was placed on a Rothberg Restrainer (Phipps and Bird, Inc., Richmond, Virginia), and allowed to come out of anesthesia. Throughout the experimental period, the animals were given small amounts of water by mouth. Sacrifice of surviving animals was by an overdose of sodium pentobarbital given 48 h after injury. Following sacrifice the hemispheres were analyzed separately for water, sodium, potassium, chloride and iron according to methods previously described [9]. The uptake of Evans blue and I^{131} iodinated serum albumin (RISA), given just prior to injury, was also determined [8]. The values were compared to those in a sample of peripheral blood obtained just prior to sacrifice. The lesion size was determined from a template of the surface area.

The first set of experiments was designed to test the proposition that the response to steroids is related to the size of the lesion. Lesions smaller than our standard size were produced in 21 animals (Group 1). Nine of these were produced by the modified technique and the remainder by the standard technique. Eleven of these animals were treated with dexamethasone. Treatment was begun 30 min after injury and continued until sacrifice. The dosage was 4 mg per day given in four divided doses by the intramuscular route.

The second set of experiments was designed to test the proposition that the response to steroids is related to pretreatment with the drug. Standard sized lesions were produced in 19 animals (Group 2). Nine of these were treated with dexamethasone in the same dose as the above groups but therapy was begun 48 h prior to injury and continued until the time of sacrifice. The brains of animals dying spontaneously were fixed in formalin and studied morphologically.

The thymi of all animals were studied histologically.

2. Clinical

Paraffin blocks from cases of human metastatic brain tumors studied in our laboratory for the past 5 years were obtained. Cases with multiple mass involvement, such as seen in melanomas, cases with single small nodules, and instances of meningeal spread were excluded. Sections were stained by the following methods: hematoxylin-eosin, luxol fast blue-hematoxylin-periodic acid Schiff (PAS), Gomori trichrome, Gridley reticulum stain, Holtzer stain, and the gold sublimate technique for astrocytes [1]. The slides were graded blindly for the following points: type and degree of edema, necrosis of tumor, inflammation, glial response and mesenchymal response. After the cases were tabulated, the clinical charts were studied in order to determine if the patients had received steroids and if a good clinical response was present at the time of death. In one case of bronchogenic carcinoma, which was originally thought to have a primary brain tumor, we were able to study a biopsy of the metastatic tumor before therapy had been begun.

In the past 3 years we have also been able to obtain quantitative data in patients with unilateral disease. The brains were fixed in 20 % formalin – 1 % acetic acid which results in a minimal change in weight [1]. After fixation the hemispheres were weighed separately. The tumor was then removed by gross dissection and also weighed.

Results

1. Experimental

There were no spontaneous deaths in Group 1 (smaller lesions). In Group 2 there were 3 spontaneous deaths in the untreated group; all occurred later than 24 h after injury. In the group pretreated with the steroid there were also 3 spontaneous deaths but these all occurred during the first 24 h after injury.

There were no gross or histological differences between the brains of animals receiving the steroid and those of the controls. All animals receiving the steroids showed necrosis of the thymic lymphocytes. This was absent in the controls and the treated cases were easily distinguishable by blind sorting. This finding demonstrates that an adrenal cortical steroid effect was obtained in these animals by the use of dexamethasone.

There were no morphological or chemical differences in the lesions produced by the standard and modified techniques. The results will, therefore, be presented together in the chemical tables.

The findings for the undamaged right hemisphere are recorded in Table 1, in terms of the mean ($\bar{x}$) and standard error ($S\bar{x}$). The apparently higher RISA value in the Group 2 pretreated animals is due to the presence of a higher serum level of the tracer (683 as compared to 483 ctts/min/0.1 ml). When expressed as serum equivalents [6], the values are the same. This is also seen in the next table. The Group 1 control figures are based on ten observations and the treated on eleven observations. Except for the sodium in the group pretreated with dexamethasone, the values in each subgroup are statistically the same and are also the same as those previously reported for the undamaged hemisphere [8]. The sodium is significantly lower than the corresponding control group. This is viewed as a effect of the drug. The assumption will be made that a similar change occurs in the undamaged portion of the left hemisphere.

The findings for the damaged hemisphere in terms of mean increments are given in Table 2. These means are calculated by comparing the value in each animal with its own control undamaged hemisphere. The Group 2 pretreated animals are based on 6 animals and the control on 7 animals, with exception of the dye, RISA and iron which are based on 6 observations. All values are statistically significant at the 1 % level of probability. Within each group, the means for animals given steroids are the same as those for the untreated animals. This table demonstrates the lack of an effect of the steroid on the edema associated with the cryogenic lesion in these experiments.

In Figure 1 the weight increase in the damaged hemisphere of individual animals is plotted against the lesion size in these animals. All the control figures greater than 9 cm² represent animals in Group 2. The higher mean weight increment is a reflection

Table 1. The mean weight and concentrations of substances expressed in terms of dry weight of the undamaged right hemisphere

	Group 1 Control		Treated		Group 2 Control		Pretreated	
	$\bar{x}$	$S\bar{x}$	$\bar{x}$	$S\bar{x}$	$\bar{x}$	$S\bar{x}$	$\bar{x}$	$S\bar{x}$
Weight								
gms	36.9	0.9	35.3	0.9	35.6	0.7	33.8	0.9
Water								
gms/100 gms	329.0	2.9	337.3	3.9	333.8	5.2	327.6	6.5
Sodium								
mEq/100 gms	23.7	0.8	34.7	0.4	25.3	0.8	21.6[a]	1.1
Chloride								
mEq/100 gms	16.9	0.4	16.6	0.4	16.9	0.5	16.3	0.4
Potassium								
mEq/100 gms	41.0	0.8	42.0	0.7	43.3	0.7	42.6	1.5
Iron								
mg/100 gms	10.9	0.4	11.2	0.6	11.0	0.8	11.9	0.6
RISA								
ctts/min/0.1 gm	286	71	293	40	180	18	351	32
RISA								
serum equivalents gm/100 gms	0.37	0.04	0.37	0.02	0.36	0.04	0.39	0.02

[a] Significantly different at the 5% level of probability.

Table 2. The lesion size and mean increments in the damaged left hemisphere expressed in terms of dry weight

	Group 1 Control		Treated		Group 2 Control		Pretreated	
	$\bar{x}$	$S\bar{x}$	$\bar{x}$	$S\bar{x}$	$\bar{x}$	$S\bar{x}$	x	$S\bar{x}$
Lesion Size								
cm^2	7.2	0.2	6.8	0.4	10.5	0.4	10.4	0.4
Weight								
gms	4.9	0.2	4.7	0.2	6.9	0.4	6.8	0.5
Water								
gms/100 gms	29.8	3.0	30.5	2.9	44.7	3.8	46.4	2.6
Sodium								
mEq/100 gms	7.5	0.8	6.5	0.4	10.0	0.7	11.4	1.9
Chloride								
mEq/100 gms	4.4	0.5	4.9	0.4	8.0	0.7	7.3	0.7
Potassium								
mEq/100 gms	—3.1	0.8	—2.4	0.6	—3.5	1.3	—7.5	2.1
Iron								
mg/100 gms	6.5	1.1	5.9	0.6	4.3	0.8	7.2	1.5
Evans blue								
mg/100 gms	16.0	1.3	13.8	1.1	20.5	1.4	22.3	3.2
RISA								
ctts/min/mg	45.2	8.2	41.4	5.6	45.7	4.8	81.7	6.9
RISA								
serum equivalents gm/100 gms	7.2	0.6	6.4	0.4	8.7	0.6	10.4	0.8

160

of the larger lesion in this group as compared to Group I. There is a reasonably good correlation between the variables. This is described by the least square line. The slope and intercept are given in terms of the mean and standard error. It is again quite apparent that the groups given dexamethasone cannot be separated from the control groups.

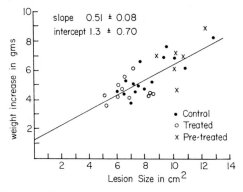

Fig. 1. Relationship between the lesion size and the weight increase in the damaged hemisphere

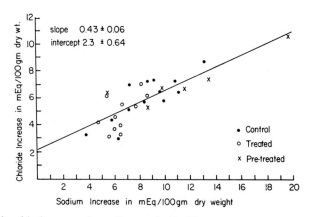

Fig. 2. Relationship between the sodium and chloride increase in the damaged hemisphere

In Figure 2 the sodium increase for individual animals is plotted against the chloride increase as above. This was the only good correlation between the chemical variables which we were able to define. This figure demonstrates that the relationship between these variables has not been influenced by steroid therapy.

2. Clinical

The mean weight of the grossly normal male cerebral hemisphere based on 16 brains is 572 g with a standard deviation (S.D.) of 56 g. The mean difference is 6 g with a S.D. of 6 g. For the female the figures were 515 g, S.D. 50 g, n = 16. The mean difference was 2 g with an S.D. of 2 g.

Data on cases with unilateral metastases are given in Table 3. There is a greater degree of swelling due to the accumulation of edema fluid in those cases which did not show a favorable clinical response to steroids. The last case represents a very rare instance of cerebral metastasis from a malignant thymoma.

Table 3. Patients with unilateral cerebral hemisphere metastases. The degree of swelling is calculated from the weights of the edema fluid and the uninvolved hemisphere

Case	Primary	Tumor gms	Edema Fluid gms	Swelling %	Response to Steroids
70611	lung	83	0	0.0	+
70036	kidney	36	21	4.1	+
70372	lung	37	32	6.0	+
70431	lung	10	46	6.7	+
70055	lung	46	43	7.4	+
66419[a]	pancreas	50	55	8.5	+
71455	uterus	10	53	9.0	0
70019	lung	3	53	10.6	0
72160	thymus	25	74	12.8	0

[a] Figures based on fresh tissue weights

The histologic changes in and around metastatic lesions proved, in general, to be uniform for a given case. There was no correlation between the clinical response to steroids and the degree of edema judged histologically or the chemical character of the edema fluid as judged by its PAS staining characteristics [7]. There also was no correlation between this and the mesenchymal response to the tumor as judged by vascular proliferation, collagen production or macrophage response nor was there any correlation with the degree of astrocytosis and glial scarring. A correlation was seen with the degree of inflammation, acute or chronic. These results are given in Table 4. Those cases showing a favorable clinical response to steroids showed less inflammation. The results are significant at the 5 % level of probability. Although there appeared to be a correlation between the presence of necrosis in the tumor and inflammation, in terms of the clinical response to steroids, this was not statistically significant.

Table 4. Number of patients showing a favorable clinical response to steroid therapy in relation to the presence of significant inflammation and necrosis in the metastatic nodules

	Present	Absent	Chi-square	
Response	1	11	6.4	Inflammation
No response	8	4		
Response	9	3	0.3	Necrosis
No response	11	1		

The case in which a clinical diagnosis of primary brain tumor was made, underwent a craniotomy with removal of a right frontal metastatic lesion. This proved to be an epidermoid carcinoma with extensive chronic inflammation and necrosis of the tumor. The patient was placed on steroids and showed a slight but definite improvement in clinical symptoms. The clinical response, however, lasted only for a period of 6 weeks at which time he developed a grand mal seizure and lapsed into a semicomatous state. The patient remained in this state until his death 4 weeks later, showing no further response to steroids. At autopsy two additional lesions were demonstrated. One of these involved the vermis of the cerebellum and the other the left parietal lobe. Both showed a degree of inflammation and necrosis comparable to that seen in the original frontal lesion.

Discussion

1. Cryogenic Lesions

At the time that the experiments involving pretreatment with steroids were conducted, it had not been demonstrated that the edema associated with cryogenic lesions could be treated with steroids, only that it could be prevented [30, 31]. We, therefore, reasoned that pretreatment with steroids could in some way modify the injury resulting in less edema and that this might be the explanation of our negative results [8]. It was subsequently shown that this edema could be both prevented and treated with steroids [23, 29]. This, together with the negative results herein reported, clearly shows that the failure to pretreat the animals does not explain our negative results.

Another possible explanation for the failure of our lesions to respond to steroids lies in their qualitative character. The cryogenic lesions which have been reported as responding to steroids have all been produced by the Klatzo technique or some modification thereof [13, 23, 29, 30, 31]. These lesions incite a macrophage response and resolve as glial scars [19]. Lesions produced by our technique, on the other hand, are associated with an intense acute inflammation and resolve as collagenous scars [35]. Even small cryogenic lesions produced by liquid nitrogen in rabbits have been reported to resolve as collagenous scars [4]. Cryogenic lesions produced in our laboratory in rabbits using carbon dioxide as the refrigerant are not associated with an acute inflammatory response and resolve as glial scars [16]. Such lesions have shown a favorable clinical response to steroids used in combination with systemic hypothermia [34]. These considerations suggest that the type of exudative and proliferative response associated with the lesion determines its response to steroids and was the rationale for our (unsuccessful) attempt to produce a different type of lesion using solid carbon dioxide in place of liquid nitrogen.

Another explanation for the failure of our lesions to respond to steroid therapy lies in their quantitative character, i.e. the relative degrees of necrosis and edema [36]. As judged by gross illustrations, lesions produced by the Klatzo technique, which respond to steroids, are not essentially different in size from our smallest lesions [24]. It would appear, therefore, that lesion size is not the factor accounting for our negative results.

2. Metastatic disease

It was the attempt to unravel the relative roles of necrosis and inflammation in this process which led us to study human metastatic disease. The histology of the cerebral

163

edema associated with this condition is quite similar to that seen with the cryogenic lesion, as are the ultrastructural characteristics [2, 21, 26]. Pathogenetic similarities have also been defined [17]. The finding of less cerebral edema in patients showing a good clinical response to steroids is in keeping with data reported on cerebral biopsies in primary and metastatic brain tumors [25]. It would appear that inflammation is the prime factor involved in the response to steroids of the edema associated with metastases. It must be borne in mind that even if one accepts the proposition that the presence of inflammation adversely affects the response to steroids, this does not mean that inflammation *per se* is the factor responsible for this. It may be that the inflammation merely reflects a tissue factor which is primary, but this would not appear to be necrosis as judged by ordinary histologic techniques. It may be, however, that necrosis associated with inflammation is chemically different from necrosis not associated with inflammation.

The only specific experimental investigation of this question of which we are aware involves melanomas implanted into the brains of mice [20]. The authors failed to demonstrate suppression of edema by steroids but attributed the alleviation of symptoms and prolongation of life in treated animals to a steroid induced diminution of tumor size. These results are not in keeping with the clinical data presented above. This may be related to the unsuitability of the experimental model. The cerebral edema associated with tumors is essentially a disease of white matter and the rodent cerebral hemisphere contains very little white matter in proportion to the amount of grey matter.

3. Other forms of experimental cerebral edema

The cerebral edema associated with radiofrequency lesions responds to steroid management [36]. This we view as being pathogenetically related to the edema associated with our lesions. Necrosis is relatively less in the radiofrequency lesions but inflammatory changes also were not described.

The pathogenesis of the edema associated with the intracerebral implantation of psyllium seeds has in our opinion not been well-defined. It may be that this experimental model reproduces the factor of slowly progressive growth seen in human brain tumors, as the cryogenic lesion reproduces the factor of focal vascular hyperpermeability [17]. In any case, this edema responds to steroids [24]. It is associated with little inflammation and essentially no necrosis [5]. The closely related edema associated with extradural balloon implantation also responds to steroids [24].

It has been reported that the cerebral edema associated with triethyl tin intoxication responds to steroid management [37]. In this condition the fluid accumulates within the myelin sheath and neither inflammation nor necrosis have been described [27].

The cerebral edema associated with the intracarotid injection of Hypaque is diminished following pretreatment with dexamethasone [14]. This paper did not include a histological evaluation. On the other hand, no suppression of edema with steroids was reported for intracarotid Urokon [15]. Histologically, some petechial hemorrhages were observed in the brains of these animals. It is of interest that animals given intra-aortic injections of Urokon and allowed to survive for several weeks showed extensive necrosis of the spinal cord [28].

The transient cerebral edema associated with convulsions is also responsive to steroid management [12]. Although histologic studies were not included, the absence of necrosis and inflammation may be assumed.

The necrosis associated with anoxic-ischemic injury in the rat is not associated with significant inflammatory changes [22, 32], and the cerebral edema seen in this condition does not respond to steroids [33]. The edema associated with LASER beam injury is also accompanied by a great deal of necrosis without inflammation and fails to respond to steroids [3].

The experimental disturbances in vascular permeability and cerebral fluid balance reviewed above have in common the fact that cerebral edema in the absence of significant necrosis and inflammation is diminished by steroid therapy. In addition there are two instances of necrosis without significant inflammation in which negative results were obtained and one instance of negative results with steroids [15] in which necrosis might have been demonstrated if the experimental period had been prolonged [28]. These findings suggest that the degree of necrosis associated with cerebral edema is the factor which determines the response to steroids. The data which we have presented both on the cryogenic lesion in monkeys and metastatic lesions in humans indicate that the presence or absence of cellular inflammation is the determining factor in this response.

References

1. Adachi, M., Rosenblum, W. I., Feigin, I.: Hypertensive disease and cerebral edema. J. Neurol. Neurosurg. Psychiat. **29**, 451–455 (1966).
2. Aleu, F., Samuels, S., Ransohoff, J.: The pathology of cerebral edema associated with gliomas in man. Amer. J. Path. **48**, 1043–1061 (1966).
3. Benson, V. M., McLaurin, R. L., Foulkes, E. C.: Traumatic cerebral edema. Arch. Neurol. **23**, 179–186 (1970).
4. Brierley, J. B.: The prolonged and distant effects of experimental brain injury on cerebral blood vessels as demonstrated by radioactive indicators. J. Neurol. Neurosurg. Psychiat. **19**, 202–208 (1956).
5. Bryar, G. E., Goldstein, N. P., Svien, H. J., Sayer, G. P., Jones, J. D.: Experimental cerebral edema: vital staining with Evans blue during the developmental and regressive phases. J. Neurosurg. **30**, 391–398 (1969).
6. Clasen, R. A., Pandolfi, S., Russell, J., Stuart, D., Hass, G. M.: Hypothermia and hypotension in experimental cerebral edema. Arch. Neurol. **19**, 472–486 (1968).
7. — Sky-Peck, H. H., Pandolfi, S., Laing, I., Hass, G. M.: The chemistry of isolated edema fluid in experimental cerebral injury. In: Klatzo, I. and Seitelberger, F. (Eds.): Brain Edema, p. 536–553. Wien-New York: Springer 1967.
8. — Cooke, P. M., Pandolfi, S., Carnecki, G., Hass, G. M.: Steroid-antihistaminic therapy in experimental cerebral edema. Arch. Neurol. **13**, 584–592 (1965).
9. — — — — Bryar, G.: Hypertonic urea in experimental cerebral edema. Arch. Neurol. **12**, 424–434 (1965).
10. — Brown, D. V. L., Leavitt, S., Hass, G. M.: The production by liquid nitrogen of acute closed cerebral lesions. Surg. Gynec. Obstet. **96**, 605–616 (1953).
11. Ducker, T. B., Hamit, H. F.: Experimental treatments of acute spinal cord injury. J. Neurosurg. **30**, 693–697 (1969).
12. Eisenberg, H. M., Barlow, C. F., Lorenzo, A. V.: Effect of dexamethasone on altered brain vascular permeability. Arch. Neurol. **23**, 18–22 (1970).
13. Go, K. G., van Woodenberg, F., Beekhuis, H., Schut, T., Dorrenbos, H.: The effect of cortisone on cold-induced oedema in the rat brain. Neurochir. Fort. **14**, 232–240 (1971).
14. Hammargren, L. L., Geise, A. W., French, L. A.: Protection against cerebral damage from intracarotid injection of Hypaque in animals. J. Neurosurg. **23**, 418–424 (1965).

15. Harris, A. B.: Steroids and blood brain barrier alterations in sodium acetrizoate injury. Arch. Neurol. **17**, 282–297 (1967).
16. Hass, G. M., Taylor, C. B.: A quantitative hypothermal method for the production of local tissue injury. Arch. Path. **45**, 563–580 (1948).
17. Hindo, W. A., Clasen, R. A., Rayudu, G. V. S., Pandolfi, S.: Technetium in cryogenic cerebral injury and edema. Arch. Neurol. (in press).
18. Hooshmand, H., Dove, J., Houff, S., Suter, C.: Effects of diuretics and steroids on CSF pressure, a comparative study. Arch. Neurol. **21**, 499–509 (1969).
19. Klatzo, I., Piraux, A., Laskowski, E. J.: The relationship between edema, blood-brain barrier and tissue elements in a local brain injury. J. Neuropath. exp. Neurol. **17**, 548–564 (1958).
20. Kotsilimbas, D. G., Meyer, L., Berson, B. A., Raylor, J. M., Scheinberg, L. C.: Corticosteroid effect on intracerebral melanomata and associated cerebral edema. Some unexpected findings. Neurology **17**, 223–227 (1967).
21. Lee, J. C., Bakay, L.: Ultrastructural changes in the edematous central nervous system. II. Cold-induced edema. Arch. Neurol. **14**, 36–49 (1966).
22. Levine, S.: Anoxic-ischemic encephalopathy in rats. Amer. J. Path. **36**, 1–17 (1960).
23. Long, D. M., Maxwell, R. E., French, L. A.: The effects of glucosteroids on experimental cold-induced brain edema. Ultrastructural evaluation. J. Neuropath. exp. Neurol. **30**, 680–697 (1971).
24. — Hartmann, J. F., French, L. A.: The response of experimental cerebral edema to glucosteroid administration. J. Neurosurg. **24**, 843–854 (1966).
25. — — — The response of human cerebral edema to glucosteroid administration. An electron microscopic study. Neurology **16**, 521–528 (1966).
26. — — — The ultrastructure of human cerebral edema. J. Neuropath. exp. Neurol. **25**, 373–395 (1966).
27. Magee, P. N., Stoner, H. B., Barnes, J. M.: The experimental production of oedema in the central nervous system of the rat by triethyltin compounds. J. Path. Bact. **73**, 107–124 (1957).
28. Margolis, G., Tarazi, A. K., Grimson, K. S.: Contrast medium injury to the spinal cord produced by aortography, pathologic anatomy of the experimental lesion. J. Neurosurg. **13**, 261–277 (1956).
29. Maxwell, R. E., Long, D. M., French, L. A.: The effects of glucosteroids on experimental cold-induced brain edema. Gross morphological alterations and vascular permeability changes. J. Neurosurg. **34**, 477–487 (1971).
30. Palleske, V. H., Herrmann, H. D., Kremer, G.: Verlaufsuntersuchungen über Veränderungen des Elektrolyt- und Wassergehaltes des Gehirns im experimentellen Hirnödem und deren therapeutische Beeinflußbarkeit durch Dexamethason. Zbl. Neurochir. **31**, 31–38 (1970).
31. Pappius, H. M., McCann, W. P.: Effects of steroids on cerebral edema in cats. Arch. Neurol. **20**, 207–216 (1969).
32. Plum, F., Posner, J. B., Alvord, E. C.: Edema and necrosis in experimental cerebral infarction. Arch. Neurol. **9**, 563–570 (1963).
33. Plum, B., Alvord, E. C., Posner, J. B.: Effect of steroids on experimental cerebral infarction. Arch. Neurol. **9**, 571–573 (1963).
34. Raimondi, A. J., Clasen, R. A., Beattie, E. J., Taylor, C. B.: The effect of hypothermia and steroid therapy on experimental cerebral injury. Surg. Gynec. Obstet. **108**, 333–338 (1959).
35. Rosomoff, H. L., Clasen, R. A., Hartstock, R., Bebin, J.: Brain reaction to experimental injury after hypothermia. Arch. Neurol. **13**, 337–345 (1965).
36. Rovit, R. L., Hagen, R.: Steroids and cerebral edema: the effects of glucocorticoids on abnormal capillary permeability following cerebral injury in cats. J. Neuropath. exp. Neurol. **27**, 277–299 (1968).
37. Taylor, J. M., Levy, W. A., Herzog, I., Scheinberg, L. C.: Prevention of experimental cerebral edema by corticosteroids. Neurology **15**, 667–674 (1965).

Effect of Antioxidants on Experimental Cold-Induced Cerebral Edema

Bienvenido D. Ortega, Harry B. Demopoulos, and Joseph Ransohoff

Departments of Neurosurgery and Pathology, New York University Medical Center, New York, NY 10010, USA

With 1 Figure

Summary. Cerebral edema was produced by local cortical freezing in untreated and treated animals. Treated animals received p-Ethoxyphenol (pEOP) and N,N'-diphenyl-p-phenylenediamine (DPPD). A daily dose of 100 mg/kg in pre-treated animals and 500 mg/kg of DPPD in post-injured animals showed a significant reduction in cerebral edema as demonstrated in gross and coronal specimens, histologic study and differences in white matter weights. A similar dose of 100 mg/kg of DPPD given 1 h after injury was ineffective, while a large dose of 1000 mg/kg was lethal in this experimental model. The effect of pEOP was not significant. The beneficial effect of DPPD, an antioxidant, is postulated to be in the prevention or inhibition of free radical peroxidative mechanisms. It is postulated that membrane lipids may be the principle molecules undergoing free radical damage. The hypothesis is advanced that steroids, by intercalating into membranes in a specific configuration may prevent the radical initiation and chain reactions that damage the fatty acids of membrane phospholipids. The molecular mechanism of cerebral edema is harmonious with other mechanisms that are at the cellular and subcellular level.

Introduction

Although glucocorticoids have received wide acceptance in clinical practice based on extensive data from several clinics [5, 13, 18, 19, 20, 21, 24, 30, 36, 48, 49, 51, 52, 54], the mechanisms whereby they alter cerebral edema are still obscure. Experimental investigations have been largely contradictory. Some workers have claimed beneficial results [6, 7, 15, 22, 28, 34, 35, 40, 43, 45, 50, 53, 58, 59], while others have reported no effective results from the use of steroids on experimental cerebral edema [10, 42, 44, 47].

Various procedures have also been used in the experimental production of cerebral edema [9, 14, 25, 27, 31, 32, 39, 55, 60, 63, 64]. In spite of the intense study, it is not yet clear how edema is brought about. It has been suggested that the cerebral edema which follows a traumatic cerebral injury is largely due to abnormal vascular permeability [2, 3, 4, 11, 12, 16, 23, 27, 28, 29, 34, 40, 56]. It is therefore possible that steroids exert their effect by their capacity to stabilize membranes that have been perturbed by the injury to develop altered transport mechanisms [37, 61, 62].

Supported by: U.S. Army Medical Research and Development Command, Office of the Surgeon General under Contract DA-49-93-MD-2232; National Institutes of Health, N.I.N.D.S. Grant 5-PO1-NSO4257-08/09.

The use of steroids, as well as other agents with known inhibitory properties, is a valid, although indirect method, for studying molecular and subcellular mechanisms. Cellular and myelin membranes contain lipids that are vulnerable to degradation by free radical peroxidative mechanisms [12, 26]. Metal complexes, such as iron and copper complexes, are known to initiate and catalyze this process [57]. In Wilson's disease, copper complexes have been implicated in the pathogenesis of its brain lesions [33].

Antioxidants have long been used to prevent free radical reactions in both chemical and biologic studies. Two of these agents were used to test the hypothesis that radical reactions in membrane lipids are involved in the production of brain edema induced by experimental cold-injury in the cat.

Materials and Methods

General Procedure: Mature, healthy cats on standard diet, weighing 1.5–4.0 kg were employed in this study. All animals were anesthetized with intravenous sodium pentobarbital in the range of 30 mg/kg and were kept lightly anesthetized. The head was fixed on a head rest and prepared in an aseptic technique. An intravenous normal saline infusion was started to keep a vein open for the purpose of administering the indicator dye utilized to delineate the spread of edema. The I.V. drip was maintained slowly and discontinued soon after the dye was given. Through a midline incision, a 16 × 16 mm left fronto-parietal craniectomy was performed using a hand trephine. The dura was opened widely.

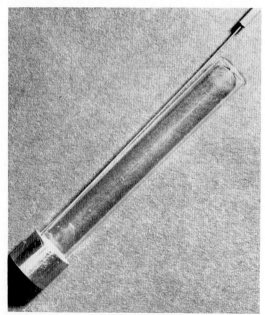

Fig. 1. Freezing disc with mounted test tube and microthermocouple

Cerebral edema was produced utilizing a modification of Klatzo's technique [27]. A test tube filled with dry ice and acetone was used to cool a flat-bottom circular metal disc measuring 12 × 12 mm in diameter (see Fig. 1). The disc, cooled to

—50 $\pm$ 2° C, was then applied on the left marginal and middle suprasylvian gyri for 30 sec. At the time of application, an assistant administered 2.5 cc/kg of 2% Evans blue intravenously. The disc was loosened from the pia by irrigating with room-temperature physiologic saline. The dura was returned in place and covered with silastic. The trephine button was replaced and the wound closed with silk sutures and skin clips. The animals were maintained without special care for periods up to 72 h. The lesion produced was fairly constant. Animals that received a freezing temperature outside the range of —50 $\pm$ 2° C were eliminated from the study.

Two antioxidants were used: p-Ethoxyphenol (pEOP) (Eastman 4803; $C_2H_5OC_6H_4OH$; MW 138.17) and N,N'-diphenyl-p-phenylenediamine (DPPD) (Eastman p5689; $C_6H_5NHC_6H_4NH_6H_5$; MW 260.34).

Group I : 18 cats were subjected to cold-injury as described. One-half received pEOP subcutaneously in the dose of 50 mg/kg body weight. The drug was suspended in Dextrose 5% in water at concentrations of 50 mg/cc, warmed until dissolved. Treatment was given daily, starting one day prior to the cold-injury. The other 9 animals were left untreated. The cats were sacrificed at 24, 48 and 72 h, 3 cats per time period, for each treated and untreated group, by intracardiac 10% formalin perfusion under sodium pentobarbital anesthesia. The brains were removed and photographed and stored in containers of 10% buffered formalin. After additional fixation for 24 h, the brains were serially sectioned at 5 mm intervals in the coronal plane. The lesion was divided into thirds. The extravasation of Evans blue dye into the white matter was estimated grossly and recorded by photographs. The anterior third of the lesion was sent for histologic study. The stains utilized included Hematoxylin-Eosin, Luxol Fast Blue-PAS and Bodian.

Group II : 36 cats were employed in this part of the study and were subjected to cold lesions. 9 animals received subcutaneous treatment of pEOP in 100 mg/kg given a day prior to surgery and daily until the day of sacrifice at 24, 48 and 72 h, 3 cats per time period. 9 animals received intramuscular injections of DPPD in the dose of 100 mg/kg, starting the day before cold application, until the day of sacrifice at 24, 48 and 72 h, 3 cats per time period. 9 cats were given varying daily dosages of DPPD, 100, 500 and 1000 mg/kg at 1 h after cold injury until sacrifice at 48 h. DPPD was dissolved in Tween 20 (100 mg/cc). 9 cats served as untreated controls.

All of these animals were sacrificed by intrathoracic exsanguination. The brains were immediately removed and sectioned to remove a coronal slice of the middle third of the lesion. This slice was utilized for wet and dry weight determinations. Separate matching samples of injured and contralateral cerebral white and grey matter were removed from this coronal slice by sharp dissection and placed in separate aluminium containers and promptly weighed. They were then dried in an oven at 100° C to constant weight for 24 h and reweighed. Calculations of wet and dry weights between matching samples, and between groups, were made. The remaining tissue was stored in 10% buffered formalin solution and sectioned coronally and studied in the same manner as in Group I.

Results

An occasional animal had to be rejected from these studies because the desired temperature was not obtained.

Group I : All the animals were awake, withdrawn and tended to ignore their food. None had motor weaknesses. Grossly, cold injury produced a localized area of cortical necrosis, corresponding to the area of disc application. There was edema surrounding the lesion and extravasation of blue dye. Coronal slices showed widened gyri, cortical necrosis limited to the surface of the gryi, widening of the underlying white matter and flattening of the ipsilateral ventricle. Dye extended into the subjacent gyral white matter at 24 h, and the deep white matter at 48 h. It appeared to be diminished at 72 h. These changes were seen in both the pEOP pre-treated and untreated control animals.

Microscopically, the cortical surface showed complete cell disintegration. There were areas of punctate hemorrhage within the necrotic area and subjacent white matter. The white matter edema was represented by areas of rarefaction. Myelinated fibers were separated as demonstrated by the Luxol fast blue-PAS and Bodian stain sections. There was no microscopic evidence of fragmentation and degeneration of nerve fibers to any significant extent. There was no apparent correlation between the extent of the hemorrhage and the degree of edema formation.

Treatment with pEOP showed no convincing evidence of diminished edema histologically.

Group II : The DPPD treated animals, except 3 that received the dose of 1000 mg/kg, were awake and less withdrawn than the untreated and pEOP treated groups. The 3 animals that remained stuporous died before 24 h.

The effect of the antioxidants on the wet and dry weights of cerebral tissue were studied in this group (see Table 1). The effect of pEOP on experimental cold injury in cats was barely appreciable. There appeared to be a reduction of about 29 % in the amount of edema in the white matter, compared with the control at 48 h. There was no significant difference in weights at 24 and 72 h after production of the lesion.

Table 1. Effects of antioxidants on water content of injured versus contralateral cerebral tissue

Time	Tissue	Control	Pre-treated		Post-trauma treated N,N′-diphenyl-p-phenylenediamine		
			pEOP	DPPD			
			0.1 gm/kg	0.1 gm/kg	0.1 gm/kg	0.5 gm/kg	1.0 gm/kg
24 h	Grey	0.44	0.09	0.33			0.53[b]
	White	0.97	1.04	0.46			0.21[b]
48 h	Grey	0.32	0.33	0.35	0.32	0.25	
	White	1.12	0.79	0.45	1.00	0.41	
72 h	Grey	0.14	0.24	0.22			
	White	0.68	0.59	0.46			

Each group, control, pEOP, DPPD pre-treated, DPPD post-treated, contained 3 cats. The calculation for water content was as follows: (gm wet wgt.) — (gm dry wgt.) = gm H_2O content; $\dfrac{gm H_2O\ content}{gm\ dry\ wgt.} = X$; $X_L - X_R$ = difference between left (L), which is the injured side, and right (R), contralateral cerebral tissue; $X_L - X_R$ was determined individually in each cat. The values shown represent the averages of the three animals in each group. Ranges were narrow and are not given.

[b] All three animals died between 12–24 h post injury.

Animals that were pre-treated with DPPD, 100 mg/kg, and those that received 500 mg/kg 1 h following the lesion showed a highly significant reduction in the weight of the injured hemisphere. This was demonstrated by a 60% and 30% reduction in white matter weights at 48 and 72 h, respectively, in the pretreated animals. There was a 63% difference between untreated cats and the group that received 500 mg/kg post-injury. The 3 animals that received a dose of 1000 mg/kg of DPPD showed a more profound reduction in edema but this can not be relied upon since none of these animals survived more than 24 h. This large dose appeared to be the lethal dose of DPPD in cats. Post-injury treatment of 100 mg/kg DPPD was ineffective in altering the amount of brain edema an hour after the injury.

The topography of the untreated and pEOP treated animals was similar to that described in the first group. DPPD-treated animals, on the other hand, in general, showed less edema grossly. In the coronal slices, there was no widening of the white matter and edema was localized to the white matter of the involved gyri. The blue tracer dye did not extend to the deep white matter nor to the white matter of non-injured, adjacent gyri.

Microscopically, the untreated and pEOP-treated animals were similar to those described in the first group. DPPD-treated animals, except for the 100 mg/kg dose, showed demonstrable reduction of brain edema histologically.

Discussion

The use of antioxidants, primarily DPPD, decreases experimental cold-induced cerebral edema in the cat. The beneficial effect of antioxidants suggests that free radical mechanisms may be one of the factors involved in the formation of cerebral edema.

Cellular and myelin membranes, because of their lipid composition are susceptible to degradation by free radical peroxidative mechanisms [12, 26]. This is the classical "rancidity" of fats. This process can be initiated and catalyzed by metal complexes such as iron and copper complexes [57]. These may be derived from extravasated red blood cells and from metal complexes that are dislocated from their normal locations in the electron transport chains of mitochondria and endoplasmic reticulum.

Although antioxidants as used in this study suggest free radical mechanisms are operative in the formation of brain edema, such a mechanism is not in conflict with other proposals. It rather dove-tails with data that point to altered vascular permeability and destabilized membranes. Free radical mechanisms may be the molecular basis, while other proposals explain edema at subcellular, and cellular levels.

The relationship between the present data, which shows the beneficial effects of antioxidants, and the data of others demonstrating the variable efficacy of steroids may be explicable as follows.

Steroids may function to prevent the early spread of radical reactions through a membrane by forming close hydrophobic associations with the fatty acids in membrane phospholipids that are susceptible to radical attack [38]. Specifically, the alpha methylene carbons in unsaturated fatty acids lose their hydrogens very readily and result in radical centers on the carbon. This is the first step chemically in lipid peroxidation. Steroids are bulky and form tight hydrophobic associations, which physically may hinder the loss of hydrogen from alpha methylene carbons [38]. In this way, peroxidative chain reactions may be prevented.

171

The variable efficacy of steroids in different conditions may be explicable on the basis of how far peroxidative damage to membranes has progressed by the time steroids are started. In trauma, which includes hemorrhage as well as dislocated electron transport metal complexes, the radical damage might be expected to progress rapidly because metal complexes catalyze lipid peroxidation by 3–5 orders of magnitude [57]. The rapid peroxidation induced by trauma explains the greater efficacy of DPPD when used in a pre-treatment regimen. A dose of 100 mg/kg was effective before, but not after, injury. Post-trauma, it was necessary to go to much higher levels, 500 mg/kg, to diminish brain edema.

If membranes are already severely damaged, there would be a loss of the "archways" normally formed by unsaturated fatty acids within membrane phospholipids [41]. It is within such "archways" that steroids fit when they intercalate into membranes [38]. Catalyzed lipid peroxidation quickly destroys such archways and literally leaves no sites for steroid intercalation.

If free radical reactions are progressing at a slow rate, it may be possible for steroids to actually protect against the spread of radical chain reactions, because as they fit into the "archways" of unsaturated fatty acids, they protect the alpha methylene carbons, which are present within the "arch". It is these carbons that are initially attacked in peroxidation.

Antioxidants prevent or stop radical reactions in different ways. They may prevent the initiation of radical reactions, quench radicals already formed, or chelate metal complexes that are responsible for catalysis [1, 8]. DPPD, which was shown to be highly effective in the present studies, is a powerful antioxidant. It has been used in numerous biologic studies to elucidate the participation of free radical reactions, including the prevention of encephalomalacia in the vitamin E-deficient chicks [46]. Although generally considered a safe antioxidant, a dose of 1000 mg/kg proved uniformly fatal in cats. Potential application of the beneficial effects of antioxidants may be in the conjoint use of several antioxidants at low concentrations. They would have additive chemical protective effects against free radical damage, and the low concentrations would minimize undesired toxic effects.

Acknowledgements. The authors gratefully thank the assistance of Dr. James B. Campbell and his technical staff at the Milbank Research Laboratory.

References

1. Aaes-Jorgensen, E.: Antioxidation of fatty compounds in living tissue, biological antioxidants. In: Lundberg, W. O. (Ed.): Autoxidation and Antioxidants, Vol. II, pp. 1045 to 1094. New York: Interscience 1961.
2. Bakay, L.: The movement of electrolytes and albumin in different types of cerebral edema. In: DeRobertis, E. D. P., Carrea, R. (Eds.): Progress in Brain Research. Amsterdam: Elsevier 1965.
3. Bakay, L., Hague, I. V.: Morphological and chemical studies in cerebral edema. I. Cold induced edema. J. Neuropath. Exper. Neurol. 23, 393–418 (1964).
4. Bakay, L., Lee, J. C.: In: Cerebral edema. Springfield, Ill.: Charles C. Thomas 1965.
5. Bernard-Weil, E., David, M.: Pre-operative hormonal treatment in cases of cerebral tumor. J. Neurosurg. 20, 841–848 (1963).
6. Blinderman, E.: Effect of dexamethasone on mitochondria in anoxic brain. Arch. Neurol. 12, 278–283 (1965).
7. Blinderman, E. E., Graf, C. J., Fitzpatrick, T.: Basic studies in cerebral edema: its control by cortico-steroid (Solu-medrol). J. Neurosurg. 19, 319–324 (1962).

8. Chipault, J. R.: Antioxidants for use in foods. In: Lundberg, W. O. (Ed.): Autoxidation and Antioxidants, Vol. II, pp. 477–682. New York: Interscience 1961.
9. Clasen, R. A., Brown, D. V. L., Leavitt, S., *et al.*: The production by liquid nitrogen of acute closed cerebral lesions. Surg. Gynec. Obstet. **96**, 605–616 (1953).
10. Clasen, R. A., Cooke, P. M., Pandolfi, S., *et al.*: Steroid-antihistamine therapy in experimental cerebral edema. Arch. Neurol. **13**, 584–592 (1965).
11. Cutler, R. W. P., Watters, G. V., Barlow, C. F.: I^{125}-labelled protein in experimental brain edema. Arch. Neurol. **11**, 225–238 (1964).
12. Demopoulos, H. B., Milvy, P., Kakari, S., Ransohoff, J.: Molecular aspects of membrane structure in cerebral edema. In: Reulen, H. J., Schürmann, K. (Eds.): Steroids and brain edema. Berlin-Heidelberg-New York: Springer 1972.
13. Dyken, W., White, P. T.: Evaluation of cortisone in the treatment of cerebral infarction. J. Amer. med. Ass. **162**, 1531–1534 (1956).
14. Edström, R. F. S., Essex, H. E.: Swelling of the brain induced by anoxia. Neurology **6**, 118–124 (1956).
15. Elliott, K. A. C., Jasper, H.: Measurement of experimentally induced brain swelling and shrinkage. Amer. J. Physiol. **157**, 122–129 (1949).
16. Elliott, K. A. C., Yrarrazaval, S.: An effect of adrenalectomy and cortisone on tissue permeability in vitro. Nature (London) **169**, 416–417 (1952).
17. Feigin, I., Popoff, N.: Neuropathological observation on cerebral edema. The acute phase. Arch. Neurol. **6**, 151–160 (1962).
18. French, L. A., Galicich, I. H.: Use of steroid for control of cerebral edema. Clin. Neurosurg. **10**, 212–223 (1966).
19. Galicich, J. H., French, L. A.: Use of dexamethasone in the treatment of cerebral edema resulting from brain tumors and brain surgery. Amer. Practit. **12**, 169–174 (1961).
20. Galicich, J. H., French, L. A., Melby, J. C.: Use of dexamethasone in treatment of cerebral edema associated with brain tumors. J. Lancet **81**, 46–53 (1961).
21. Gårde, A.: Experiences with dexamethasone treatment of intracranial pressure caused by brain tumors. Acta neurol. scand. Suppl. **13**, 439–443 (1965).
22. Grenell, R. G., McCawley, E. I.: Central nervous system resistance. III. The effect of adrenal cortical substances on the central nervous system. J. Neurosurg. **4**, 508–518 (1947).
23. Hammargren, L. L., Geise, A. W., French, L. A.: Protection against cerebral damage from intracarotid injection of hypaque in animals. J. Neurosurg. **23**, 418–424 (1965).
24. Hume, D. M., Moore, F. D.: The use of ACTH, cortisone and adrenal cortical extracts in surgical patients. Proceedings of the Second Clinical ACTH Conference. Mote, J. R. (Ed.), Vol. 2, pp. 289–309. London: J. A. Churchill Ltd. 1951.
25. Ishii, S., Hayner, R., Kelly, W. A., *et al.*: Studies of cerebral swelling. II. Experimental cerebral swelling produced by supratentorial extradural compression. J. Neurosurg. **16**, 152–166 (1959).
26. Jacob, H. S., Lux, S. E.: IV. Degradation of membrane phospholipids and thiols in peroxide hemolysis. Studies in Vitamin E deficiency. Blood **32**, 549–569 (1968).
27. Klatzo, I., Miquel, H., Otenasek, R.: The application of fluorescein labeled serum proteins (FLSP) to the study of vascular permeability in the brain. Acta neuropath. (Berl.) **2**, 144–160 (1962).
28. Klatzo, I., Piraux, A., Laskowski, E. S.: The relationship between edema, blood-brain barrier, and tissue elements in a local brain injury. J. Neuropath. exp. Neurol. **17**, 548–564 (1958).
29. Klatzo, I., Wisniewski, H., Smith, D. E.: Observations on penetration of serum proteins into the central nervous system. In: DeRobertis, E. D. F., Carrea, E. (Eds.): Progress in brain research, pp. 73–88. Amsterdam: Elsevier 1965.
30. Kotsilimbas, D. G., Meyer, L., Berson, M., *et al.*: Corticosteroid effect on intracerebral melanomata and associated cerebral edema. Neurology **17**, 223–227 (1967).
31. Lee, J., Oslzewski, J.: Permeability of cerebral blood vessels in healing of brain wounds. Neurology **9**, 7–14 (1959).
32. Levine, S., Zimmerman, H. M., Weak, E. J., *et al.*: Experimental leukoencephalopathies due to implantation of foreign substances. Amer. J. Path. **42**, 97–110 (1963).

173

33. Lindquist, R. R.: Studies on the pathogenesis of hepatolenticular degeneration. III. The effect of copper on rat liver lysosomes. Am. J. Path. **53**, 903–916 (1968).
34. Lippert, R. G., Svien, H. J., Grindlay, J. H., *et al.*: The effect of cortisone on experimental cerebral edema. J. Neurosurg. **17**, 583–589 (1960).
35. Long, D. M., Hartmann, J. F., French, L. A.: The response of experimental cerebral edema to glucosteroid administration. J. Neurosurg. **24**, 843–854 (1961).
36. Long, D. M., Hartmann, J. F., French, L. A.: The response of human cerebral edema to glucosteroid administration. Neurology **16**, 521–528 (1966).
37. Long, R. A., Hruska, F., Gesser, H. D.: Membrane condensing effect of cholesterol and the role of its hydroxyl group. Biochem. biophys. Res. Commun. **41**, 321–327 (1970).
38. Lucy, J. A.: Theoretical and experimental models for biological membranes. In: Chapman, D. (Ed.): Biological Membranes, pp. 233–288. New York: Academic Press.
39. Magee, P. N., Stoner, H. G., Barnes, J. M.: The experimental production of edema in the central nervous system of the rat by triethyltin compounds. J. Path. Bact. **73**, 107 to 124 (1957).
40. Maxwell, R. E., Long, D. M., French, L. A.: The effects of glucosteroids on experimental cold-induced brain edema. I. Gross morphological alterations and vascular permeability changes. J. Neurosurg. **34**, 477–487 (1971).
41. O'Brien, J. S.: Cell membranes. Composition. Structure. Function. J. theor. Biol. **15**, 307–324 (1967).
42. Pappius, H., Gulati, D. R.: Water and electrolyte content of cerebral tissues in experimentally induced edema. Acta neuropath. (Berl.) **2**, 451–460 (1963).
43. Pappius, H., McCann, W. P.: Effects of steroids on cerebral edema in cats. Arch. Neurol. **20**, 207–216 (1969).
44. Plum, F., Alvord, E. C., Jr., Posner, J. B.: Effect of steroids on experimental cerebral infarction. Arch. Neurol. **9**, 571–573 (1963).
45. Prados, M., Strowger, B., Feindel, W.: Studies on cerebral edema. II. Reaction of the brain to exposure to air; physiologic changes. Arch. Neurol. Psychiat. **54**, 290–300 (1945).
46. Privett, O. S.: Oxidative deterioration and its prevention in miscellaneous products. In: Lundberg, W. O. (Ed.): Autoxidation and Antioxidants, Vol. II, pp. 985–1044. New York: Interscience 1961.
47. Raimondi, A. J., Clasen, R. A., Beattie, E. J., *et al.*: The effect of hypothermia and steroid therapy on experimental cerebral injury. Surg. Gynec. Obstet. **108**, 333–338 (1959).
48. Rasmussen, T., Gulati, D. R.: Cortisone in the treatment of postoperative cerebral edema. J. Neurosurg. **19**, 535–544 (1962).
49. Roberts, H. J.: Supportive adrenocortical steroid therapy in acute and subacute cerebrovascular accidents with particular reference to brain stem involvement. J. Amer. Geriat. Soc. **6**, 686–702 (1958).
50. Rovit, R. L., Hagan, R.: Steroids and cerebral edema: the effects of glucocorticoids in abnormal capillary permeability following cerebral injury in cats. J. Neuropath. exp. Neurol. **27**, 277–299 (1968).
51. Ruderman, N. B., Hall, T. C.: Use of glucocorticoids in the palliative treatment of metastatic brain tumors. Cancer **18**, 298–306 (1965).
52. Russek, H. L., Russek, A. S., Zohman, B. L.: Cortisone in immediate therapy of apoplectic stroke. J. Amer. Med. Ass. **159**, 102–105 (1955).
53. Scialabba, D. A., Shulman, K.: Use of steroids in clinical and experimental cerebral edema. Surg. Forum, **XV**, 426–427 (1964).
54. Sparacio, R. R., Lin, T., Cook, H. W.: Methylprednisolone sodium succinate in acute craniocerebral trauma. Surg. Gynec. Obstet. **121**, 513–516 (1965).
55. Sperl, M. P., Jr., Svien, H. J., Goldstein, N. P., *et al.*: Experimental production of local cerebral edema by an expanding intracranial mass. Proc. Mayo Clin. **32**, 744–749 (1957).
56. Stern, W. E.: The contribution of the laboratory to an understanding of the cerebral edema: A Review of Recent Progress. Neurology **15**, 902–912 (1965).
57. Tappel, A. L.: Biocatalysts: Lipoxidase and hematin compounds. In: Lundberg, W. O. (Ed.): Autoxidation and Antioxidants, Vol. I, pp. 325–366. New York: Interscience 1961.

58. Taylor, J. M., Levy, W. A., Herzog, I., *et al.*: Prevention of experimental cerebral edema by corticosteroids. Neurology **15**, 667–574 (1965).
59. Taylor, J. M., Levy, W. A., McCoy, G., *et al.*: Prevention of cerebral edema induced by triethyltin in rabbits by corticosteroids. Nature **204**, 891–892 (1964).
60. Weed, L. H., McKibben, P. S.: Experimental alteration of brain bulk. Amer. J. Physiol. **48**, 531 (1919).
61. Weissman, G., Thomas, L.: Studies on lysosomes. II. Effect of cortisone on release of acid hydrolases from large granule fracture of rabbit liver, induced by excess of vitamin A. J. clin. Invest. **42**, 661–669 (1963).
62. Weissman, G.: Studies on lysosomes. VI. Effect of neutral steroids and bile acids on lysosomes in vitro. Biochem. Pharmacol. **14**, 525–535 (1965).
63. White, J. C., Brooks, J. R., Goldthwait, J. C., *et al.*: Changes in brain volume and blood content after experimental concussion. Ann. Surg. **118**, 619–634 (1943).
64. Yanagihara, T., Goldstein, N. P., Svien, H., *et al.*: Experimental cerebral edema: enzyme-histochemical study. Neurology **17**, 669–679 (1967).

175

Steroids and the Blood-Brain Barrier with Special Reference to Astrocytic Cells

Keiji Sano, Hiroshi Hatanaka, and Shuji Kamano

Department of Neurosurgery, University of Tokyo, Japan

With 1 Figure

Summary. Effects of corticosteroids in different doses on the blood-brain barrier in oil-emboli-induced cerebral edema were studied by means of RISA. Initial doses of hydrocortisone and prednisolone should be about 10 mg/kg and 2 mg/kg respectively to protect or repair the blood-brain barrier which is impaired in case of cerebral edema, and smaller doses may not exhibit significant effect. Effects of prednisolone on the cellular membrane were examined by employing cultured astrocytoma cells. Swelling and vacuole-formation of astrocytoma cells in media of low osmolarity were prevented by addition of prednisolone to that medium. It is suggested that steroids are concerned with permeability of the cellular membrane, thus exerting protective effects upon the blood-brain barrier.

Introduction

In most types of brain edema which we clinically encounter, all the substances which appear in the edematous tissue after the onset of the edema, such as surplus water, serum albumin [3] and others, can be regarded to have entered the brain tissue through the impaired blood-brain barrier. Therefore, if one could defend or repair the so-called barrier by applying some certain medicaments, this would succeed in preventing or treating brain edema.

I. Assay of the Protective Effects of Various Medicaments on the Blood-Brain Barrier by means of Radioactive Iodinated Serum Albumin (RISA)

Most of this part was published by us in 1963 [1, 4]. Adult mongrel dogs, 9–16 kg in weight, were anesthetized by intravenous sodium pentobarbital (25 mg/kg of body weight). The carotid arteries were exposed. RISA (8μCi/kg) was injected intravenously. Then, the medicaments to be tested were given intravenously. These were prednisolone (2 mg/kg, in the form of water-soluble prednisolone hemisuccinate), beta-methasone (0.2 mg/kg in the form of phosphate), ε-aminocaproic acid (1 g/kg), Venostasin (30 mg/kg) and α-chymotrypsin (0.5 mg/kg). 15 min later 0.1 ml/kg of sesame oil was injected into the left common carotid artery, in order to produce cerebral embolism and cerebral edema. The dogs were sacrificed 2 h later by infusing 200 ml of 10–15 % formalin into the carotid arteries and by aspirating the blood from the external jugular vein. The brain was deprived of the pia mater. 2 blocks were taken

177

from the gyrus lateralis and gyrus ectosylvius of the left cerebral hemisphere and their radioactive emission was measured with the aid of a scintillation counter.

As shown in Table 1, prednisolone (2 mg/kg) was demonstrated to have a remarkable prophylactic effect on the blood-brain barrier. When injected 15 min prior to the embolism production, prednisolone decreased the amount of RISA which invaded the brain tissue to less than one-tenth of that of control.

Table 1. Defence of the blood-brain barrier by various medicaments

	RISA-invasion (counts/g/min)	Standard deviation	Number of dogs
Non-treated group	13,540	5,381	7
Prednisolone (2 mg/kg)	1,093	728	6
Betamethasone (0.2 mg/kg)	5,687	2,610	9
Venostasin (30 mg/kg)	8,423	4,862	6
ε-Amino-caproic acid (1 g/kg)	11,273	5,542	7
α-Chymotrypsin (0.5 mg/kg)	13,364	4,760	4

Betamethasone, which is believed to be effective with one-tenth dosage as that of prednisolone, did not show the equivalent effect to that of prednisolone with the dosage one-tenth of prednisolone. This may imply that betamethasone must be used in a larger amount than one-tenth of that of prednisolone to prevent brain edema. Venostasin, ε-aminocaproic acid and α-chymotrypsin were not effective as far as defence of the blood-brain barrier was concerned.

In order to confirm the prophylactic effect of prednisolone and also various dosages of hydrocortisone on the blood-brain barrier, the same experiment was repeated in another series of mongrel dogs, this time dogs being sacrificed 3 h after the cerebral embolism. The results are shown in Table 2. Hydrocortisone (10 mg/kg) and prednisolone (2 mg/kg) were effective by a significant degree ($p < 0.01$) in protecting the blood-brain barrier, whereas hydrocortisone (5 mg/kg and 2 mg/kg) being not effective.

Table 2. Blood-brain barrier and corticosteroids

	Number of dogs	RISA-invasion (counts/g/min)
Hydrocortisone[a] (10 mg/kg)	12	5,263
Hydrocortisone (5 mg/kg)	5	11,648
Hydrocortisone (2 mg/kg)	5	11,520
Prednisolone[a] (2 mg/kg)	9	4,503
Control	11	12,311

[a] Effective by a significant degree ($p < 0.01$).

In clinical practice, steroids are administered usually after the blood-brain barrier has been impaired. Therefore, reparative effect of prednisolone on the damaged blood-brain barrier was tested as shown in Table 3.

Table 3. Reparation of the blood-brain barrier

I. Prednisolone 4 mg/kg 5 min after the impairment of B.B.B., RISA 8 μc/kg 15 min later than prednisolone	
No. 1	7,510
2	7,510
3	1,830
4	6,840
5	5,310
6	4,975
average	5,664 ($\sigma = 1,980$, $\sigma^2 = 3,920,400$)
II. Control	
No. 1	11,690
2	8,690
3	15,500
4	3,740
average	9,780 ($\sigma = 4,481$, $\sigma^2 = 20,079,361$)

5 min after the cerebral embolism production, prednisolone (4 mg/kg) was intravenously administered and then 15 min after the administration, RISA (8 μCi/kg) was intravenously injected. The dogs were sacrificed 2 h later. It seems prednisolone has a considerable reparative effect on the blood-brain barrier, although its prophylactic effect is more remarkable.

As previously reported elsewhere [4], succinic dehydrogenase activity of the nerve cells in the prednisolone-treated group was almost normal, whereas that in the nontreated group was fairly depressed in the same oil-embolism experiment in the dog. DPN- or TPN-diaphorase activity of the glial cells which markedly increased in the edematous brain tissue, was not so marked in the treated group as that in the nontreated. In a word, in the steroid-treated group, these enzymatic activities were kept within the normal limits. In these experiments prednisolone (4 mg/kg) was given 30 min after the oil-embolism formation, then prednisolone (2.5 mg/kg) was given daily for a week and then the animal was sacrificed. Therefore these findings support the conclusion that steroids are effective for brain edema, not only prophylactically, but also therapeutically.

Electron-microscopic findings also support this. Namely, alterations of the capillary endothelium (disruption and vesiculation), swelling of the basement membrane of the capillary and the astrocytes which were seen in the edematous brain of the control, were practically not observed in the steroid-treated group [4].

II. Differences of Therapeutic Effects of Steroid in Relation to the Time of Administration

Head injury was produced in the female rat, 100–110 g in weight, using Tedeschi's method [5]. As seen in Figure 1, the rat fixed in the cervical and lumbar region fell on a iron block, hit in the parietal region, the energy being about 0.9 joules. Almost all rats showed generalized convulsions and became unconscious, but recovered within a few minutes. About 20 % of rats died within a few minutes. These were excluded from the experiment. The other survived rats were kept in a room, 21–23° C in temperature and were observed for 7 days. They were divided into 4 groups.

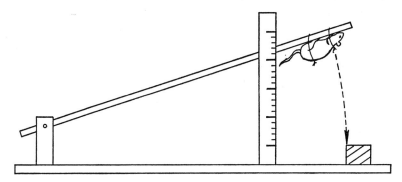

Fig. 1. Apparatus for experimental head injury

Group 1 (93 rats): Immediately after the injury, prednisolone sodium hemisuc-cinate (5 mg/kg) was administered intraperitoneally and then every 6 h intramuscularly (therefore 20 mg/kg per day). From the second day to the 7th day, prednisolone (5 mg/kg) acetate was given intramuscularly two times a day.

Group 2 (34 rats): The initial administration of prednisolone was 1 h after the injury. Subsequent injections were the same as in Group 1.

Group 3 (36 rats): The initial administration of prednisolone was 6 h after the injury. Subsequent injections were the same as in Group 1 and 2.

Group 4 (74 rats): Control. Prednisolone was not administered. Numbers of rats dead every day and in the total are listed in Table 4. This shows that the earlier the administration, the better are the results.

Table 4. Effects of steroid on head injury

Administration of prednisolone (5 mg/kg) started	Nos. of rats	Numbers of rats dead									Total	Mortality %
		0–1 h	1–6 h	1st day	2nd day	3rd day	4th day	5th day	6th day	7th day		
Without interval	93	(1)	(4)	13	4	2	4	6	5	2	36	39
1 h after injury	34	—	(2)	6	2	1	1	4	2	0	16	47
6 h after injury	36	—	—	8	2	3	2	4	1	0	20	55
Control	74	(3)	(3)	17	8	6	3	4	3	0	41	55

III. Assay of Protective Effects of Steroid on Cultured Astrocytic Cells Against low Osmolarity

It is known that the astrocytes especially the pericapillary astrocytes easily show changes even in the early stage of brain edema and the plasma protein infiltrates into

180

the astrocytes in case of edema. Therefore we experimented on the astrocytes. As the model of the astrocytes, cultured cells of fibrillary astrocytoma was used, using the trypsinization-monolayer method.

As seen in Table 5, there were 5 groups [2].

Group 1: Prednisolone was added to the culture medium in the concentration of 1 μg/ml, and at the same time, distilled water was added to dilute the culture medium.

Group 2: Prednisolone was added to the culture medium in the concentration of 1 mg/ml, and at the same time, distilled water was added to dilute the culture medium.

Group 3: Prednisolone was added to the culture medium in the concentration of 1 μg/ml, 30 min before diluting the medium with water.

Group 4: Prednisolone was added to the culture medium in the concentration of 1 mg/ml, 30 min before diluting the medium with water.

Group 5: Control. No prednisolone.

Osmolarity of the medium in each group was lowered by diluting it with water, to $1/3$, $1/5$ and $1/10$. 30 min after dilution, cells were stained with Giemsa and at least 200 cells of each group were observed under a microscope.

Table 5 shows percentage of cells showing swelling and vacuole formation in each group and each dilution. The percentage increases proportionately to lowering of osmolarity. Addition of prednisolone, however, apparently lowers this percentage.

Table 5. Vacuolization of astrocytes

Doses of prednisolone added (per ml)	Timing of addition	Rate of dilution 3× (%)	5× (%)	10× (%)
1 μg	simultaneously	17.2	23.1	100.0
1 mg	simultaneously	7.4	21.3	99.4
1 μg	30 min previously	5.1	15.6	95.6
1 mg	30 min previously	4.3	13.4	31.7
Control	—	19.8	33.9	99.3

For example, in the control group, the percentage was about 20%, 34% and 100% in the dilution of 3×, 5× and 10×, respectively, whereas in the Group 4, the percentage was 4%, 13% and 32% respectively. The data show the protective effects of prednisolone on the astrocytic cells against low osmolarity.

Furthermore, in the same experiment, when H^3-prednisolone was added, silver grains were observed on the surface of the cells or in the cytoplasm by means of autoradiography [2].

It may be suggested that steroids are concerned with permeability of the cellular membrane or active transport of the membrane, thus exerting protective effects upon the blood-brain barrier.

References

1. Hatanaka, H., Sano, K., Kitamura, K., Kamano, S., Masuzawa, H.: Steroids and cerebral edema. Brain & Nerve **15**, 624–633 (1963) (In Japanese).
2. Kamano, S.: Basic studies in cerebral edema in relation to corticosteroid therapy. Advances in Neurological Sciences **15**, 968–976 (1971) (In Japanese).
3. Klatzo, I., Miquel, H., Otenasek, R.: The application of fluorescein labeled serum proteins (FLSP) to the study of vascular permeability in the brain. Acta neuropath. (Berl.) **2**, 144–160 (1962).
4. Sano, K., Hatanaka, H., Kamano, S., Masuzawa, H.: Steroids and the blood-brain barrier with special reference to treatment of brain edema. Neurol. med.-chir. **5**, 21–43 (1963).
5. Tedeschi, C. G.: Cerebral injury by blunt mechanical trauma, special references to the effects of repeated impacts of minimal intensity. Observations on experimental animals. Arch. Neurol. Psychiat. **53**, 333–354 (1954).

Adrenal Cortical Response to Neurosurgical Problems, Noting the Effects of Exogenous Steroids

WILLIAM F. BOUZARTH, HENRY A. SHENKIN, and PAUL GUTTERMAN

Department of Neurosurgery, Episcopal Hospital, Philadelphia, PA 19125, USA

With 4 Figures

Summary. Adrenal cortical response has been studied in 238 patients with various types of neurosurgical problems, with the exception of those with pituitary lesions. The height and prolongation of plasma cortisol could usually be correlated with the severity of the clinical picture, and this was confirmed by cortisol production studies. However, there were examples where this correlation failed. After 24 h, diurnal rhythm (08.00 and 21.00 h) usually was restored. A reversal thereafter most often, but certainly not always, could be explained by a complication in the clinical course. Midline shift of the cerebral hemisphere, either acute or chronic, does not diminish the stress response and may enhance it. After uncomplicated brain surgery, accidental trauma, or hemorrhagic stroke, the adrenal cortical output had its most marked decline between the 24th and the 48th h, a time when cerebral edema appears to be gaining momentum. This suggests that exogenous steroids may exert a beneficial influence because cerebral edema evokes little or no protective adrenal cortical output. Dexamethasone suppresses adrenal cortical output following a somewhat more controlled form of cerebral trauma, craniotomy for brain tumor. This suppression is dose dependent.

Adrenocortical response to cerebral trauma, whether caused by a blow on the head, craniotomy for tumor, or spontaneous intracranial hemorrhage, can be measured by many parameters. Eosinopnea was one of the early clinical laboratory tests used to document the stress response. Although this eosinopnea also occurred as a result of adrenalin injection or ACTH, being the basis for the Thorn test [43], it soon gave way to more sophisticated procedures. Cortisol can be measured as a chromagen in the plasma [28], or urinary excretion of the 17-hydroxy-corticosteroids (17-OHCS) in a 24 h period can be used as a gauge of adrenocortical output [30]. Renal function must be adequate for this test to be valid; also, urinary excretion is only a rough guide to adrenal function as it varies both with the psychological state and with body size [32]. In our laboratory, it has not been possible to correlate urinary 17-OHCS excretion with the clinical picture. The Silber-Porter method measures other chromagens, so this test is not a reliable indicator for 17-OHCS especially during starvation [42] or when the patient is near death [34]; however, 17-OHCS can be measured by a fluorometric method which is more reliable, although corticosterone is also measured

Supported in part by U.S. Public Health Service Research Grant NS-04996.

[33]. The level of circulating 17-OHCS varies according to the time of day or night (circadian rhythm) with the 08.00 level being greater than at 21.00 h. A reversal of this diurnal variation has been used as a guide to the stress response; this will be discussed later. The level of circulating free plasma cortisol also relates to liver function [44], cellular uptake, amount of globulin binding (transcortin) [29], serum dilution, and renal clearance as well as to its production. The ratio of bound and free cortisol has been used to study the stress response [2]. An isotopic dilution technique which reflects cortisol production by way of its renal excretion has been advocated [9]. Thus, there is no single test that adequately reflects the total adrenocortical response to stress, but all the tests mentioned serve as a guide.

Most clinical reports deal with non-neurosurgical disease, which is surprising since the centers for the stress response reside within the skull. However, diurnal variation of plasma 17-OHCS was reported to be abolished in subjects with severe brain damage [10]. This was confirmed [15, 24], but others [21, 27] noted the persistence of diurnal rhythm in patients with cerebral neoplasm or epilepsy. In 1959, urinary 17-OHCS were reported to be increased after neurosurgical procedures in 5 patients [12]. Later, seven patients with tumor involving the diencephalon demonstrated less excretion of 17-OHCS than eight with tumor not involving the hypothalamic pituitary region [35]. 14 patients with intracranial extrasellar lesions simulated primary pituitary disease [18], but the majority of pathology involved the diencephalon. It had been our concern that brain pathology at a distance from pituitary gland could affect the hypothalamo-hypophyseal tracts since the infundibular stalk and its portal system represent the final common pathway from the brain to the pituitary gland. When a supratentorial mass shifts the cerebral midline structures, the infundibular stalk undergoes physical stress, acting as a checkrein to maintain the floor of the third ventricle nearly in the midline (Fig. 1). In this circumstance 4 types of stress response can be expected: 1) normal, 2) exaggerated, 3) depressed, or 4) perverted. We wish to report our findings in 238 patients with neurosurgical disease or injury, many with marked midline displacement.

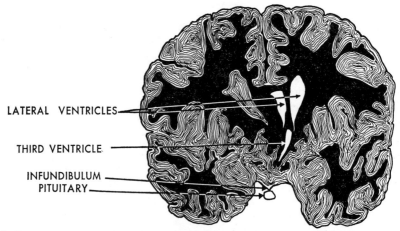

LATERAL VENTRICLES
THIRD VENTRICLE
INFUNDIBULUM
PITUITARY

Fig. 1. Demonstration of the floor of the third ventricle being maintained nearly in the midline when a hemispheral mass lesion shifts the lateral ventricle and the roof of the third ventricle; the infundibular stalk serves as a checkrein

Over a decade ago, pharmacologic doses of corticosteroids were suggested for the treatment of cerebral edema in neurosurgical problems [3, 13]. The rationale was the previous observations [16, 31] that replacement therapy for pituitary tumors significantly reduced the mortality rate with minimal evidence of post-operative cerebral edema. In our study, 42 patients with brain tumor were treated with either cortisone, hydrocortisone, and/or ACTH. An equal number of untreated patients served as controls. Needless to say, the patients treated with steroids, overall, did better than the control patients. In addition, daily morning eosinophil counts were obtained in both groups of patients. If the chamber count was below five on the first and the second post-operative day, the patient was doing well. A count above 25 generally correlated with a stormy post-operative course. We next reported the benefit of hydrocortisone in 14 neurosurgical patients with altered levels of consciousness and sudden collapse of the circulation [36].

In light of this experience it appeared desirable to evaluate the natural adrenocortical response (glucocorticoids) in neurosurgical patients (Fig. 2). 66 hospitalized patients with no brain disease but with somatic pain had higher morning (08.00) and evening (21.00) plasma cortisol levels than our healthy, non-hospitalized subjects [37]. 14 patients undergoing hemilaminectomy for lumbar discs were used as the standard for comparison with patients who had undergone brain surgery. On the operative day, evening values were increased over the preoperative morning levels in the majority with a trend towards normal in both a.m. and p.m. samples over the next 5 days; the averages remained above the preoperative value. Except in 3 instances out of 46 observations the diurnal variation was preserved [41]. Two additional patients undergoing extensive laminectomy had a much greater and more prolonged response. Thus, it appears that neurosurgical patients who did not have brain disease had elevation of plasma cortisol proportional to the severity of the neurosurgical procedure. As such, they did not differ from general surgical patients.

A study of eight older patients undergoing retrogasserian rhizotomy revealed that patients suffering from tic douloureux had a higher preoperative level of circulating

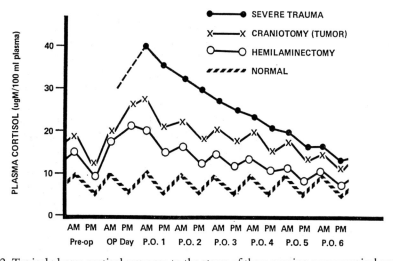

Fig. 2. Typical plasma cortisol response to the stress of three varying neurosurgical problems

17-OHCS, which made the post-operative elevations less apparent. None of these patients had normal levels by the sixth post-operative day. This prolongation was greater than that seen in general surgical patients, but similar to the 2 patients undergoing extensive laminectomy [6].

In a study of the adrenocortical response to craniotomy for brain tumor, the urinary excretion of 17-OHCS was noted to be increased during the first three post-operative days returning to normal by the 7th day [26]. Plasma levels were not reported. In our series (Fig. 2) of 32 patients undergoing craniotomy for brain tumor [41], the preoperative plasma cortisol values were found to be elevated 30% above normal with the diurnal variation persisting. This indicates that despite a midline shift, which was present in the majority of patients, adrenal cortical secretion was increased. On the evening of the operative day plasma cortisol levels were increased 125% above the preceding evening, being 23% higher than those of the laminectomy group. The highest plasma cortisol was on this evening and/or the next morning. Thereafter, plasma cortisol levels decreased and reached normal usually by the ninth postoperative day. This response is of greater duration than observed after general surgical procedures [1] or laminectomy, but similar to that observed after retrogasserian rhizotomy. On the whole, diurnal variation was maintained preoperatively and reversed on the day of operation. Thereafter, it was maintained 85% of the time. We had anticipated that reversals in the circadian rhythm would correlate with the clinical course and thus predict a complication or a poor prognosis. No such correlation could be made in 5 of the 12 observed reversals.

It was particularly interesting that there was a tendency for a sudden rise in plasma cortisol levels, both morning and evening, on the 5th or 6th day. This does correlate with an unexpected naturesis and chloruresis that was found to occur rather consistently in the same post-operative period [39]. While there is no obvious explanation for these late post-operative observations the fact that they were noted independently, thus confirming one another, indicates that an unrecognized metabolic phenomenon must take place at that time.

61 patients presented with cranial injury, minimal body trauma and no known pre-existing disease were graded on a 1–10 scale and their adrenocortical response studied in detail, including cortisol production [5]. Of the 22 who were judged to have severe injuries (Fig. 2), 7 died. 18 were considered to have moderately severe injury, and 12 had only minimal damage. 9 additional patients were operated on for chronic lesions such as subdural hydromas or hydrocephalus two or more weeks after the trauma. Slightly more than 50% of the patients in this series required surgery, 14 within 3 days of injury. The degree of elevation of plasma cortisol and the amount of cortisol produced in 24 h, as determined by the isotopic dilutional technique [9], was greatest in patients with severe craniocerebral injuries and was minimal in those with mild injury. In the moderately severe group there was great variability in the glucocorticoid response. It is not certain if this is due to the inability to grade properly the mid-zone of cranial injury. A later study [20] of 13 head injured patients confirmed our findings that plasma cortisol levels are greater in severe and less in mild trauma, but they, too, could not correlate the degree of trauma to the adrenocortical response. In war injuries, plasma cortisol elevation did not correlate to somatic trauma [7]. Further work should be done in this regard, for it may be that the glucocorticoid response serves as a reliable guide to the severity of injury.

The prolongation of the elevation of plasma cortisol also correlated to the severity of the initial injury. This is similar to that observed in the group operated on for brain tumor. Reversal of the diurnal rhythm of plasma cortisol on the days after injury occurred infrequently, being observed 33 times out of 175 observations (19 %). Usually a surgical procedure or a clinical complication, such as protracted convulsions or infection, accounted for the reversal, but as with the brain tumor group, no reason for reversal could be found in 8 patients.

A surprising fact was noted in the group which underwent neurosurgical procedures after trauma. The height of the plasma cortisol elevation depended upon the interval between injury and operation. The earlier a corrective procedure was performed, the greater was the response and the longer the elevation lasted. Patients operated on 14 or more days after injury had a minimal response but their operative procedures were generally more benign, compared to those who were operated on early.

10 patients exhibiting decerebrate rigidity were studied in the subacute or chronic phase [14]. Intravenous metopirone tests were performed in four. These patients demonstrated a similar elevation of plasma cortisol level in the acute phase as did the severely injured patients without decerebrate posturing. 4 patients with acute decerebration also showed an increase of two-fold or greater in the 24 h urinary 17-OHCS output following intravenous infusion of metopirone. Another patient, studied two months after injury, exhibited a four-fold increase in his urinary 17-OHCS. These results indicate an intact adrenal cortex and an intact feedback mechanism. However, other observers [25] performed the metopirone test in 11 severely head injured patients and found a failure to respond in 4 (3 with cortical damage and 1 with apparent brain stem damage). That these 4 patients also failed to respond adequately to dexamethasone suppression is evidence suggesting disturbance in the hypothalamic-pituitary-adrenal feedback mechanism. Although we did not perform formal dexamethasone suppression tests, 2 patients were treated with pharmacological doses of dexamethasone (4 mg every 4 h), and they showed greater than 50 % reduction in their previously elevated cortisol levels. Our results differ and suggest that the negative feedback control by the level of circulating plasma cortisol does not require a normally functioning brain stem, and this has been reported by others [19].

29 patients [38] with hemorrhagic stroke had increased cortisol, an average elevation on the first day of 50 % over normal. After that, there was a steady decline towards normal during the next week. Diurnal reversals occurred in at least one half of these patients, usually without obvious cause. (Another report of 18 patients noted abnormal diurnal variations in 11 [17].) When surgery was performed, there was a marked elevation in the height of that response depending on the timing of the operation similar to that observed in the trauma group [4]. In the non-operative cases the plasma cortisol in subsequent weeks remained either abnormally high or approached normal, generally paralleling the clinical course.

Although it is difficult to assess cerebral edema in vivo, it is generally accepted that this develops over the first few days after a cerebral insult. The rapid early decline of plasma cortisol after uncomplicated but severe head injury or after craniotomy for tumor suggests that cerebral edema evokes little or no stress reaction because circulating glucocorticoids were found to be diminishing at the time that the cerebral edema was considered to be clinically increasing (Fig. 3). This may be an explanation of the beneficial effect of exogenous glucocorticoids in these patients. Also, the variability of cortisol output in the moderately injured group, indicates that some patients will have a low cortisol output even though they appear to be moderately severely injured and, hence, may be in need of exogenous steroids as compared to the others who do not.

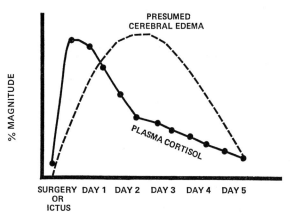

Fig. 3. Daily plasma cortisol levels after cerebral trauma compared with the presumed course of cerebral edema

Seven other patients with neurosurgical disorders had, in addition, acute gastrointestinal bleeding [40]. At the time of bleeding the mean plasma cortisol (Silber-Porter) and the transcortin binding capacities were 36.0 and 12.5 μg/100 ml respectively as compared to 30 and 17.8 μg/100 ml in 144 patients who did not bleed. It can be assumed that the amount of free (or active) cortisol was unusually high, and this fact may account for erosion and bleeding. This possibility should always be kept in mind with patients whose preexisting disease may lead to low serum protein, especially if exogenous steroids in pharmacological doses are contemplated.

Effect of Dexamethasone

Having described the adrenocortical response to neurosurgical problems, the next step is to note the effect of dexamethasone. This synthetic steroid is well known to suppress ACTH release and lower 24 h urinary 17-OHCS [22]. Rather than measure urinary 17-OHCS, 24 h cortisol production was determined by an isotopic dilutional technique [9]. Plasma cortisol was also obtained at 08.00 and 21.00 h. 19 patients undergoing craniotomy were divided into 3 groups. Group I did not receive dexamethasone; patients in Group II were given 12 mg of dexamethasone intravenously prior to surgery and were maintained on 4 mg administered intramuscularly every 4 h until the seventh post-operative day; and Group III patients received half of the above dose on the same schedule. Cortisol production in the post-operative period was considered to be suppressed if it was lower than the preoperative level in the same patient. Also, post-operative cortisol production in those patients receiving dexamethasone was considered to be relatively suppressed if it was less than the average production in the untreated group. The results are summarized in Figure 4.

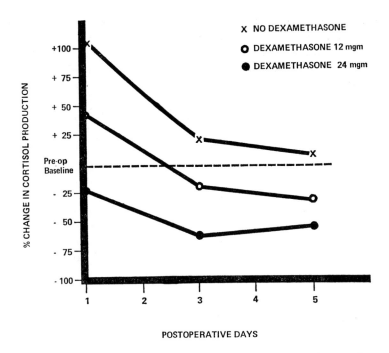

Fig. 4. Dexamethasone suppression of cortisol production after craniotomy for tumor

There was no significant difference in average preoperative cortisol production studies in the 3 groups. Cortisol produced in the first 24 h post-operative period by patients not treated with dexamethasone was increased to a level more than twice that of the preoperative level. From this elevation, a steady decline occurred by the fifth post-operative day to preoperative levels. On the first post-operative day, 6 of 7 patients receiving high amounts of dexamethasone (Group II) showed a reduction in the cortisol production below preoperative levels (an average decrease of 26 %). This differed significantly from the response of patients not receiving the steroid ($p < 0.01$). On the third post-operative day cortisol production was further suppressed in all patients in Group II (an average decrease of 67 % below preoperative levels). This was again noted to differ significantly from the response of Group I patients ($p < 0.01$). On the fifth post-operative day cortisol production remained suppressed in 6 of 7 patients in Group II, and average cortisol production was 55 % less than preoperative levels ($p < 0.01$).

On the first post-operative day, 5 of 6 patients receiving the lower dose of dexamethasone demonstrated an increase in cortisol production above preoperative levels (an average increase of 41 %). Nevertheless, their cortisol levels were 66 % lower than those noted in the group receiving no steroids. On the third and fifth post-operative days cortisol production was noted to be suppressed 21 % and 34 % respectively, below the preoperative levels, as compared to increases in cortisol production in the patients of Group I. The suppression of cortisol production below preoperative levels by dexamethasone was noted in both groups, but was more marked in the group given 24 mg dexamethasone daily. Failure to suppress cortisol production below preoperative levels with massive steroid doses was associated with clinical deterioration in both of the 2 instances out of 21 in Group II and 7 of 18 instances in the patients treated with half the amount of dexamethasone (Group III).

Isotopic cortisol production studies showed a relatively greater increase after craniotomy than did plasma cortisol levels in the nontreated group. The rise in mean cortisol production was more than three times the rise in plasma cortisol on the first post-operative day. This difference was significant ($p < 0.01$). Both the 24 h cortisol production and diurnal plasma cortisol levels then declined to preoperative levels on the third to fifth post-operative days with the fall being more precipitous in isotopic cortisol production levels. The more precipitous initial drop in cortisol production can also be noted in Groups II and III.

Under normal conditions a negative feedback mechanism regulates hypothalamic-anterior pituitary-adrenocortical function by which a small dose of dexamethasone given on the night preceding surgery may suppress plasma cortisol [8]. Failure of suppression with daily doses of dexamethasone up to 32 mg has been reported in patients with pituitary hypersecretion, adrenal hyperplasia, or adrenal tumor [23]. This may be due to the unusually high setting of the control mechanism for ACTH secretion or autonomous secretion of cortisol from an ectopic source. Under conditions of stress produced by surgery there is a marked elevation of plasma ACTH levels despite initially elevated cortisol levels, causing a further rise in the plasma cortisol levels. It has been hypothesized that the negative feedback mechanism still functions under these circumstances but that the "thermostat" is set at a higher level [45].

The adrenocortical response to laparatomy in patients receiving dexamethasone was similar to that of control patients [1]. It was concluded that the negative feedback mechanism does not function during major stress which corroborates a previous report [11]. Large doses of dexamethasone produced a decrease in urinary 17-OHCS levels in 85% of patients following craniotomy for brain tumor which is indirect evidence of suppression [26]. Our results demonstrate that 24 mg and 12 mg of dexamethasone daily cause definite suppression of cortisol production, the magnitude of which, with the present evidence, appears to be directly dose dependent. This suppression occurs even though our previous observations indicate that adrenocortical response to craniotomy is more prolonged and intense than the response to general surgical procedures [41]. Cortisol production studies revealed a more intense initial response to craniotomy than noted in diurnal plasma cortisol levels as well as a greater degree of suppression in the post-operative period.

Conclusions

1. There is no single, simple laboratory method which accurately reflects adrenal cortical response to neurosurgical problems. Plasma 17-OHCS determined by a non-chromagen technique [33] obtained at 08.00 and 21.00 h, as well as urinary secretion of labeled cortisol to denote 24 h production [9], serve as useful guides to the stress response.

2. When lumbar laminectomy is used as a standard operation, brain surgery for tumor evokes a greater and more prolonged cortisol output indicating that displace-

190

ment of the brain across the midline and/or increased intracranial pressure does not diminish the general stress response; in fact, may enhance it.

3. Acute neurosurgical lesions, such as trauma or spontaneous intracranial bleeding, evoke a stronger steroid response when the patient is severely damaged and a lesser one in milder problems. This observation does not always hold for those patients judged to fall into the mid-zone of injury. (Whether this is due to the inadequate clinical testing or to a varied stress response is not certain.)

4. During uncomplicated recovery the most rapid decline in cortisol output occurs between the 24th and 48th h, a time when clinical evidence suggests cerebral edema to be accelerating. Perhaps this indicates that cerebral edema, per se, evokes little or no response from the adrenal gland; whereas, surgery during this same time produces an exaggerated response.

5. After the acute phase, endocrine studies in patients with brain stem damage manifested by decerebrate rigidity indicate that an intact brain stem is not required for the negative feedback mechanisms of cortisol control.

6. Diurnal variations occur in the majority of post-operative or post-traumatic days, and reversals usually predict an obvious cause. Either the morning or evening values, or both, reach normal after seven days following craniotomy or serious accidental brain trauma.

7. Gastrointestinal bleeding in neurosurgical patients occurs most frequently when the active or free plasma cortisol is unusually high. A more subtle cause of gastrointestinal bleeding may be the patient with pre-existing disease resulting in diminished plasma protein as measured by transcortin, which binds cortisol.

8. The administration of dexamethasone appears to diminish the expected adrenal cortical output in neurosurgical patients. The degree of suppression is dose dependent.

9. From this study of neurosurgical patients with apparent normal pituitary and adrenal function, glucocorticoid administration in pharmacological doses may be used in: a) all patients with moderate to severe cerebral trauma; b) during the phase of cerebral edema after elective craniotomy; and, c) whenever surgery is delayed for chronic traumatic lesions. Obviously, this treatment is contraindicated in patients with peptic ulcer disease or those patients with pre-existing plasma protein deficiency.

References

1. Asfeldt, V. H., Elb, S.: Hypothalamo-pituitary-adrenal response during major surgical stress. Acta endocr. (Kbh.) **59**, 67 (1968).
2. Beisel, W. R., DiRaimondo, V. C., Forsham, P. H.: Cortisol transport and disappearance. Ann. intern. Med. **60**, 641 (1964).
3. Bouzarth, W. F.: The effect of cortisone, hydrocortisone and ACTH in cerebral function following craniotomy. In: A. S. Marrazzi, Aprison, M. H. (Eds): Studies of Function in Health and Disease, Galesburg, Ill.: Galesburg State Hospital Press. 1960.
4. — Feldman, W., Shenkin, H. A.: Corticosteroid response to acute cerebral injury and subarachnoid hemorrhage. Trans. Coll. Phycns Philad. **35**, 32 (1967).
5. — Shenkin, H. A., Feldman, W.: Adrenocortical response to craniocerebral trauma. Surg. Gynec. Obstet. **126**, 995 (1968).
6. — — Unpublished data.
7. Carey, L. C., Cloutier, C. T., Lowery, B. D.: Growth hormone and adrenal cortical response to shock and trauma in the human. Ann. Surg. **174**, 451 (1971).

8. Connolly, C. K., Gore, M. B. R., Wills, S. N.: Single dose dexamethasone suppression in normal subjects and hospital patients. Brit. med. J. **2**, 665 (1968).
9. Cope, C. L., Black, E. G.: The production rate of cortisol in man. Brit. med. J. **1**, 1020 (1958).
10. Eik-Nes, K., Clark, I. D.: Diurnal variation of plasma 17-hydrocorticosteroid in subjects suffering from severe brain damage. J. clin. Endocr. **18**, 764 (1958).
11. Estep, H. L., Island, D. P., Ney, R. L., Liddle, G. W.: Pituitary adrenal dynamics during surgical stress. J. clin. Endocr. **23**, 419 (1963).
12. Fisher, R. G., Copenhaver, J. H., Jr., Naukkarinen, I.: Adrenal cortical hormone output in cerebral injury and neoplasm. Surg. Forum **9**, 683 (1959).
13. Galicich, J. H., French, L. A.: Use of dexamethasone in the treatment of cerebral edema resulting from brain tumors and brain surgery. Amer. Practit. **12**, 169 (1961).
14. Gutterman, P., Bouzarth, W. F., Shenkin, H. A.: Unpublished data.
15. Halasz, B., Vernikos-Danellis, J., Gorski, R. A.: Pituitary ACTH content in rats after partial or total interruption of neural afferents to the medial basal hypothalamus. Endocrinology **81**, 921 (1967).
16. Ingraham, F. D., Matson, D. D., McLaurin, R. L.: Cortisone and ACTH as an adjunct to the surgery of craniopharyngiomas. New Engl. J. Med. **246**, 568 (1952).
17. Jenkins, J. S., Westlake, S., Buckell, M., Carter, A. B.: Diurnal variations after subarachnoid hemorrhage. Brit. med. J. **4**, 707 (1969)
18. Kahana, L., Lebovitz, H., Lush, W., et al.: Endocrine manifestations of intracranial extrasellar lesions. J. clin. Endocrinol. **22**, 304 (1962).
19. Kendall, J. W., Allen, C., Greer, M. A.: ACTH secretion in midbrain-transected rats. Endocrinology **77**, 1091 (1965).
20. King, L. R., McLaurin, R. L., Lewis, H. P., Knowles, H. C., Jr.: Plasma cortisol levels after head injury. Ann. Surg. **172**, 975 (1970).
21. Krieger, D. T., Krieger, H. P.: Circadian variation of the plasma 17-hydroxycorticosteroids in central nervous system disease. J. clin. Endocr. **26**, 929 (1966).
22. Liddle, G. W.: Tests of pituitary adrenal suppressability in the diagnosis of Cushing's Syndrome. J. clin. Endocr. **20**, 1539 (1960).
23. Linn, J. E., Bowdoin, B., Farmer, T. A., Meador, C. K.: Observations and comments on the failure of dexamethasone suppression. New Engl. J. Med. **277**, 403 (1967).
24. Mason, J. W.: Central nervous system regulation of ACTH stimulation. In: Jasper, H. H. (Ed.): Reticular Formation of the Brain, Boston: Little, Brown and Co. 1958.
25. McCarthy, C. F., Wills, M. R., Keane, P. M., et al.: The Su-4885 (methopyrapone) response after head injury. J. clin. Endocr. **24**, 121 (1964).
26. Nakamura, K.: Pituitary-adrenocortical response after craniotomy for brain tumor, and its suppression with administered glucocorticoid. Nagoya J. med. Sci. **30**, 69 (1967).
27. Oppenheimer, J. H., Fisher, L. V., Jailer, J. W.: Disturbance of the pituitary-adrenal interrelationship in disease of the central nervous system. J. clin. Endocr. **21**, 1023 (1961).
28. Peterson, R. E., Karrer, A., Guerra, S. L.: Evaluation of Silber-Porter procedure for determination of plasma hydrocortisone. Anal. Chem. **29**, 144 (1957).
29. Plager, J. E., Knopp, R., Slauwhite, W. R., Jr., Sandberg, A. A.: Cortisol binding by dog plasma. Endocrinology **73**, 353 (1963).
30. Porter, C. C., Silber, R. H.: A quantitative color reaction for cortisone and related 17.21-dihydroxy-20-ketosteroids. J. biol. Chem. **185**, 201 (1950).
31. Raaf, J., Stainsby, D. L., Larson, W. L. E.: The use of ACTH in conjunction with surgery for neoplasms in the parasellar area. J. Neurosurg. **11**, 463 (1954).
32. Rose, R. M., Poe, R. O., Mason, J. W.: Factors affecting corticosteroid excretion. Arch. intern. Med. **121**, 406 (1968).
33. Rudd, B. J., Sampson, P., Brooke, B. N.: A new fluorometric method of plasma cortisol assay with a study of pituitary adrenal function using metapyrone. J. Endocr. **27**, 317 (1963).
34. Sandberg, A. A., Eik-Nes, K., Migeon, C. J., Samuels, J. T.: Metabolism of adrenal steroids in dying patients. J. clin. Endocr. **16**, 1001 (1956).
35. Sawada, K.: Alterations in Total Urinary 17-OHCS and serum ADS following surgical operations of the brain. Tohoku J. exp. Med. **87**, 262 (1956).

36. Shenkin, H. A.: Acute hypotension treated successfully with hydrocortisone. New Engl. J. Med. **264**, 645 (1961).
37. — The effect of pain on the diurnal pattern of plasma corticoid levels. Neurology (Minneap.) **14**, 1112 (1964).
38. — Bouzarth, W. F., Feldman, W.: Plasma cortisol values in spontaneous intracranial hemorrhage. Circulation **34**, 216 (1966).
39. — — Tatsumi, T.: Analysis of body water compartments in postoperative craniotomy patients. I. Effect of craniotomy alone. J. Neurosurg. **28**, 417 (1968).
40. — Feldman, W.: Plasma cortisol binding globulin levels in gastro-intestinal bleeding of stress origin. J. clin. Endocr. **28**, 15 (1968).
41. — Gutterman, P., Bouzarth, W. F.: The adrenocortical response to craniotomy for brain tumor. J. Neurosurg. **34**, 657 (1971).
42. Schultz, A. L., Kerlow, A., Ulstrom, R. A.: Effect of starvation on adrenal cortical function of obese subjects. J. clin. Endocr. **24**, 1253 (1964).
43. Thorn, G. W.: The Diagnosis and Treatment of Adrenal Insufficiency. Springfield, Ill.: Charles C. Thomas 1949.
44. Tyler, F. H., Schmidt, C. D., Eik-Nes, K., *et al.*: The role of the liver and the adrenal in producing elevated plasma 17-hydroxycorticosteroid levels in surgery. J. clin. Invest. **33**, 1517 (1954).
45. Yates, F. E., Leeman, S. E., Glenisten, D. W., Dallman, M. F.: Interaction between plasma corticosterone concentration and adrenocorticotrophic releasing stimuli in the rat: Evidence for the reset of an endocrine feedback control. Endocrinology **69**, 67 (1961).

Physiological and Biochemical Findings in the Central Nervous System of Adrenalectomized Rats and Mice*

Alexander Baethmann** and Anthonie Van Harreveld

Institute for Surgical Research, Dept. Surgery, University Munich and Division of Biology, California Institute of Technology, Pasadena, CA 91109, USA

With 5 Figures

Summary. Adrenalectomy produces in rats and mice a water and Na^+ accumulation in the CNS which is similar to changes found in metabolic forms of brain edema. In adrenalectomized animals the cerebral water content is in close correlation with the tissue/plasma Na^+- and K^+-concentration gradient and, furthermore, appears to be a function of the external sodium supply. Impedance measurements and results obtained from electron-microscopy suggest that the fluid is not intracellularly localized but probably distributes within the extracellular space. Tissue concentration levels of energy-rich phosphate compounds or of lactate and pyruvate revealed no changes after adrenalectomy. Changes of metabolic activity as demonstrated by a decreased activity of NADP-dependent ICDH, GLDH and GOT may, however, participate in the mechanisms which produce the cerebral Na^+ and water influx.

Studies on corticosteroid deprivation of the CNS, experimentally produced by adrenalectomy, may enhance the understanding of the mechanism of the effects of these hormones on brain edema. Clinical and experimental observations indicate that adrenalectomy affects the CNS in various ways. The electroshock seizure threshold as a measure of brain excitability is found to be reduced in adrenal insufficient rats [6]. Reports concerning electrolyte changes in the cerebral tissue are not uniform however. Increases of the cerebral water and Na^+ content, with the K^+ remaining unchanged, or K^+ decreases and Na^+ remaining unchanged, as well as a lack of electrolyte changes, have been found in cerebral tissue of adrenalectomized animals [2, 6, 7, 16, 17]. Different experimental conditions are probably responsible for these conflicting results, e.g., the use of female rats [7] which are shown to display alterations of the cerebral water content during the estrous cycle [10]. Usually no attempts were made to test the total surgical removal of all adrenal tissue.

The interest of this laboratory in possible steroid effects on the water and electrolyte composition of the central nervous system derived from observations on brain edema. A possible involvement of corticosteroid activity was suggested by characteristically changed electrolyte patterns, such as a reduced Na^+ and increased K^+ excretion in the urine of animals with experimental traumatic brain edema [14]. Corresponding clinical results confirmed these findings in patients with severe head

---

* Dedicated to Prof. R. Zenker for his 70th birthday.

** Member of Sonderforschungsbereich 51, 4 BE.

Supported in part by USPHS Grants, 1FO5TW01688 and NB-07658, and by the Deutsche Forschungsgemeinschaft Ba 452/1.

injury or after major intracranial surgery [5, 21]. In order to obtain more information concerning an interaction along the CNS-adrenal axis in brain edema, a variety of investigations were carried out dealing with physiological and biochemical changes in the CNS after adrenalectomy. In some instances, studies of substitution with different steroid hormones were included. Due consideration was given to the surgical removal of all adrenal tissue, applying a water retention test. The studies here reported, include measurements of the cerebral electrolyte and water content, determinations of the labile energy-rich phosphate compounds, and, of the activity of enzymes related to the tricarboxylic acid cycle which in other organs were shown to be sensitive to aldosterone [8, 9, 11], finally, attempts to assess possible changes of the cerebral water distribution with physiological methods and electronmicroscopy.

Figure 1 shows the sodium and potassium content in the CNS and plasma of controls and adrenalectomized animals, without and with substitution with various steroids. Adrenalectomy produces a significant increase of the cerebral water and sodium content, similar to that observed in metabolic forms of brain edema [1, 15]. The plasma-Na^+ and K^+ changes are typical for adrenal insufficiency. Corticosteroids with different properties such as aldosterone, dexamethasone, or desoxy-corticosterone were more or less identical in preventing these changes.

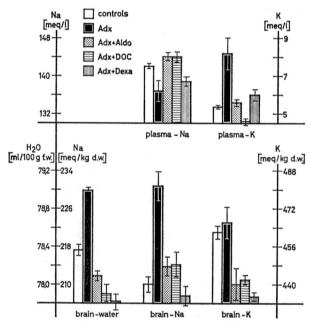

Fig. 1. Cerebral water and electrolyte content (mean ± SEM) of controls and adrenalectomized rats without and with substitution with various corticosteroids (bottom). On top the corresponding plasma electrolyte concentration (mean ± SEM). Adx = adrenalectomized; Aldo = aldosterone (0.1 mg/kg/day); DOC = desoxycorticosteroneacetate (10 mg/kg/day); Dexa = dexamethasone (0.4 mg/kg/day); f.w. = fresh weight; d.w. = dry weight

Figure 2 is a diagram which shows the relationship between the brain water and the sodium or potassium gradient, respectively. Since the intracellular electrolyte concen-

196

trations were not known the real intra-exctracellular Na$^+$ and K$^+$ gradient cannot be calculated. Therefore the ratio of the respective brain and plasma electrolyte concentrations was used as a measure for this entity. This graph implies that in adrenalectomy the brain water is correlated with the electrolyte gradient between brain and plasma. Furthermore the external sodium supply apparently has an influence on these parameters. In adrenalectomized animals maintained on a high sodium regimen a lower cerebral water content combined with a higher electrolyte gradient was found, as compared to adrenalectomized animals on a low sodium diet. The observation of a protective effect of a Na$^+$-rich diet on the excessive water accumulation in the brain of adrenalectomized animals may, at least in part, explain the beneficial effects of a high sodium regimen in adrenal insufficiency, e.g., a longer survival time, etc.

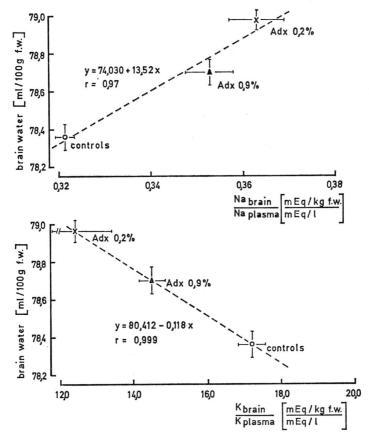

Fig. 2. Correlation diagram of the brain water and the Na$^+$ (or K$^+$) tissue/plasma distribution ratio. The electrolyte distribution ratio may be considered as a measure of the tissue/plasma gradient. An increase along the abscissa signifies for K$^+$ an increase of the gradient, and for Na$^+$ a decrease of the gradient. Adrenalectomized animals received a 0.2% NaCl solution (Adx 0.2%) or a 0.9% NaCl (Adx 0.9%) solution as drinking fluid

In studies concerned with the distribution of the fluid accumulation in the CNS the sodium- or chloride-spaces are often considered [17]. In view of the probability that the distribution of the electrolytes themselves may be subject to changes after adrenalectomy, this procedure appears to be questionable. In investigations made in Munich in collaboration with Horsch and Steude [4] the technique of ventriculo-cisternal perfusion of the brain with an extracellular label was applied in adrenalectomized rats. This technique is designed to circumvent the blood-brain barrier.

Preliminary results of ventriculo-cisternal perfusion in adrenalectomized animals are shown in Figure 3, in which the tissue/perfusate ratio and the tissue/plasma ratio of labeled Na-thiosulfate on the ordinate is plotted against the time on the abscissa. The distribution space in the tissue was calculated both using the marker concentration of the plasma and of the artificial cerebro-spinal fluid as reference value. Compared to control animals, in which a distribution space of about 12 % was obtained, the marker distribution appears to be somewhat smaller after adrenalectomy, especially when calculated from the tissue/perfusate ratio. The computed distribution space using the perfusion fluid as reference probably reflects more faithfully the real distribution due to a less restricted access of the marker to the tissue.

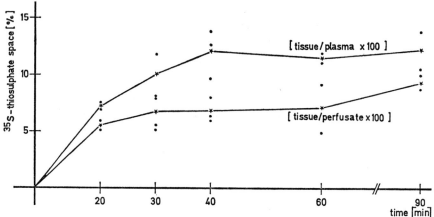

Fig. 3. S-35-thiosulphate distribution space after ventriculo-cisternal perfusion in the brain of adrenalectomized rats. The space is computed as follows:

$$\frac{\text{tissue activity [IPM/g w.w.]}}{\text{plasma (or perfusate) activity [IPM/g]}} \times 100.$$

The corresponding thiosulphate space computed as [tissue-activity/perfusate-activity] × 100 of controls (not shown here) is about 12% after 60 min perfusion time [4]. IPM = impulses per minute

However, according to more recently published observations, the ventriculo-cisternal perfusion as a method employed to study the extracellular space may suffer some shortcomings, due to a concentration gradient from the ependymal surface to the subarachnoidal space, which persists over a long experimental period [12, 13]

Two different approaches for an estimate of the extracellular space were used at the California Institute of Technology; the measurement of the specific electrical resistance of the cortical tissue in adrenalectomized animals and electron-microscopy of freeze-substituted material in which the fluid distribution in the central nervous system was shown to be preserved more faithfully [19]. The tissue impedance was measured between two surface silver–silverchloride electrodes by means of an equal ratio impedance bridge. The electrodes were placed on the exposed cortical surface of

198

rats, which had been adrenalectomized approximately 10 days prior to the experiment. Using a low frequency (1000 cps) alternating current, the tissue impedance, or its reciprocal, the conductivity, can be considered as a function of the abundance of extracellular material [18]. Circulatory arrest was induced in control and experimental animals by severing the major abdominal vessels just below the diaphragm. As previously shown by Van Harreveld [20], asphyxiation of the cerebral tissue causes typical fluid and electrolyte shifts from the extra- to the intracellular compartment accompanied by a drop in conductivity. The magnitude of the asphyxial conductivity change observed over a certain time period, therefore may be related to the amount of extracellular material present before the asphyxiation. We analyzed the asphyxial drop in conductivity in controls and after adrenalectomy as shown in Table 1. As seen, the initial conductivity in adrenalectomized animals is slightly higher compared to controls, indicative for a somewhat larger volume of extracellular space; the difference, however, does not attain statistical significance.

Table 1. Conductivity [mho $\times$ 10^6] before and 10 min after circulatory arrest in controls and adrenalectomized animals given as mean value $\pm$ SEM

	Conductivity before circulatory arrest	Latency (sec)	Conductivity after 10 min circulatory arrest	Asphyxial conductivity change
Controls n = 8	580 $\pm$ 15	111 $\pm$ 8	282 $\pm$ 17	298 $\pm$ 14
Adrenalectomized n = 13	620 $\pm$ 22	59 $\pm$ 6	309 $\pm$ 14	311 $\pm$ 19
p	n.s.	< 0.001	n.s.	n.s.

The latency, the time elapsing between circulatory arrest and onset of the precipitous drop in conductivity, is significantly reduced in adrenalectomized animals. No significant differences between controls and experimental animals were established for the 10 min conductivity change, as well as the conductivity at the end of the 10 min observation period.

Electronmicrographs were obtained of control and adrenalectomized mouse cerebellum, prepared by freeze substitution. Only the tissue surface up to 10–15 microns deep can be used, since in deeper regions the tissue structures are severely damaged by ice-crystal formation, resulting from a less rapid cooling rate. The morphology of the tissue structures in adrenalectomized animals is not essentially different from control preparations, e.g., no swelling of cellular elements is detectable, however, the extracellular space surrounding axonal fibres, or, some areas immediately under the pia-glia membrane appear occasionally somewhat enlarged. The extracellular space was in some experiments not uniformly enlarged, but rather formed here and there extended gaps which were scattered over the section.

According to the results obtained from the impedance measurements and the electronmicroscopy, the excess fluid, accumulated in the CNS after adrenalectomy, is probably not intracellularly localized. The results rather permit the conclusion that the fluid is taken up into the extracellular compartment.

Finally, I would like to mention briefly some biochemical investigations in the CNS of adrenalectomized rats. The increased sodium and water uptake in the CNS of adrenalectomized animals may be the consequence of metabolic disturbances resulting from a lack of stimulation of certain steps of the intermediary metabolism by corticosteroids. This may, for example, cause an insufficient production of energy which is supposed to fuel ion-pumps maintaining transmembraneous electrolyte concentration gradients. According to this concept, alterations of the energy metabolism in one way or the other, should be found in the brain after adrenalectomy.

Studies of the energy-rich phosphate compounds ATP, ADP and AMP or of the lactate and pyruvate concentration did not reveal a conclusive difference in adrenalectomized animals as compared with controls. No changes in tissue concentrations of these metabolites were found. This negative result could imply either that no changes at all in the rate of metabolic energy production occur, or, that the balance of metabolic energy production and utilization has been stabilized at a new, lower level, without affecting the absolute metabolite concentration in the tissue.

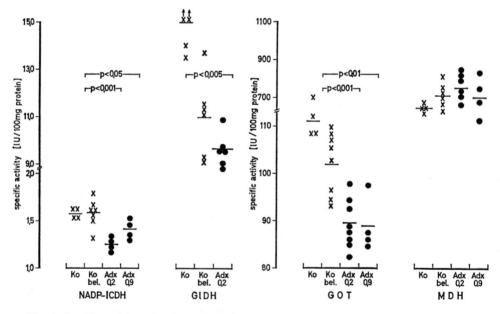

Fig. 4. Specific activity of NADP dependent isocitric dehydrogenase, glutamate dehydrogenase, glutamate-oxalacetate transaminase and malate dehydrogenase in the cortical grey matter of intact controls (Ko), controls orally loaded with a 0.45% NaCl-solution (Ko bel.), and adrenalectomized animals (Adx) maintained on a 0.2% NaCl- or a 0.9% NaCl-solution as drinking fluid

In collaboration with Wesemann [3] the activity of enzymes related to the citric acid cycle were determined in the grey matter, which were shown in the kidney to be sensitive to aldosterone stimulation. Figure 4 shows the results. The activity of the

NADP dependent isocitric dehydrogenase (ICDH), glutamate dehydrogenase (GLDH) and glutamate-oxalacetate transaminase (GOT) were found significantly reduced in adrenalectomy, whereas malate dehydrogenase and glycolysis enzymes, such as, lactate dehydrogenase and pyruvic acid kinase remained unchanged.

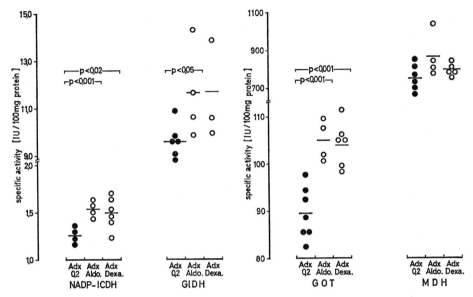

Fig. 5. Specific activity of citric acid cycle enzymes in the cortical grey matter of adrenalectomized rats and after daily administration (i.m.) of 100 μg/kg d-aldosterone (Adx Aldo) or 400 μg/kg dexamethasone (Adx Dexa). The treated adrenalectomized animals as well as the untreated ones were maintained on a 0.2% NaCl solution as drinking fluid

Since the enzyme activity is computed as specific activity, the decrease of the respective enzymes is not due to a dilution by the fluid taken up in the brain of adrenalectomized animals. In Figure 5 the effect of corticosteroid substitution on the enzyme activity is shown. As seen, aldosterone as well as dexamethasone is able to prevent almost entirely the effect of adrenalectomy. The activity of the NADP, ICDH, GLDH and GOT is almost normal. It has to be mentioned again, that, as in the case of the cerebral water and electrolyte content, the effect of the mineralocorticosteroid and glucocorticosteroid appears to be identical.

Acknowledgement. The technical assistance of Miss E. Hungbaur, Miss B. Alzner, Mrs. Jane Sun is gratefully acknowledged.

References

1. Baethmann, A., Reulen, H.-J., Brendel, W.: Die Wirkung des Antimetaboliten 6-Aminonikotinamid (6-ANA) auf Wasser- und Elektrolytgehalt des Rattenhirns und ihre Hemmung durch Nikotinsäure. Z. ges. exp. Med. **146**, 226–240 (1968).
2. — Koczorek, Kh. R., Reulen, H. J., Wesemann, W., Hofmann, H. F., Angstwurm, A., Brendel, W.: Die Beeinflussung des traumatischen Hirnödems durch Aldosteron, Aldosteronantagonisten und Dexamethason im Tierexperiment. In: Bücherl, E. S., *et al.* (Ed.): Postoperative Störungen des Elektrolyt- und Wasserhaushaltes, pp. 163–175. Stuttgart-New York: F. K. Schattauer 1968.

3. Baethmann, A., Wesemann, W., Brendel, W.: Enzymaktivitäten in der Großhirnrinde von adrenalektomierten Ratten und ihre Beeinflussung durch Aldosteron und Dexamethason. Pflügers Arch. ges. Physiol. **300**, R 37 (1968).
4. — Steude, U., Horsch, S., Brendel, W.: The Thiosulphate (^{35}S) Space in the CNS of Rats After Ventriculo-Cisternal Perfusion. Pflügers Arch. Europ. J. Physiol. **316**, 51–63 (1970).
5. Brilmayer, H., Marguth, F.: Störungen im Zwischenhirn-Hypophysensystem bei Hirntumoren. Dtsch. Z. Nervenheilk. **176**, 441–448 (1957).
6. Davenport, V. D.: Relation between Brain and Plasma Electrolytes and Electroshock Seizure Thresholds in Adrenalectomized Rats. Amer. J. Physiol. **156**, 322–327 (1945).
7. Ebel, H., Wolff, J. R., Dorn, F., Günther, Th.: Wirkung von Hormonen auf Elektrolytgehalt, ATPase und endoplasmatisches Retikulum im Rattenhirn. Z. klin. Chem. **9**, 249–256 (1971).
8. Fimognari, G. M., Porter, G. A., Edelmann, I. S.: The Role of the Tricarboxylic Acid Cycle in the Action of Aldosterone on Sodium Transport. Biochim. biophys. Acta (Amst.) **135**, 89–99 (1967).
9. Kinne, R., Kirsten, R.: Der Einfluß von Aldosteron auf die Aktivität mitochondrialer und cytoplasmatischer Enzyme in der Rattenniere. Pflügers Arch. ges. Physiol. **300**, 244–254 (1968).
10. Litteria, M., Schapiro, S.: Brain Water: Regional Changes During the Estrous Cycle in the Rat. Proc. Soc. exp. Biol. **136**, 73–74 (1971).
11. Losert, W., Sitt, R., Senft, G., v. Bergmann, K., Schultz, G.: Untersuchungen zum Wirkungsmechanismus des Aldosterons. Naunyn-Schmiedeberg's Arch. exp. Path. Pharmak. **257**, 309–311 (1967).
12. Pollay, M., Kaplan, R. J.: Effect of Cerebrospinal Fluid Sink on Sucrose-Diffusion Gradients in Brain. Exp. Neurol. **30**, 54–65 (1971).
13. Rall, D. P.: Transport Through Ependymal Linings. Progr. Brain Res. **29**, 159–167 (1968).
14. Reulen, H.-J., Hofmann, H. F., Baethmann, A.: Die Beeinflussung des experimentellen traumatischen Hirnödems bei der Ratte mit einer Nikotinsäuretheophyllin-Verbindung. Z. ges. exp. Med. **138**, 246–256 (1964).
15. — Baethmann, A.: Das Dinitrophenol-Ödem. Ein Modell zur Pathophysiologie des Hirnödems. Klin. Wsch. **45**, 149–154 (1967).
16. Stern, T. N., Cole, V. V., Bass, A. C., Overmann, R. R.: Dynamic Aspects of Sodium Metabolism in Experimental Adrenal Insufficiency Using Radioactive Sodium. Amer. J. Physiol. **164**, 437–449 (1951).
17. Timiras, P. S., Woodbury, D. M., Goodman, L. S.: Effect of Adrenalectomy, Hydrocortisone Acetate and Desoxycorticosterone Acetate on Brain Excitability and Electrolyte Distribution in Mice. J. Pharmacol. exp. Therap. **112**, 80–93 (1954).
18. Van Harreveld, A., Murphy, T., Nobel, K. W.: Specific Impedance of Rabbit's Cortical Tissue. Amer. J. Physiol. **205**, 203–207 (1963).
19. — Crowell, J., Malhotra, S. K.: A Study of Extracellular Space in Central Nervous Tissue by Freeze-Substitution. J. Cell Biol. **25**, 117–137 (1965).
20. — "Brain Tissue Electrolytes". Molecular Biology and Medicine Series. Washington (D.C.): Butterworth 1966.
21. Wesemann, W., Pia, H. W.: Aldadiene-Kalium in der Neurochirurgie. In: Bücherl, E. S., et al. (Ed.): Postoperative Störungen des Elektrolyt- und Wasserhaushaltes, pp. 259 to 270. Stuttgart-New York: F. K. Schattauer 1968.

The Effect of Aldosterone and an Aldosterone-Antagonist on the Metabolism of Perifocal Brain Edema in Man *

Peter Schmiedek, Alexander Baethmann, Eberhard Schneider, Wolfgang Oettinger, Robert Enzenbach, Frank Marguth, and Walter Brendel

Institute for Surgical Research, Surgical Clinic and Neurosurgical Department, University of Munich, W. Germany

With 3 Figures

Summary. Pretreatment of neurosurgical patients with either spirolactone or aldosterone shows a favourable influence on perifocal brain edema, as reflected by the results of brain tissue analysis. Data derived from animal experiments provide new information concerning the mechanism of action of both substances on CNS.

Introduction

While the beneficial effects of glucocorticoids on brain edema were discussed since the middle of the forties [11] only to regain a great deal of interest during the last 10 years [4, 8, 12], the significance of mineralocorticoids in this regard has been pointed out for the first time not longer than 5 years ago [2, 7]. Fortunately enough, Dr. Koczorek and Dr. Baethmann who are both very much responsible for this new concept are contributing to this meeting. Therefore, I think, I don't have to recall clinical and experimental findings in detail which finally resulted in the hypothesis that aldosterone probably plays an important role in preventing brain edema. Until that time, aldosterone was supposed rather to be a factor able to enhance the development of brain edema in analogy to its renal sodium and water retention ability. The finding that spirolactone, a compound with antimineralo-corticoid action did also show a favourable influence on brain edema, which did seem at first not to fit into this concept, was interpreted by the same authors as a result of an increased aldosterone production induced by the antagonist [2, 7]. Being aware of the admittedly provocative character of this idea, it soon became obvious that additional specific data were needed to prove its validity and thereby possibly leading to a new approach to the treatment of brain edema. In contrast to some reports on the use of spirolactone in neurosurgical patients, based primarily on clinical data [9, 17], the present study was designed to investigate directly perifocal brain tissue in man as affected by spirolactone and aldosterone.

Materials and Methods

The material for this investigation was obtained from a total of 59 neurosurgical patients undergoing craniotomy for brain tumor. During operation tissue sampling was performed in a standard manner. Special care was taken to avoid coagulation or

---

* Dedicated to Prof. R. Zenker for his 70th birthday

manipulation of the tissue before sampling. Care was also taken to assure that the samples were removed from presumably edematous brain at the periphery of the tumor. Whenever possible, multiple samples were obtained from cortex and underlying white matter. A complete set of tissue samples included 5 specimens for the study of the following parameters. The first sample for analysis of labile metabolites was obtained by means of a new cryoprobe especially developed for this purpose. Details of this method have been reported elsewhere [15]. Two samples, one from cortex and one from white matter were submitted to measurement of tissue water and electrolyte content according to methods earlier described [13]. Samples from both compartments were also analysed for their content of tissue enzymes particularly those participating in oxidative metabolism.

Patients were divided in 3 groups. *Group 1 :* The 20 patients included in this series were regarded as control because no specific treatment for brain edema was given to them before operation. *Group 2 :* 21 patients received 800–1000 mg of spirolactone per day for a mean of 3 days before operation. *Group 3 :* 15 patients were treated during their preoperative course with aldosterone. The drug was given twice daily intramuscularly, starting with 5 mg on the first day, then increasing the dose to 10 mg per day and in 2 cases even to 15 mg per day. Except 2 patients pretreated for only 2 days, all others were treated for a mean of 4 days, not included 2 patients who stayed on this medication for 9 days. Following the operation administration of spirolactone or aldosterone was continued for several days depending on the patients postoperative condition. In all patients belonging to group 2 and 3 and in most patients of the control group electrolytes in serum and urine as well as input and output were measured daily. In 5 patients of group 3 regional cerebral blood flow studies with the ^{133}Xe clearance method and 16 detectors were performed in addition to other preoperative routine diagnostic procedures.

Results

Water content : In Fig. 1 tissue water content of cortex and white matter is given for the control group in the left and for the two groups either pretreated with spirolactone or aldosterone. Though no reference values for water content in normal human brain tissue are available in our series, the means of 27 and 25 samples obtained from patients without pretreatment, certainly reflect edema in the sense of high tissue water content. This is also supported by a considerable variation of individual values, especially in the white matter compartment. On the other hand, when compared with control values water content of cortex and white matter is markedly diminished following pretreatment with spirolactone or aldosterone. This is most pronounced in the aldosterone group, with the difference being highly significant in both compartments, whereas after pretreatment with spirolactone only water content of cortex is significantly reduced but not to the same extent in white matter.

Electrolytes : Fig. 2 shows the values for sodium and potassium, as measured after extraction of the dry residue of cortex and white matter samples with 10% trichloric acetic acid. Because only too few analyses were done for white matter in the aldosterone group, the result was found to be not representative and therefore omitted here. In cortex sodium content is reduced in both groups treated before operation when compared with control values. Here, sodium is lowest in the spirolactone group,

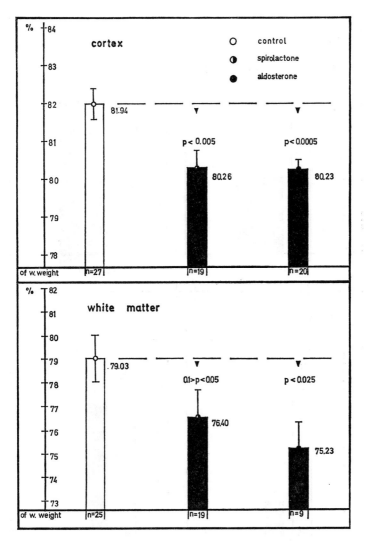

Fig. 1. Water content in % of wet weight (means ± SEM) in samples from perifocal cortex and white matter, left control; middle pretreated with spirolactone; right pretreated with aldosterone

whereas the difference between the aldosterone and the control group is not as striking as might have been expected from the corresponding water figures. Potassium which does not reveal any marked change when the control and the spirolactone group are considered, reveals a significant increase in the aldosterone group. In white matter the comparison between control and spirolactone is in good agreement with that found for cortex: decrease of sodium, with only slight changes of potassium.

Enzymes : In Fig. 3 results of enzyme studies in cortex and white matter are compared for the 3 groups. While the overall changes are not too impressive, elevated enzyme levels in the spirolactone group may be interpreted as evidence for enzyme

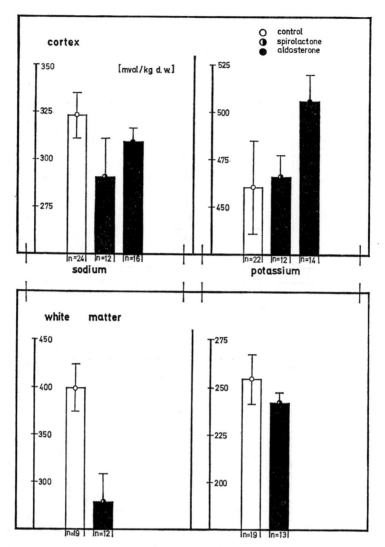

Fig. 2. Electrolyte content in mEq/kg of dry weight (means ± SEM) in cortex and white matter in the 3 groups

induction due to administration of this drug. Condensing enzyme (C.E.), isocitrate-dehydrogenase (IDH), glutamate-dehydrogenase (GLDH) and malate-dehydrogenase (MDH) are, among those studied here, the ones to be particularly affected. In the samples from patients pretreated with aldosterone the enzyme pattern does not show the same consistent picture. Again, there are some enzymes with higher levels than in the control group, but only in the case of MDH values exceed those found in the spirolactone group.

Metabolites : As indicated in Table 1, tissue metabolites in cortex are showing virtually no grossly evident change in the 3 groups. This is true when considering energy-rich phosphate compounds on the left, and also concerning the degree of

206

glycolysis as reflected by lactate and the lactate/pyruvate ratio which all fall in the same range.

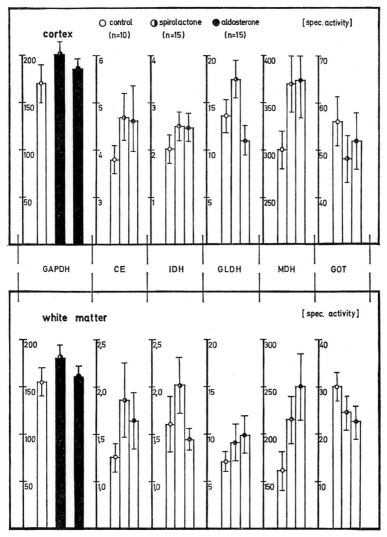

Fig. 3. Comparison of enzymes in cortex and white matter in the 3 groups (specific activity; means ± SEM)

Discussion

When this investigation was started 2 years ago, there were some experiments done in rats, there was a clinical study in patients presenting with what has been called pseudo-tumor cerebri whose symptoms largely disappeared when they were given spirolactone, and then there was a very attractive hypothesis on brain edema, aldosterone and spirolactone as outlined briefly in the introduction. According to this theory it would

207

have been only logical, to start with aldosterone. The reason for not trying this direct approach is very simple. To be honest, we were afraid to lose our first patient treated with aldosterone from iatrogenic brain edema, and to bury a good theory at the same time. With the spirolactone group then completed, a twofold result became evident.

Table 1. Metabolites in samples from cortex in μmoles/g of wet weight

	CP	ATP	ADP	AMP	Pyr.	Lact	L/P-R
control	3,30	1,66	0,55	0,19	0,29	4,24	16
(n = 20)	± 0,22	± 0,08	± 0,05	± 0,04	± 0,04	± 0,70	
spirolactone	2,89	1,55	0,51	0,12	0,22	2,66	14
(n = 10)	± 0,32	± 0,14	± 0,07	± 0,02	± 0,02	±0,32	
aldosterone	3,30	1,62	0,65	0,27	0,20	3,40	17
(n = 8)	± 0,27	± 0,12	± 0,08	± 0,04	± 0,03	± 0,60	
				- μmoles / g w. wt. -			

The decrease of water content paralleled by a reduction of sodium as compared to control suggested a beneficial effect on edematous brain tissue, or in other words, a step towards a causal therapy of brain edema. In addition to this, especially the finding of increased enzyme levels following pretreatment with spirolactone seemed to be consistent with the assumption that, indeed, aldosterone was the active principle, since similiar changes of enzyme pattern are reported from experiments with aldosterone alone [3, 6]. Experimental work gave further support to this [14]. When adrenal glands from dogs given spirolactone for several days, were examined microscopically, there was a significant enlargement of the zona glomerulosa, which, with a reasonable degree of certainty, is indicative of an increased aldosterone production. But there were other findings and observations being in less good agreement. With the aid of the ventriculo-cisternal perfusion method and ^{3}H-labeled spirolactone, it was possible to demonstrate the penetration of activity from the blood into the perfusate [16]. Subsequent analysis of the perfusate by fluorimetric assay revealed the activity to be identical with spirolactone and its main metabolite canrenone. Moreover, 24 h after i.v. application of the tracer, activity in brain tissue was found to be considerably higher than either in CSF or serum. This, though not being conclusive, did suggest the possibility of an aldosterone independent action of spirolactone on central nervous system. The observation that 2 patients in our series treated with spirolactone developed transient seizure episodes immediatedly following the administration of the drug, caused another experimental investigation concerning EEG changes induced by spirolactone in dogs [10]. The preliminary results showing characteristic dose dependent alterations of the EEG, in our opinion, speaks very much in favour of a specific influence of this drug on the brain. The relevance of this remains to be clarified. The results obtained in 15 patients pretreated with aldosterone in large doses for several days, do need some comments as well. To begin with a negative statement, aldosterone can no longer be regarded as a brain edema producing or enhancing factor. On the contrary, from the present data there is clear evidence for a favourable influence of this hormone on perifocal brain edema, as indicated by a significant decrease of water and sodium in samples excised from perifocal cortex and white matter. Unlike the spirolactone group, there is in addition an increase in potassium, at least in the studied samples from cortex. This finding is in agreement to what has been shown by Woodbury and Koch [18] years ago for normal rat brain after aldosterone administration. Concerning the enzymes or study of metabolites, data are as yet too few as to allow any definite conclusions. Instead of going into speculation, I would prefer to mention very briefly clinical data from the 2 treated groups especially on aldosterone since only very limited information is available from the literature concerning the clinical use of aldosterone [1, 5]. First of all aldosterone, even in the large doses used in this study proved to be an extremely safe medication. The only side effects were weight gain during the first days of treatment, rarely more than 1 kg, and a drop of serum potassium which could be easily corrected for by oral supplement. During the postoperative course patients on aldosterone did surprisingly well, showing in most cases full responsiveness soon after the end of the operation, without signs of deterioration during the following days. Postoperative need for dehydrating therapy, as mannitol or renal diuretics could be considerably reduced in this group. In the spirolactone group, about 50 % of the patients did show side effects, as nausea, vomiting, and as mentioned, in 2 patients episodes of fits. Interestingly enough, these side effects seemed to be more pronounced in the preoperative phase, and often disappeared completely following the operation in spite of a continued medication. The conclusion from this, that aldosterone represents a better drug for the treatment of brain edema than spirolactone would be an oversimplification. We are not dealing here just with drugs, their effectiveness or side effects. This investigation was primarily initiated, to provide information with regard to the significance of mineralocorticoids in brain edema. The data presented suggest that the hypothesis offered by Koczorek and Baethmann is essentially correct: both aldosterone and spirolactone do act on edematous brain tissue resulting in an amelioration of this pathological condition. But very likely – in contrast to the original concept – we must differentiate between the effects induced by aldosterone and those induced by spirolactone, since there is now increasing evidence that spirolactone itself influences brain tissue.

Acknowledgement. This study was supported by Sonderforschungsbereich 51 – Medizinische Molekularbiologie.

Technical assistance was provided by Miss A. Gruber and Mrs. R. Hößl.

References

1. August, J. T., Nelson, D. H., Thorn, G. W.: Response of normal subjects to large amounts of aldosterone. J. clin. Invest. 37, 1549–1555 (1958).
2. Baethmann, A., Koczorek, Kh. R., Reulen, H. J., Wesemann, W., Hofmann, H. F., Angstwurm, A., Brendel, W.: Die Beeinflussung des traumatischen Hirnödems durch Aldosteron, Aldosteronantagonisten und Dexamethason im Tierexperiment. In: Bücherl, E. S. (Ed.): Postoperative Störungen des Elektrolyt- und Wasserhaushalts. Stuttgart-New York: Schattauer 1968.
3. Fimognari, G. M., Porter, G. A., Edelman, I.: The role of the tricarbocylic acid cycle in the action of aldosterone on sodium transport. Biochim. Biophys. Acta (Amst.) 135, 89 (1971).

4. Galicich, J. H., French, L. A., Melby, J. C.: Use of dexamethasone in treatment of cerebral edema associated with brain tumors. Lancet **81**, 46–53 (1961).
5. Hetzel, B. S., McSwiney, R. R., Mills, I. H., Prunty, F. T. G.: Observations on the effects of aldosterone in man. J. Endocr. **13**, 112–124 (1956).
6. Kinne, R., Kirsten, R.: Der Einfluß von Aldosteron auf die Aktivität mitochondrialer und cytoplasmatischer Enzyme in der Rattenniere. Pflügers Arch. ges. Physiol. **300**, 244 (1968).
7. Koczorek, Kh. R., Angstwurm, A., Baethmann, A., Engelhardt, D., Reulen, H. J., Schmiedek, P., Vogt, W., Simon, B., Frick, E., Brendel, W.: Aldosteronausscheidung beim Pseudotumor cerebri – einer klinischen Form des Hirnödems unbekannter Ursache. In: Bücherl, E. S. (Ed.): Postoperative Störungen des Elektrolyt- und Wasserhaushalts. Stuttgart-New York: Schattauer 1968.
8. Long, D. M., Hartmann, J. F., French, L. A.: The response of experimental cerebral edema to glucosteroid administration. J. Neurosurg. **24**, 843–854 (1966).
9. Mansuy, L., Fischer, G., Bret, P., Ravon, R.: Oedème cérébrale et hyperaldostéronisme. Presse méd. **54**, 2431 (1970).
10. Mertin, J., Simon, O., Schmiedek, P.: EEG-Veränderungen unter Aldadiene-Kalium (in preparation).
11. Prados, M., Strowger, B., Feindel, W. H.: Studies on cerebral edema: II. Reaction of the brain to exposure to air; physiologic changes. Arch. Neurol. Psychiat. **54**, 290–300 (1945).
12. Rasmussen, T., Gulati, D. R.: Cortisone in the treatment of postoperative cerebral edema. J. Neurosurg. **19**, 535–544 (1962).
13. Reulen, H. J., Medzihradsky, F., Enzenbach, R., Marguth, F., Brendel, W.: Electrolytes, fluids and energy metabolism in human cerebral edema. Arch. Neurol. (Chic.) **21**, 517 to 525 (1969).
14. Rohrschneider, I., Schmiedek, P., Schinko, I., Wetzstein, R.: Licht- und elektronenmikroskopische Untersuchungen an der zona glomerulosa der Nebennierenrinde des Hundes nach Gabe von Spirolactone (in preparation).
15. Schmiedek, P., Baethmann, A., Enzenbach, R.: The estimation of cerebral metabolites for the purpose of assessing the results of treatment on cerebral oedema. Proc. Germ. Soc. Neurosurg., Excerpta Medica, Amsterdam 1971.
16. Schmiedek, P., Baethmann, A., Sadée, W.: Cerebral uptake of ^{3}H-spirolactone in the dog (in preparation).
17. Wesemann, W., Pia, H. W.: Aldadiene-Kalium in der Neurochirurgie. In: Bücherl, E. S. (Ed.): Postoperative Störungen des Elektrolyt- und Wasserhaushalts. Stuttgart-New York: Schattauer 1968.
18. Woodbury, D. M., Koch, A.: Effects of aldosterone and desoxycorticosterone on tissue electrolytes. Proc. Soc. exp. Biol. (N. Y.) **94**, 720 (1957).

Discussion to Chapter III see page 274

Chapter IV

Effects of Steroids on Brain Edema in Man

The Effects of Steroids on Brain Edema in Man

Joseph Ransohoff

Department of Neurosurgery, New York University, School of Medicine, New York, NY, USA

Edema would appear to represent the major primary central nervous system response to all types of trauma whether it be physical, infectious or ischemic. Whereas the mechanisms which lead to the development of edema may vary somewhat depending on the precipitating etiological agent, the process, from a clinical point of view, is mainly a white matter phenomenon characterized by the accumulation of extracellular fluid with relative resistance on the part of the arcuate zone and the corpus callosum [6]. It is of interest that these latter areas have been demonstrated to contain higher water content in the non-edematous state [1]. Our electron microscopic studies of human edema [2] associated with gliomas and cerebral trauma confirm the indistinguishable nature of the process no matter what the etiology, at least as far as the end product is concerned. The earlier divergence of opinion between the light and electron microscopists relative to the site of the edematous fluids has now been resolved with general agreement that at least in the white matter it accumulates in the extracellular space [5].

The site of the patho-physiological process leading to CNS edema is still, however, under debate whether it be through altered blood vessel walls directly or indirectly through damaged astrocytic membranes, or possibly both. We tend to favor the latter possibility particularly in those situations characterized by normal serum osmolality. If Lumsden's concept [8] that the astrocyte has the function of fluid transport in the brain is accepted, it seems inconsistent not to assume that this is also not the case under pathological conditions unless the injury inducing the edema has the specific effect of disrupting the close relationship between astrocytes and blood vessels. In instances associated with tissue damage, as in severe trauma, both mechanisms may occur and account for observed differences in the clinical responsiveness of post-traumatic edema.

In 1965 we reported [10] on the profiles of 100 fatal and non-fatal acute closed head injuries utilizing computer storage analysis and retrieval of all pertinent information as our first application of special data processing techniques devised by Randt and Korein [7] at New York University. The ultimate goal of this method being the construction of stochastic models of disease validated by clinical experience leading eventually to increased predictability and the ability to test new therapeutic hypothesis. Correlation of ten variables with forty others in the form of a matrix resulted from the computer search and retrieve program. From this data comparison of factors of possible clinical significance was extracted (Table 1).

211

Table 1. Analysis of fatal and non-fatal head injuries

	Survivals %	Deaths %
Coma on admission	50	75
Focal neurological deficit	30	70
Skull fracture	30	75
Subdural hematoma	25	85
Subarachnoid hemorrhage	70	90
Pupillary inequality	20	25
Angiographic shift	20	20

Coma on admission, focal neurological deficit, and skull fracture were variables which demonstrated a high correlation with fatal outcome. Of especial interest to us was the 85 % instance of acute subdural hematoma in the deaths as compared to 25 % in the survivals. This was particularly provocative in view of the non-correlation of pupillary inequality and angiographic shift with death and survival.

Pathological findings served, however, to provide us with a partial answer to this apparent enigma. Massive bilateral cerebral edema was the most common finding in the fatal cases who had not developed significant hematoma. These cases were associated with the usual bilateral herniations of uncal and hippocampal complexes with associated mid-brain hemorrhages. In fatal cases with significant unilateral hematomas, massive unilateral edema with similar secondary herniations and mid-brain hemorrhages were commonly seen at autopsy. These observations led us logically to two subsequent studies.

In critically ill acute closed head injury patients without evidence of angiographic shift or significant clots, but with documented increase in intracranial pressure (lumbar puncture or intracranial monitoring) a double blind study of massive steroid therapy was conducted by Drs Randt and Wood [11] (Table 2, 3). Although the use of cortico-steroids in the treatment of head injuries and subarachnoid hemorrhage in humans is prevalent, there has been a poverty of clinical investigations designed to demonstrate its efficacy in these conditions. Sparachio *et al.* reported an increased survival rate in acute brain injured patients treated with cortico-steroids. These studies, however, did not contain control groups of patients. Therefore, the observed mortality rate in acute subdural hematoma of 63 % as compared to earlier mortality rates of 85 % is of questionable validity and significance. Several investigators have affirmed the efficaciousness of steroids in acute cerebral trauma but did not publish any data to support this conclusion. Others, again in unpublished data, have not observed significant improvement in the mortality rate or morbidity rate of patients with acute cranio-cerebral trauma treated with cortico-steroids.

This double blind study was an attempt to further define the role of cortico-steroids in patients with acute cranio-cerebral trauma. It was designed to evaluate the effects of short-term steroid therapy on the mortality rate and morbidity rate in the acutely head injured patient and to document the incidence of complications associated with this mode of treatment (Table 2, 3).

212

Table 2. Random steroid studies

I. Placebo vs. steroids

    (A) Placebo :   Total 18
    (1) Deceased   =   13
    (2) Survived   =   5
    (3) S.R.   =   27.7%

    (B) Steroid Group : Total 17
    (1) Deceased   =   9
    (2) Survived   =   8
    (3) S.R.   =   53%

II. Decerebrate (A) vs.

non-decerebrate (B)

    (A) Decerebrate :   Total 17
    (1) Placebo: Total 10
        (a) Deceased =   9
        (b) Survived   =   1
        (c) S.R.   =   10%
    (2) Steroid: Total 7
        (a) Deceased =   5
        (b) Survived   =   2
        (c) S.R.   =   28.6%

    (B) Non-decerebrate : Total 18
    (1) Placebo: Total 8
        (a) Deceased =   4
        (b) Survived   =   4
        (c) S.R.   =   50%
    (2) Steroids: Total 10
        (a) Deceased =   3
        (b) Survived   =   7
        (c) S.R.   =   70%

Table 3. Survival time in days

(A) Placebo	*(B) Steroids*
(1) Mean = 29 days	(1) Mean = 48.2 days
(2) Median = 17 days	(2) Median = 24 days
(3) Range = 1–76	(3) Range = 3–163

The patients in our study were classified relative to the severity of their head injury as manifested by responses to painful stimuli and/or the presence of significant focal neurological deficit. Methylprednisolone, 125 mg every 6 h for 4 days, was instituted, usually at the time of admission or within 24 hours of admission. The patients were observed for the development of significant electrolyte disturbances, infections, fluid retention, and or GI hemorrhage.

Concerning complications of the steroid therapy, there was no significant difference in the incidence of GI bleeding, pulmonary or urinary tract infections between the treated and control groups. Arterial blood gases were monitored closely in all the patients. It was observed that hypoxia was almost invariably associated with the decerebrate state. Its incidence in the non-decerebrate patients was varied. There was no statistically significant difference in the incidence of hypoxia between the control and treated group.

The syndrome of inappropriate ADH excretion was observed not infrequently. Invariably, this occurred after the third week of the study. This may be related to the study protocol since patients were actually maintained on IV fluid during the initial first two weeks of the study period. During this period, fluid intake was restricted to 1500 to 2000 cc's. Interestingly, those patients who subsequently developed the inappropriate ADH syndrome showed no significant recovery from their injuries or died. Therefore, the development of this syndrome usually represented a poor prognosis. The incidence of this syndrome was not significantly different between the two groups.

These investigators concluded that whereas there was a distinct trend towards a better survival rate in the steroid treated group as compared to the controls, this was not statistically significant at a "p" value of 0.2. The quality of survival also appeared to be better in the treated patients, but did not reach statistical significance. Of anecdotal interest only was the fact that the ward personnel could predict by a high percentage whether indeed the patients were receiving steroids or placebos.

A second study was stimulated in those patients with unilateral hematomas in whom surgery was required in the first 24 h after injury as a life saving procedure. Our computer analysis had shown us the significance of the massive unilateral edema even after prompt operative clot removal. Indeed, the previously reported experience with surgery of acute subdural hematoma has been associated with a mortality rate as high as 80–90 %. A clinical program was therefore developed to approach this problem by an improved surgical procedure which would afford not only complete clot removal, adequate hemostasis, but also provision for decompression of the inevitable brain edema which followed. The procedure was that of a unilateral hemicraniectomy with a wide dural opening and a careful skin closure without replacement of the bone flap. The initial series already reported [9] in which manitol was utilized during the preoperative studies, but steroids were withheld, a 50 % mortality rate was achieved and a 25 % good to excellent salvage rate was probably of even greater significance. It is important to stress once again that all these patients were operated on within the first twenty-four hours after injury, or were comatose and demonstrated either unilateral or bilateral decerebration and pupillary vital sign changes. All patients "utilized" the hemicraniectomy decompression and postoperative angiography demonstrated the cortical vessels often to be several centimeters beyond the predicted outline of the skull for as long as a week to ten days after surgery. Simultaneous apnea and bilateral pupillary dilatation, a hematoma over 300 cc's, a $CMRO_2$ of under 1.5 and an age of over 60 were all factors which were synonymous with non-survival. Subsequent to this initial group, steroid therapy has been added to the regime, but our clinical impression is that the steroid therapy has not made a very significant difference in the overall results of the surgical procedure. Accurate monitoring of intracranial pressure and cerebral blood flow studies with the use of the mass spectrometer are currently under way and may shed further light on this type of severe unilateral post-traumatic edema, particularly as it may relate to loss of cerebral vascular auto-regulation and the effect of steroid on this phenomenon.

214

Autopsy findings in the non-surviving group of patients subjected to hemicraniectomy demonstrate a pot-pourri of pathological findings. Frontal and temporal contusions, frank cerebral lacerations and widespread subarachnoid hemorrhage are all seen and the presence of a pure culture of simple or uncomplicated edema is rarely found. It is interesting to note that the effect of osmotic diuretics i. e. manitol, in this group in the early hours after injury (during workup and angiography) is usually quite effective in reversing the rapid downhill course of these patients. In contrast is the lack of dramatic clinical improvement seen later in the postoperative period when manitol is used either in a similar large bolus or a slow drip administration period. Here, while a very tight compression can often soften and intracranial pressure recordings confirm a drop in levels, there is little correlation seen in terms of clinical improvement as compared to that noted shortly after injury. We interpret these differences in the manitol effects to indicate that early after injury when a large clot is actively compressing as yet non-edematous brain, the osmotic diuretic is efficient. After cerebral edema is fully developed, dehydration of the non-edematous brain may reduce intracranial pressure but is not associated with much evidence of clinical improvement.

In the clinical situation, therefore, we are forced to conclude that following severe trauma, central nervous system tissue edema is moderately unresponsive to the effect of steroids. It also would appear that osmotic diuretics are effective early in the posttraumatic period, particularly when edema has not yet fully developed, or when still relatively normal brain is being compressed by an intracranial clot. These clinical impressions might have been suspected based on our current understanding of the effects of osmotic diuretics. It is generally held that these agents reduce intracranial pressure by dehydrating the normal brain tissue, and that it is ineffective in an area of membrane dysfunction which seems to be the pathophysiological substrate for cerebral edema.

Laboratory studies in our department indicate, however, that steroids have a distinct beneficial effect on the post-traumatic edema which develops several hours after experimental spinal cord trauma. The progress of cord dissolution has been carefully documented and can be seen to develop over a 24 h period following a 20 cm/g injury to the exposed feline spinal cord [4]. The initial pathological changes develop in the central grey matter in the form of a hemorrhagic necrosis which reaches its peak in 2 to 3 h after injury. Subsequent to this, white matter edema becomes rampant and the process progresses to severe degeneration of the cord within 24 h. Steroids administered intravenously 1 h after injury sharply reduce the post-traumatic white matter demolition although they do not significantly affect the hemorrhagic grey matter necrosis. We have recently reported the beneficial effect of an antifibrolytic agent (epsilon aminocaproic acid) [3], which if added to the steroid therapy can effect an even higher salvage rate of fairly normal appearing cords by reducing the hemorrhagic component of the process. Other investigators have demonstrated the salutary effects of steroids on brain edema in experimental models and there is no reason to believe that spinal cord edema differs basically from that seen in cerebral tissue.

Brain edema occurring in response to a non-traumatic intracranial mass lesion, particularly tumor or chronic abscess, has often a far more dramatic response to steroids than that seen following head injury. It is not uncommon to find a drowsy and hemiparetic patient become alert and almost neurologically intact after 24–36 h of massive steroid therapy. We do not believe, however, the basic process is different in these clinical situations. Edema occurring in juxtaposition to a tumor mass develops more slowly than that following trauma, and it generally is far more circumscribed. The process is probably a purer culture of edema uncomplicated by hemorrhage and laceration of brain matter. The phenomenon of rapidly developing intracranial pressure with concomitant loss of vascular auto-regulation rarely occurs in association with tumor edema. Once autoregulation is lost, the vascular bed responds in a passive fashion to increasing blood pressure and an added factor leading to the development of further edema is probably at work. These parameters may "explain" the infrequency of the almost magical steroid response in trauma as compared to that seen in tumoral edema.

In a similar fashion, edema occurring in patients with ruptured intracranial aneurysms and secondary vasospasm is not as responsive to steroid therapy as is the tumor model. The presence of blood and blood breakdown products may play an important part in the severity and resistance of this type of edema similar to that seen in the post-traumatic process.

The statement has often been made that steroids "stabilize the blood-brain barrier". I, for one, have not until recently had any practical or theoretical basis for making this statement. In the past two years, however, our department has been working in intimate cooperation with the free radical pathology group at our center. I believe we now have experimental evidence to indicate the role of free radicals in the edema process as has been reported earlier at this conference, and at least a working hypothesis concerning the methods by which steroids may reverse or inhibit the edema process both in cerebral and spinal cord tissue. The theoretical mechanisms raised by Demopoulos at this meeting in an earlier paper may explain the differential efficacy of steroids in traumatic versus tumoral edema, namely the presence of relatively large quantities of metal complexes introduced suddenly by trauma, in contrast to the slower leakage of radicals and electron transport factors from tumors. The rate of free radical damage to membranes during trauma would be great and there probably would be too much alteration of the seemingly vital archways created by the fatty acids of the membrane phospholipids. If these molecular structures are destroyed, there is no easy way for steroids to intercalate into membranes. With slower rates of free radical damage, as with tumors, there is probably sufficient preservation of membrane structure for steroid intercalation. If enough steroid molecules enter the membrane, then they can actually serve to protect the fatty acids from free radical damage, as cited in Demopoulos' initial presentation at this symposium.

A final point that has not been discussed at this meeting is the phenomenon of the steroid dependent brain. It should be "saying something" to us relative to the relationship of these agents and CNS membrane function. First described in children receiving high dose-long term steroid therapy for dermatological conditions it has now also been seen in primary CNS problems. Our own experience is related to patients referred to us, who had been placed on steroid therapy for misdiagnosed gliomas, and had been sent home to die on large steroid doses. Once the offending lesion is removed one cannot simply carry the patient through the usual 10 to 14 day steroid taper. This regimen will often result in a rapid elevation of intracranial pressure, and even the appearance of papilledema with hemorrhages, as well as coma if unrecognized. Reinstitution of the prior maintenance dose reverses the situation, and subsequently a very slow taper with careful evaluation of endogenous adrenal cortical function will be successful. I do not want to get into the relationship of the endocrine aspects of the problem as I believe they are all secondary to the adrenal cortical suppression. It is of great interest however that cerebral membrane stability can obviously become steroid dependent for its "normal" functioning, whether this be vascular, astrocytic, neither, or both! Long term administration of steroids to primates with a study of the withdrawal phenomenon should be an interesting model for study.

References

1. Adachi, M., Feigin, I.: Cerebral Edema and the Water Content of Normal White Matter. J. Neurol. Neurosurg. Psychiat. **29**, 446–455 (1966).
2. Aleu, F., Samuels, S., Ransohoff, J.: Pathology of Cerebral Edema Associated With Gliomas in Man. Amer. J. Path. **48**, 1043–1061 (1966).
3. Campbell, J. B., DeCrescito, V., Tomasula, J. J., Demopoulos. H. F., Ortega, B. D.: Experimental Treatment of Acute Spinal Cord Contusion. Presented at the meeting of The American Association of Neurological Surgeons, April 17, 1972, Boston, Massachusetts.
4. — Goodkin, R.: Sequential Pathologic Changes in Spinal Cord Injury. A Preliminary Report. Surg. Forum (55th Annual Clin. Cong.) **20**, 430–432 (1969).
5. Feigin, L.: Sequence of Pathological Changes. In: Klatzo, I., Seitelberger, F. (Eds.): Brain Edema, pp. 128–151. Berlin-Heidelberg-New York: Springer 1967.
6. — Popoff, N.: Neuropathological Observations on Cerebral Edema. Arch. Neurol. **6**, 151–160 (1962).
7. Korein, J., Tich, L. J., Woodbury, M. A., Cady, L. Goodgold, A. L., Randt, C. T.: Computer Processing of Medical Data by Variable Field-Length Format. J. Amer. med. Ass. **196**, 132–140 (1963).
8. Lumsden, C. E.: Proceed. 2nd Intl. Cong. Neuropath. London, Excerpta Med. Found. pp. 373–376. Amsterdam 1955.
9. Ransohoff, J., Benjamin, M. V., Gage, E. L., Jr., Epstein, F.: Hemicraniectomy in the Management of the Acute Subdural Hematoma. J. Neurosurg. **34**, 70–76 (1971).
10. — Randt, C. T.: Profiles of Fatal and Non-Fatal Closed Head Injury. Proceed. III Intl. Cong. of Neurolog. Surg. Excerpta Med. Found. pp. 137–142. Copenhagen 1965.
11. Wood, D., Randt, C. T.: Personal Communication.

The Clinical Effects of a Synthetic Gluco-Corticoid used for Brain Edema in the Practice of Neurosurgery

Robert E. Maxwell, Don M. Long, and Lyle A. French

Department of Neurosurgery, University of Minnesota, Health Science Center, Minneapolis, MN 55455, USA

With 2 Figures

Summary. The clinical effect of dexamethasone, a potent, synthetic gluco-corticoid, was studied in a large series of neurosurgical patients with brain edema seen over a 12 year period. A protocol was established at the beginning of the study to evaluate the severity of the edema and its clinical response to steroid therapy. The results showed that the treatment of brain edema with dexamethasone was highly effective in patients with focal lesions where edema production persists or progresses with time, as is the case particularly with brain tumors and abscesses. Patients with metastatic tumors, glioblastomas and abscesses responded better to steroid therapy than patients with low grade infiltrating astrocytomas and meningiomas. This correlated well with the relative severity of the edema associated with these respective tumors. Steroid administration proved least effective in patients with generalized brain lesions of acute onset as seen in severe closed head injuries. The prevention of severe operative and post-operative edema in patients started on dexamethasone prior to brain surgery was apparent. This was particularly emphasized in the group of patients who had craniotomies for the excision of large meningiomas and the pathophysiology of this response was discussed. Steroid therapy proved to be safe when administered for the brief period of time usually necessary in neurosurgical problems. Gastrointestinal bleeding was not a serious problem except in very ill patients who were either comatose and on the respirator, or moribund following severe head injuries with brain stem involvement.

Introduction

It seems especially appropriate that the "Workshop on the Effect of Steroids on Brain Edema" is being held in the general geographic setting where the concept of brain edema arose and where its importance in clinical medicine and neurosurgery was first recognized. The awareness of this pathological entity occurred gradually during the latter part of the nineteenth century, particularly in the German literature, and cannot be ascribed to any single investigator [22]. Kocher, in 1901, however, was able to discuss "Hirnödem" as if it were a familiar process and he concluded that edema was secondary to a transudation of fluid from distended capillaries and veins [19]. Interest remained keen among German neuropathologists over the next 30 years concerning the relation between brain tumors, cerebral swelling, and edema. Prior to 1930 numerous papers were published by Stengel, Spatz, and Fünfgeld, and others who concluded that brain swelling was common with cerebral neoplasms and an important cause of increased intracranial pressure [8, 36, 37].

This research was supported in part by USPHS Grants No. NBO7341 and NSO5546

As physicians and surgeons working with the central nervous system became more familiar with this concept, the high mortality associated with brain swelling was appreciated and attempts were made to discover methods for its relief. The rational therapy of brain edema was initiated in 1919 when Weed introduced the use of hypertonic solutions for the reduction of brain bulk [44]. Short of surgical decompression, this turned out to be the primary method for controlling increased intracranial pressure due to edema for 40 years. The hypertonic solutions proved effective in reducing the bulk of the swollen brain because of their osmotic properties, but as experience grew with the use of these agents, two undesirable features became apparent. The effect was of brief duration and there could be an exaggerated rebound in brain swelling and intracranial pressure after a period of time which often surpassed that present when therapy was initiated.

Then in 1930, about 75 years after Thomas Addison described the effects of bilateral adrenal disease and Rokitansky and Virchow began talking about tissue edema, F. A. Hartman and Brownell reported the preparation of a potent extract from the adrenal gland [13]. Swingel and Pfiffner reported similar success the same year [38]. Almost immediately Hartman began giving his newly prepared extract to humans with nervous system impairments because of the neurological involvement often associated with Addison's disease. He treated a 54 year old physician in 1930 who had noted increasing weakness of the shoulder girdle muscles and radicular pain shooting into the right hand. The patient also noted cramps of his quadriceps and abductor muscles on leg stretching. A lumbar puncture was performed which precipitated a quadriparesis associated with "diarrhea". Physical examination revealed atrophy and weakness in the upper extremities and spastic weakness in the lower extremities. Sensory examination suggested a segmental distribution involving C3, C4, and C5 bilaterally and loss of vibration in the lower extremities. The patient was given 225–500 g of adrenal cortical extract daily in divided doses for 17 days. After three days, the patient reported that he was feeling quite well. The cramps in his legs stopped as did the "diarrhea". One week after initiation of therapy, the previously absent left biceps jerk returned and he was able to walk with a greater degree of flexibility and agility and was able to go up and down stairs with ease. The patient was enthusiastic about the effective treatment, but the cortin therapy was discontinued because he decided to go South for the winter. He subsequently became worse again and all the old symptoms returned. He then underwent a laminectomy and an arachnoid cyst was found compressing the spinal cord at the fourth cervical segment [14]. This case was reported in 1933 but was never acknowledged or referred to in the subsequent literature on the role of steroids in brain and spinal cord edema, and its possible significance was apparently missed.

Shortly thereafter, investigators concerned with the physiology of shock called attention to the role of cortin in the prevention of interstitial edema in dogs in vasogenic shock [39]. 6 years later, Menkin found that adrenal cortical extract prevented the increase in capillary permeation normally caused by tissue injury products such as leukotaxine in rabbits [25]. In 1941, Freed and Lindner reported that desoxycorticosterone, which is more concerned with salt and water metabolism, was unable to prevent an increasing capillary permeability under conditions where the adrenal cortical extracts were effective [6]. They also found that corticosterone, which had relatively little effect on salt and water metabolism, was quite capable of neutralizing the leukotaxine action of increasing the permeability of skin capillaries and causing edema. They therefore concluded that the activity of adrenal cortical extract was due to its content of corticosterone. In 1945, Prados, Strowger, and Feindel exposed part of the hemisphere of cat brains to air and found brain swelling associated with increased capillary permeability. They also noted marked hypothalamic involvement in these animals [29]. They were aware of the earlier studies of Menkin, Freed, and Lindner and also the observation of Cope and his associates that the protein content of dog lymph was almost doubled after adrenalectomy. On this basis, a group of animals were pretreated with ACTH prior to the exposure procedure and this pretreatment effectively prevented many of the changes interpreted as cerebral edema. Prados postulated that the ACTH administration helped the adrenals to maintain capillary tone in the presence of a relative hypothalamic-pituitary insufficiency [30]. Two very limited studies shortly thereafter supported Prados' findings. Aird and his associates referred to a clinical study they did in which adrenal cortical extracts appeared to have some beneficial effects on the post-concussional state [1]. Aware of the findings of Prados and Aird, Grenell and McCawley then injected cortin into a man with a post-traumatic concussion syndrome. They noted "that by the third day of therapy his incessant headache had disappeared. An electroencephalogram taken 2 weeks after treatment was begun showed no abnormality whatsoever and the slowing and irregularity seen before treatment was no longer in evidence" [12]. They acknowledged that although it was possible that the patient's electroencephalogram would have recovered in any case, they suggested that further work of this nature was indicated. In view of the reports of the effectiveness of this treatment, it is surprising to discover that these findings were not transposed to the clinical situation immediately. It is interesting, however, that these papers of Prados, Aird, and Grenell suggesting the efficacy of steroid treatment for cerebral edema, preceded by two to four years the report in 1949 of Hench and Kendall that ACTH and cortisone were effective in ameliorating the symptoms of rheumatoid arthritis and rheumatic fever [15]. This discovery was later said to "have incited a revolution in clinical thought and to have been an event proclaimed by certain usually undemonstrative observers, as comparable with the advent of anesthesia and the enunciation of the germ theory of disease" [40].

Hume and Moore in 1951 noted relief of the signs and symptoms of increased intracranial pressure in one patient with a metastatic tumor treated with ACTH [16]. Then 6 more years elapsed before Kofman and his associates reported a series of patients with intracranial neoplasms treated with prednisolone and prednisone. 19 of these patients had metastatic tumors and one had a craniopharyngioma, and another an acoustic neurinoma. The majority of these patients showed an improvement in their signs and symptoms of increased intracranial pressure and neurological deficit [20]. In the meantime, reports occurred in the literature recommending the use of corticoids as supplemental therapy in patients having craniotomies for lesions in and around the sella [17, 31, 41, 42]. The emphasis in these reports was on the replacement value of the steroid as prophylaxis against the complications of operative trauma to the hypothalamus and pituitary gland. Ingraham did state, however, that a particularly desirable effect of cortisone and ACTH was their beneficial action on the development of cerebral edema. None of these reports, however, stimulated the use of corticosteroids for the control of increased intracranial pressure due to brain edema.

During this time, and going back to the early 1940's the Department of Neurosurgery at the University of Minnesota Health Sciences Center was concerned with problems related to cerebral edema. The use of sodium fluorescein to differentiate tumor from adjacent brain tissue at the operating table was an early by-product of this work [26]. The concept was then developed of using radioactive sodium diiodo-fluorescein in the detection of brain tumors by an external counting technique. This technique was later refined by the use of other gamma emitting agents and improvements in the detecting systems [28]. Other laboratory studies were conducted from which methods of altering cerebral vascular permeability and producing cerebral edema were developed such as intracarotid injection of concentrated doses of hypaque, diodrast, and bile salts [24]. Subsequently, these techniques were used to help assess the effects of other substances such as corticoids on altered cerebral vascular permeability. It was with this background that the observation was made in the laboratory in 1959, during studies with experimental brain tumors, that corticoids in large doses seemed to inhibit the growth of neoplasms. A study was therefore designed to determine at the time of surgery the concentration of corticoids in neoplastic and adjacent brain tissue when the corticoid was given by carotid injection immediately after angiography. It was conceived that perhaps the hypaque used for angiography would alter cerebral vascular permeability so that the corticoid could permeate the tumor in high concentration and inhibit the neoplastic growth. When this procedure was performed on extremely lethargic, aphasic, and hemiplegic patients with suspected brain tumors, it was observed that within 24 h they were often alert, talking and stronger. The responses seemed too rapid to be related to tumor growth inhibition alone and it was realized that the steroid must have altered the peritumoral edema. Based on this finding, a large clinical study was initiated in conjunction with the laboratory program. Galicich and French reported the earliest results from this study in 1961 which showed that dexamethasone often resulted in the rapid and dramatic relief of symptoms and signs of increased intracranial pressure and neurological dysfunction associated with cerebral edema [9, 10]. It was probably no coincidence that this first really enthusiastic and unequivocal report on the efficacy of steroids in the treatment of cerebral edema followed shortly after Arth and his associates reported the synthesis of dexamethasone in 1958 [2]. This newly synthesized gluco-corticoid was shown to have a very potent anti-inflammatory effect, yet little tendency to

Table 1. Relative pharmacological potencies of the steroids in common use

Compound	Relative antiinflammatory index	Relative sodium retaining index
Dexamethasone	25.0	0.0
Betamethasone	25.0	30.0
Fludrocortisone	15.0	125.0
Triamcinolone	5.0	0.0
Methylprednisolone	5.0	0.0
Prednisone	4.0	0.8
Prednisolone	3.5	0.8
Hydrocortisone	1.0	1.0
Cortisone	0.8	0.8

promote salt and water retention when compared with cortisone (Table 1). Galicich and French recognized the potential value of these characteristics and soon other confirmatory reports appeared [11, 18, 21, 32, 33, 34, 35, 43]. The clinical study has now been in progress over 12 years and is the subject of this report (Table 2 and 3).

Table 2. Etiology of cerebral edema in 1361 patients treated with dexamethasone

Associated Disease	No. of Patients Treated for Edema
Neoplasm	815
Craniotomy { operative and postoperative edema }	194
Intracranial hemorrhage	189
Closed head injury	142
Abscess	21
Total	1361

Table 3. Histological character of cerebral neoplasms in 815 patients treated with dexamethasone

I. Primary Brain Tumors		———	635
Gliomas		——— 551	
Glioblastoma	338		
Astrocytoma	196		
Oligodendroglioma	17		
Meningiomas		——— 84	
II. Secondary Brain Tumors (metastases)		———	180

Method

Dexamethasone (16 alpha methyl – 9 alpha fluoroprednisolone) was chosen for clinical evaluation and has been used exclusively in this study. This synthetic gluco-corticoid was chosen, as mentioned, because of its potent antiinflammatory effect and low salt retaining activity. Before dexamethasone was given to human beings, a preliminary study showed that two to four mg per kilogram of the drug could be injected parenterally into dogs with no ill effects. These doses exceeded by far the dosage used in the clinical study. The first 2 patients in the series were started with a 40 mg injection of dexamethasone phosphate into the carotid artery at the time of angiography. The intravenous and intramuscular routes of administration proved to be just as effective, however, and maximum effects seemed to be achieved with a lower loading dose of 10 mg intravenously followed by 4 mg intramuscularly every 6 h. In those patients subsequently undergoing surgery, this schedule was continued for 3 to 4 days because our clinical and laboratory studies suggested that surgical edema tends to peak between 48 and 72 h. Dosage was then usually tapered over a 5 to 7 day period and where the patient's condition permitted, the orally administered free alcohol form of the drug was used. In the initial phase of the study, a controlled double blind approach was used for drug administration. The early results left so little doubt about the efficacy of steroid therapy, that this approach was soon abandoned in the best interest of patients coming under our care. During the early years of the study, aluminum hydroxide gel and anticholinergic agents were given concomitantly to combat any possible ulcerogenic effect of the corticosteroid therapy. More recently, only antacids have been used. Some of the patients received anticonvulsants and antibiotics when indicated.

A clinical method was established at the outset of the study to evaluate the severity of edema and increased intracranial pressure. During the history, it was recorded if the patient was suffering from headache, nausea, or vomiting. The patient's general level of consciousness was described in detail and a bedside psychometric evaluation conducted. The ability to perform all functions of self-care and to ambulate were noted and a detailed neurological evaluation was included. Serial fundoscopic examinations were routinely carried out and the presence or absence of papilledema noted. Treatment with a steroid was then begun and improvement or disappearance of symptoms and signs noted. The temporal relationship of clinical changes to time of therapy onset were observed in addition to the extent of improvement. In addition, whenever possible, and still consistent with the best interests of the patients, brain scans and/ or angiograms were obtained before and after treatment in an attempt to verify and account for the clinical findings. Where feasible, serum and urine electrolytes were obtained to ascertain any gross disturbances in electrolyte metabolism. Fluid intake and output were recorded along with daily weights. At the time of surgery, a qualitative estimation of the amount of edema was carried out by gross observation of the brain tissue; by evaluation of fluorescein staining around the lesion after intravenous administration of 5 cc of 20 % fluorescein; and by light and electron microscopic study of tissue selected at specific distances from the lesion. Finally, the complete hospital course of these patients was carefully compared with that of similar patients not receiving steroids.

Results and Discussion

The symptoms of increased intracranial pressure associated with cerebral neoplasms such as headache, nausea, vomiting and depression of the sensorium, were the first to respond to dexamethasone therapy. These symptoms either improved or were completely alleviated in 84 % of the patients in whom they occurred, and this improvement usually began within 12 to 24 h (Fig. 1). Supportive evidence for the relief of increased intracranial pressure was obtained from patients with recurrent tumor whose tense, protruding craniotomy flap, or bulging burr holes relaxed noticeably after 24 to 72 h of steroid therapy. Some of these patients with nonresectable, recurrent gliomas were treated for weeks with the orally administered free alcohol form of dexamethasone. The symptomatic relief achieved was sufficient that they were able to live at home and interact socially with their families long after they otherwise would have been hospitalized for pre-terminal nursing care. The response of papilledema to steroids was more difficult to evaluate and interpret in the context of this study because unless improvement was detected before surgery or other treatments were started, it was not tabulated as such. The resolution of optic nerve edema was often quite gradual and the one-third incidence of improvement with steroid treatment was probably biased on the low side by the discipline of our criteria.

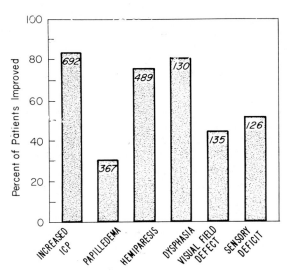

Fig. 1. Response of symptoms and signs in 815 patients with cerebral neoplasms after dexamethasone

Improvement in neurological function was related to the location of the tumor, and to some extent, to the type of tumor. Dysphasia was particularly responsive to therapy; presumably a reflection of the well recognized sensitivity of language funtion to increases in intracranial pressure. Hemiparesis also was significantly improved in better than 75 % of the cases studied. A poor response to therapy was usually associated with either a low grade infiltrating astrocytoma with only minimal weakness to begin with, or else a dense hemiplegia, later found to be associated with a particularly destructive lesion of the motor area.

The visual field defects and other sensory deficits appeared less responsive to steroid therapy. Occasionally, however, disturbances were not appreciated at the initial examination, and only after 24 to 48 h of steroid therapy did the patient's sensorium improve to levels adequate for cooperation and detailed sensory testing. It is conceivable under these circumstances that more improvement in sensory function would have been recorded by the examiner had better initial baseline evaluation of sensory function been possible. The best responses of visual field defects were seen in patients with small metastatic tumors and considerable edema located in the temporal or occipital regions of the brain. Patients with metastatic tumors showed more improvement, more rapidly, than those with glioblastomas, and these in turn responded better than patients with infiltrating astrocytomas. This finding correlates well with the severity of edema usually associated with these respective tumors [27]. The symptoms and signs caused by meningiomas responded less to steroid therapy than those secondary to high grade gliomas and metastatic tumors. The operative findings and light and electron microscopic observations on tissue obtained at surgery suggested that the clinical effects of meningiomas were better explained by the mass effect of the tumor itself, than by cerebral edema, thus accounting for less symptomatic response to steroids. The meningiomas examined by electron microscopy had many vessels with open pentalaminar junctions and large extracellular spaces which theoretically should favor edema formation. Usually, however, various combinations of pia mater, cerebral cortex, arcuate fibers, and gliosis were interposed between the extracellular tumor and the white matter. These tissues might prevent or lessen the passage of protein-rich edema fluid from tumor into white matter where the relative vulnerability to edema accumulation and spread is well appreciated [5]. Gliomas and metastatic tumors, on the other hand, were born in or adjacent to white matter and even infiltrated it and the above mentioned barriers to fluid egress from the tumor were not present. The slower growing meningiomas often reached large size before producing symptoms, presumably because of the brain's compressibility and compensability of function. This resulted in more cerebral compression than edema prior to removal of the tumor. When this ischemic, compressed brain tissue was decompressed at the time of surgery, however, edema often accumulated rapidly.

These clinical findings were supported by angiographic and radioisotope studies carried out before and 72 to 96 h after the initiation of steroid therapy. Brain scans sometimes showed reduction of radioisotope uptake around glioblastomas and metastatic tumors, when repeated after three days of therapy. Occasionally positive scans at the site of small metastatic tumors appeared almost normal when repeated. Repeat angiograms on patients with glioblastomas and metastatic tumors of the cerebral hemispheres showed less shift of the anterior cerebral artery and internal cerebral vein following steroid administration. These radiologic responses were much less obvious in cases that proved to have low grade astrocytomas and meningiomas.

The malignant edema associated with brain abscesses also responded to dexamethasone. Failure to control the edema and consequent increased intracranial pressure would have forced an operation to be performed under less than optimum conditions on many occasions. With good edema control, we were able to treat brain abscesses with systemic antibiotics and wait for them to encapsulate. This allowed us to semi-electively remove abscesses entirely in one operation or institute drainage procedures only after they were well walled off. The morbidity and mortality associated with brain abscesses were diminished considerably by this approach because the patients came to surgery with cerebral swelling under better control and there was also less opportunity for significant contamination of healthy brain and subarachnoid space. Early concern that the steroid therapy might reduce the body's resistance to infection and promote a fulminant meningo-encephalitis was not supported by our experience.

The assessment of dexamethasone therapy for edema associated with closed head injuries, intracranial hemorrhages, and craniotomies was difficult because the temporal course of these illnesses was not sufficiently stable or predictable to accept the patient as his own control. As near as we could determine, the clinical condition of patients with severe closed head injuries either improved, deteriorated, or stayed the same whether steroid was given or not. It was not uncommon to see definite improvement within 48 h after lesser head injuries, but distinguishing the influence of dexamethasone from the natural clinical course of the illness was not conclusive.

The concept of the "nonspecificity of brain edema" implies that the brain is able to react to injury in a limited fashion and therefore, the edema resulting from a variety of insults is histologically similar. The time sequence of edema formation and resolution varies, however, according to the nature of the causative lesion. Therefore, one would expect, as we have found in this study, a variation in response to steroid therapy depending upon the nature of the injury and the time therapy is initiated, relative to the onset of the injury. Our laboratory studies of various acute lesions, showed that it was important whether the animals were pretreated with steroids. The edema secondary to these experimental lesions was significantly less in animals pretreated compared with animals treated only after the injury [23]. We found in the clinical setting, where pretreatment was obviously not practical, that acute, time limited lesions such as head injuries and cerebral vascular accidents responded measurably less well than brain tumors and abscesses where there was a chronic, on-going state of continual edema production. Steroid therapy could be imposed at any time in the latter situation and a response achieved.

Another important factor was the extent of brain involvement. Wide-spread or generalized injury, whether acute or chronic, responded less well to steroid therapy than comparable focal lesions. Thus, we have found that chronic-focal lesions, like brain tumors and abscesses, responded the most, and acute-generalized lesions, such as severe closed head injuries, the least, with steroid therapy. Acute-focal processes and chronic-generalized processes fell intermediate in this therapeutic spectrum (Fig. 2).

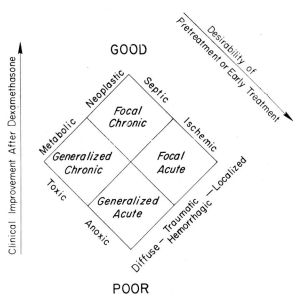

Fig. 2. Correlation of lesion characteristics with edema response after dexamethasone

Patients with various types of intracranial hemorrhage also responded less than patients with tumors to steroid therapy. Conclusive data on this group has not become available because of the rapidly changing natural clinical course of these patients and the frequent need for early institution of other supportive and definitive treatments. We have continued to give dexamethasone to patients with intracerebral and subarachnoid hemorrhages before surgery because we were impressed that the drug resulted in a smoother post-operative course. We have preferred to give steroids in preference to the osmotic diuretics to patients after subarachnoid hemorrhage from ruptured berry aneurysms for several reasons: 1) the osmotic agents cause extensive dehydration of all the brain tissues [3] which may be harmful when combined with the toxicity of the hemorrhage and the ischemia associated with cerebral vascular spasm. 2) Marked diuresis has resulted in hypovolemia and a drop in perfusion pressure through a cerebral vascular bed already constricted by spasm. 3) Osmotic diuresis can result in rapid brain shrinkage and sagging. Whether related or not, we have seen a disproportionate number of bleeds or re-bleeds occurring $1^1/_2$ to 6 h after mannitol or urea was given intravenously to patients with berry aneurysms. 4) The operative techniques we have come to depend upon rarely require the dehydrating agents for operative exposure. Steroid therapy, perhaps in conjunction with hyperventilation and/or cerebral spinal fluid drainage, has proven adequate. Moreover, we have found that during certain procedures the brain is slightly more difficult to work with because of the "toughening" of the tissue produced by the osmotic agents [7]. 5) Finally, the clinical course of these patients is erratic and difficult enough to appraise without the rebound swelling and other complications associated with osmotic agents.

We have not determined what effect, if any, steroid therapy has on the clearance rate of cells and protein from the cerebral spinal fluid of these patients. Whether steroids alter the incidence of adhesive arachnoiditis or the eventual development of communicating hydrocephalus after subarachnoid hemorrhage is currently being evaluated.

Patients initially moribund after intracerebral hemorrhage did not improve with steroid treatment and needed immediate surgery if they were to survive. Surgery should never be delayed on a deteriorating patient following an intracerebral bleed in the forlorn hope that steroids will change the clinical course. When the clinical condition of the patient permitted, however, we found that steroids could be started and surgery delayed 24 to 36 h. This approach gave the hematoma time to organize and retract so it could be delicately evacuated with less chance of fresh bleeding at the time of surgery. Better results were achieved when this latter method of management was possible.

It is apparent by now that control of operative and post-operative edema is one of the most important advantages accruing from the use of steroids in neurosurgery. Some of the early, previously reviewed reports on the use of adrenal steroids called attention to the benign post-operative course of patients undergoing craniotomy for craniopharyngioma [17, 31, 41, 42]. Galicich and French noted in one of their original papers on the subject, that post-operative edema improved characteristically within 5 to 18 h of steroid therapy [10]. It soon became apparent that brain tumor patients started on dexamethasone before surgery had unusually smooth post-operative courses. Following recovery from anesthesia, the patients were alert and active considering the extent of surgery. Furthermore, there was not as much depression of the sensorium or temporary increase in neurological deficit as was often observed during early post-operative period and usually attributed to cerebral edema. This has proven particularly true in the case of large meningiomas where we have made it an axiom that steroid therapy be started at least one day prior to craniotomy. As mentioned before, the pre-operative signs and symptoms of large meningiomas are primarily the result of the tumor mass compressing and distorting the surrounding brain. At the time of craniotomy and removal of the tumor there is a rapid decompression of this large area of compressed, ischemic brain tissue. In addition, there is surgical trauma from coagulation, exposure of the brain to air, retraction of the brain,

228

and perhaps obstruction of one or more large draining veins to the sagittal or other large sinuses causing venous congestion, stasis, and dilatation. All of these factors in combination can result in a massive edema post-operatively that may require re-operation and further surgical decompression. We have found that this sequence can be avoided by starting all suspected brain tumors on dexamethasone at least 24 h before surgery. Since this policy has been adopted, the incidence of post-operative re-exploration for brain swelling has decreased and the patients are alert and ambulating much earlier. This experience in turn has led us to begin dexamethasone before any craniotomy where we believe there is a reasonable chance that brain manipulation or retraction will be necessary.

Many of the patients treated for cerebral edema associated with surgery would have recovered without steroids, but spontaneous regression of symptoms was usually slow, extending over a period of days or even weeks. Evidence of a positive correlation between dexamethasone and symptomatic improvement came about as a result of medication being discontinued or the dosage being reduced after 2 or 3 days of therapy. The signs of edema re-appeared after a latent period of 12 to 24 h. Re-administration of the drug or increase in dosage again brought about rapid improvement. Of course, during and after surgery other means of controlling intracranial pressure and edema such as hyperventilation, fluid restriction, lumbar or ventricular drainage and occasionally osmotic agents were used when necessary and indicated.

Because the vast majority of patients in this study were treated with high doses of dexamethasone for a very short period of time, the common side effects were rarely seen. All patients were screened for any history suggesting an ulcer diathesis and this is strongly recommended. Gastro-intestinal bleeding occurred in 4.7% of the patients studied, and most of this incidence was accounted for by minor episodes of gastritis or esophagitis with small amounts of blood aspirated at one time or another from the nasal-gastric tube or else by blood found in the stomach at autopsy. Significant and serious gastrointestinal hemorrhage occurred almost exclusively in patients with severe head injuries with brain stem involvement, or in comatose patients who often were on the respirator. Five patients who died at the time of large gastrointestinal bleeds had been in the intensive care unit for a prolonged period of time, on the respirator, and the dosage of dexamethasone had been kept at 16 mg per day for 10 days or longer. All of these cases showed gastrointestinal ulceration. Others have reported a much higher incidence of gastrointestinal bleeding with steroid therapy than we have found [4]. The proportion of acute, severe head injuries is relatively low in our series, however, and we have kept the duration of therapy short. We have also been extremely compulsive about antacid coverage when the patient is taking dexamethasone. Norton and his associates had 10 of 19 patients who were comatose following severe cerebral trauma showing evidence of gastric acid hypersecretion within the week following surgery. 3 of the 10 bled from presumed stress ulcers. Their study in combination with our experience suggest that neurosurgeons treating large numbers of severe head injuries might expect more complications and less obvious symptomatic benefit from steroid therapy in that particular group of patients.

The catabolic and antifibroblastic effects of dexamethasone did not noticeably interfere with wound healing and no effort was made to treat wounds differently or leave sutures in place longer. Delayed wound healing was invariably associated with scalp that had been irradiated or was otherwise damaged. The incidence of wound infection was not greater in patients treated with gluco-corticoids and as previously mentioned, no dissemination of infection occurred after drainage or excision of intra-cerebral abscesses.

Acute rebound edema was avoided by carefully tapering the dosage over a week's time before stopping therapy. Where daily 17 – hydroxycorticosteroid excretion was monitored it was apparent that the suppression of ACTH and endogenous production of hormone could occur within 48 to 72 h. This substantiated the need for slow with-drawal from dexamethasone even after a few days of concentrated therapy.

Mild electrolyte disturbances sometimes occurred in the immediate post-operative period, though not necessarily due to the dexamethasone therapy. Mild hypochlor-emia and hyponatremia were most commonly found and these were managed without difficulty. Urinary-excretion studies were somewhat variable, but frequently showed a brief initial sodium retention followed by a sodium and water diuresis. A mild po-tassium diuresis was also seen, but hypokalemia was not a problem. The diabetogenic effect of gluco-corticoids did not cause serious problems in diabetic management, though glucosuria was occasionally recognized for the first time after steroid therapy was started and in at least three incidences was associated with noticeable diuresis.

References

1. Aird, R. B., Strait, L. A., Zealear, D., Hrenoff, M.: Neurophysiological studies on cerebral concussion. Trans. Amer. neurol. Ass. 89–92 (1947).
2. Arth, G. E., Johnston, D. B. R., Fried, J., Spooncer, W. W., Hoff, D. R., Sarett, L. H.: 16-Methylated steroids. I. 16 α-Methylated analogs of cortisone, a new group of anti-inflammatory steroids. J. Amer. chem. Soc. 80, 3160 (1958).
3. Beks, J. W. F., Walter, W. G.: Some considerations on controlling cerebral oedema. Psychiat. Neurol. Neurochir. (Amst.) 71, 9–12 (1968).
4. Cantu, R. C., Amir-Ahmadi, H., Prieto, A.: Evaluation of the increased risk of gastro-intestinal bleeding following intracranial surgery in patients receiving high steroid do-sages in the immediate post-operative period. Int. surg. Dig. 50, 325–335 (1968).
5. Feigin, I., Popoff, N.: Neuropathological observations on cerebral edema. The acute phase. Arch. Neurol. 6, 77–86 (1962).
6. Freed, S. C., Lindner, E.: The effect of steroids on the adrenal cortex and ovary on capil-lary permeability. Amer. J. Physiol. 134, 258–262 (1941).
7. French, L. A., Chou, S. N., Story, J. L., Schultz, E. A.: Aneurysm of the anterior com-municating artery. J. Neurosurg. 24, 1057–1062 (1966).
8. Fünfgeld, E.: Hirnschwellung und Hirntumor. Dtsch. Z. Nervenheilk. 114, 209–213 (1930).
9. Galicich, J. H., French, L. A., Melby, J. C.: Use of dexamethasone in treatment of cere-bral edema associated with brain tumors. J. Lancet 31, 46–53 (1961).
10. — — Use of dexamethasone in the treatment of cerebral edema resulting from brain tumors and brain surgery. Amer. Practit. 12, 169–174 (1961).
11. Gårde, A.: Experiences with dexamethasone treatment of intracranial pressure caused by brain tumors. Acta. neurol. scand. 41, Suppl. 13, Part II, 439–443 (1965).
12. Grenell, R. G., McCawley, E. L.: Central nervous system resistance. III. The effect of adrenal cortical substances on the central nervous system. J. Neurosurg. 4, 508–518 (1947).
13. Hartman, F. A., Brownell, K. A.: The hormone of the adrenal cortex. Science 72, 76 (1930).
14. — Beck, G. M., Thorn, G. W.: Improvement in nervous and mental states under cortin therapy. J. Nerv. ment. Dis. 77, 1–21 (1933).
15. Hench, P. S., Kendall, E. C., Slocumb, C. H., Polley, H. F.: The effect of a hormone of the adrenal cortex and of pituitary adrenocorticotrophic arthritis. Proc. Mayo Clin. 24, 181–197 (1949).

16. Hume, D. M., Moore, F. D.: The use of ACTH, cortisone, and adrenal cortical extracts in surgical patients. In: Mote, J. R. (Ed.): Proceedings of the Second Clinical ACTH Conference, Vol. II., pp. 289–309. London: Jr. & H. Churchill, Ltd. 1951.
17. Ingraham, F. D., Matson, D. D., McLaurin, R. L.: Cortisone and ACTH as an adjunct to the surgery of craniopharyngiomas. New Engl. J. Med. **246**, 568–571 (1952).
18. King, D. F., Moon, W. J., Brown, N.: Corticosteroid drugs in the management of primary and secondary malignant cerebral tumors. Med. J. Aust. **2**, 878–881 (1965).
19. Kocher, T.: Hirnerschütterung, Hirndruck und chirurgische Eingriffe bei Hirnkrankheiten. In: Nothnagel: Specielle Pathologie und Therapie. Wien: Holder, A., **5** (1901).
20. Kofman, S., Garvin, J. S., Nagamani, D., Taylor, S. G.: Treatment of cerebral metastases from breast carcinoma with prednisolone. J. Amer. med. Ass. **163**, 1473–1476 (1957).
21. Kullberg, G., West, K. A.: Influence of corticosteroids on the ventricular fluid pressure. Acta. neurol. scand. **41**, Suppl. 13, Part II., 445–452 (1965).
22. Long, D. M.: An electron microscopic evaluation of cerebral edema and its response to steroid administration. Thesis, University of Minnesota 1964.
23. Maxwell, R. E., Long, D. M., French, L. A.: The effects of glucosteroids upon cold-induced brain edema. I. Gross morphological and vascular permeability changes. J. Neurosurg. **34**, 477–487 (1971).
24. McIntosh, J. E., French, L. A., Peyton, W. T.: Studies on cerebrovascular permeability. Med. Bull., Univ. Minn. **28**, 250–255 (1957).
25. Menkin, V.: Effect of adrenal cortex extract on capillary permeability. Amer. J. Physiol. **129**, 691–697 (1940).
26. Moore, G. E., Peyton, W. T., French, L. A., Walker, W. W.: The clinical use of fluorescein in neurosurgery: The localization of brain tumors. J. Neurosurg. **5**, 392–398 (1948).
27. Perret, G. E., Kernohan, J. W.: Histopathologic changes of brain caused by intracranial tumors (so-called edema or swelling of the brain). J. Neuropath. exp. Neurol. **2**, 341–352 (1943).
28. Peyton, W. T., Moore, G. E., French, L. A., Chou, S. N.: Localization of intracranial lesions by radioactive isotopes. J. Neurosurg. **9**, 432–442 (1952).
29. Prados, M., Strowger, B., Feindel, W.: Studies on cerebral edema: I. Reaction of the brain to exposure to air; physiologic changes. Arch. Neurol. Psychiat. (Chic.) **54**, 163 to 174 (1945).
30. — — — Studies on cerebral edema: II. Reaction of the brain to exposure to air; physiologic changes. Arch. Neurol. Psychiat. (Chic.) **54**, 290–300 (1945).
31. Raaf, J., Stainsby, D. L., Larson, W. L. E.: The use of ACTH in conjunction with surgery for neoplasms in the parasellar area. J. Neurosurg. **11**, 463–470 (1954).
32. Rasmussen, T., Gulati, D. R.: Cortisone in the treatment of postoperative cerebral edema. J. Neurosurg. **19**, 535–544 (1962).
33. Ruderman, N. B., Hall, T. C.: Use of glucosteroids in the palliative treatment of metastatic brain tumors. Cancer **18**, 298–306 (1965).
34. Smith, R. A., Smith, W. A.: Steroid therapy of cerebral edema. J. med. Ass. Ga. **56**, 324–328 (1967).
35. Sparacio, R. R., Lin, T. H., Cook, A. W.: Methyl prednisolone sodium succinate in acute craniocerebral trauma. Surg. Gynec. Obst. **121**, 513–516 (1965).
36. Spatz, H.: Die Bedeutung der „symptomatischen" Hirnschwellung für die Hirntumoren und für andere raumbeengende Prozesse in der Schädelgrube. Arch. Psychiat. Nervenkr. **88**, 790–794 (1929).
37. Stengel, E.: Zur Pathologie der letalen Hirnschwellung (ein Beitrag zur Kasuistik der Fernwirkung von Hirntumoren). Jb. Psychiat. Neurol. **45**, 187–200 (1927).
38. Swingle, W. D., Pfiffner, J. J.: The revival of comatose adrenalectomized cats with an extract of the suprarenal cortex. Science **72**, 75–76 (1930).
39. — — Vars, H. M., Parkins, W. M.: The effect of hemorrhage on the normal and adrenalectomized dog. Amer. J. Physiol. **107**, 259–274 (1934).
40. Tapperman, J.: Adrenal Cortex. In: Drill, V. A. (Ed.): Pharmacology in Medicine, Ed. 2, p. 1057. New York: McGraw-Hill 1958.

41. Troen, P., Rynearson, E. H.: An evaluation of the prophylactic use of cortisone for pituitary operation. J. clin. Endocr. **16**, 747–754 (1956).
42. Tytus, J. S., Seltzer, H. S., Kahn, E. A.: Cortisone as an aid in the surgical treatment of craniopharyngiomas. J. Neurosurg. **12**, 555–564 (1955).
43. Verdura, J., Brown, H., White, R. J.: Use of adrenal steroids in cerebral metastasis. Case report of improvement documented by angiography. Ohio St. med. J. **50**, 693–694 (1963).
44. Weed, L. H., McKibben, P. S.: Experimental alterations of brain bulk. Amer. J. Physiol. **48**, 531–558 (1919).

Clinical Experiences with Steroids in Neurosurgical Patients

Jan W. F. Beks, H. Doorenbos and G. J. M. Walstra

Department of Neurosurgery, University Hospital, Groningen, Netherlands

Introduction

One of the most important aims in medicine is to prevent diseases or complications of necessary interventions. As you all know, one of the major problems for each neurosurgeon is the increase of intracranial pressure, caused by brain edema, that can develop after intracranial surgery.

The object of our investigations was, like Galicich and French (1961) and Rasmussen and Gulati (1962) have done before us, to study from a large number of patients, the influence of the pre-operative administration of corticosteroids on the postoperative course in patients who had intracranial surgery.

Materials and Methods

There were two groups of each 400 patients in our study, who all had intracranial surgery for different reasons.

Patients in group one, were operated upon without administration of steroids and in group two, the patients received steroids 24 h pre-operatively (Table 1 and 2).

Table 1

PATIENTS WITH STEROIDS

cause of operation	total number	pre-operative increased intra cranial pressure	
		yes	no
malignant tumor	224	198	26
benignant tumor	70	58	12
metastasis	57	51	6
aneurysm	32	–	32
pituitary tumor	17	–	17
	400	307	93

The groups were subdivided in a group of patients who had pre-operatively symptoms of increased intracranial pressure and a group, who had no signs of this

233

complication. Also was studied in both groups, in how many patients during the operation acute brain edema developed.

Table 2

PATIENTS WITHOUT STEROIDS

cause of operation	total number	pre-operative increased intra cranial pressure	
		yes	no
malignant tumor	212	193	19
benignant tumor	81	68	13
metastasis	53	47	6
aneurysm	47	–	47
pituitary tumor	7	–	7
	400	308	92

The regime of prophylactic cortisone the patients were put upon, was as follows: A patient of 70 kg body weight received the day before operation 3 × dd 100 mg cortisone-acetate intramuscularly. This dose was also given during the day of operation and the four days following operation. In the following days the dose was decreased gradually over a period of three to five days.

Because of the salt-retaining effect of cortisone-acetate and the tendency for excretion of potassium in the postoperative period, the patients were given 2 l of a 5 % glucose-infusion intravenously. KCl-supplements were added to the infusion in a dose of 40 to 60 mEq daily.

The contra-indications for the treatment with cortisone-acetate were only relative. It were those patients who had in their history gastric ulcers, diabetes and tuberculosis. This chronic infection can be activated by the use of steroids. Therefore I.N.H. was given in the postoperative period for 6 weeks.

Our criteria for the relief of postoperative cerebral edema were improvement of the pre-operative excisting papilledema, no depression of the sensorium, the lack of tension in the decompression, and no temporary increase in neurological deficit.

In our study we looked for the following complications attributed to the cortisone-acetate therapy: electrolyte-disturbances, impaired wound healing, masked postoperative clots, gastro-intestinal ulcers and bleeding, hyperglycaemia and psychotic disturbances.

The groups of patients were subdivided in:

1. Patients with malignant brain tumors
2. Patients with benign brain tumors
3. Patients with metastasis
    4 patients with subarachnoid hemorrhage
    5 patients with a pituitary tumor

Results

The use of a prophylactic cortisone regime seems as an aid in the treatment of patients who will undergo intracranial surgery.

234

Only 16 out of 400 patients had symptoms of increase of the intracranial pressure in the postoperative period. In the group of patients who were operated upon without cortisone this number was 102 (Table 3).

Table 3

COMPARISON OF INCIDENCE OF
POSTOPERATIVE CEREBRAL EDEMA WITHOUT STEROIDS AND WITH STEROIDS

cause of operation	without steroids			with steroids		
	total number	cerebral edema	percentage	total number	cerebral edema	percentage
maligne	212	51	24,1 %	224	7	3,1 %
benigne	81	18	22,2 %	70	3	4,0 %
metastasis	53	17	32,1 %	57	4	7,0 %
aneurysm	47	14	29,8 %	32	2	6,3 %
pituitary	7	2	28,5 %	17	–	0,0 %
	400	102	25,5 %	400	16	4,0 %

Also the number of patients who developed acute cerebral edema during the surgical procedure was decreased. This complication, however, was more frequent in patients who had before operation signs and symptoms of increased intracranial pressure (Table 4).

Complications of the steroid-treatment were seen in 16 out of 383 patients (Table 5).

Table 4

COMPARISON OF INCIDENCE OF
ACUTE BRAINSWELLING DURING OPERATION

Cause of operation	without steroids			with steroids		
	total number	acute swelling	percentage	total number	acute swelling	percentage
maligne	212	19	9,0%	224	3	1,3%
benigne	81	5	6,2%	70	1	1,4%
metastasis	53	6	11,3%	57	2	3,5%
aneurysm	47	2	4,3%	32	–	–
pituitary	7	–	–	17	–	–
	400	32	8,0%	400	6	1,5%

Table 5

COMPARISON OF
COMPLICATIONS OF STEROID ADMINISTRATION

cause of operation	total number		electrolyt disturb.		wound healing		wound infection		haema toma		hemorrhage intest.tract		diabetes		psych. disturb.	
	without	with	without	with	without	with	without	with	without	with	without	with	without	with	without	with
maligne	212	224	1	2	-	-	1	1	-	-	1	3	-	2	-	1
benigne	81	70	-	1	-	-	-	-	-	-	-	1	-	1	-	-
metastasis	53	57	-	1	-	-	-	1	-	-	-	2	-	-	-	-
aneurysm	47	32	-	-	-	-	-	-	-	-	-	-	-	-	-	-
	393	383	1	4	-	-	1	2	-	-	1	6	-	3	-	1

236

The patients who were operated upon for a pituitary tumor are not included in this series as a possible change in the endocrine equilibrium does not permit this. Also in this group no serious electrolyte disturbances were observed, but a deviation of the intravenous fluid administration using either saline or water in the form of 5 % glucose was necessary somewhat more often.

In none of the patients edema was observed. Retention of NaCl was not possible as it was usually not given by the intravenous route. In 7 patients serum potassium fell below 3.8 mEq/l. The lowest value observed was 3.1 mEq/l. Serum electrolytes were determined on the first five postoperative days and the i. v. fluid-administration was modified in 16 cases. In four of these cases, i. v. saline was given. In 7 cases the amount of KCl was increased. In 5 cases more than 2 l i.v. fluid was given per 24 h.

As soon as the patient was able to take oral food, salt restriction was stopped. In most cases this happened on the second postoperative day. Thus the salt content of the food taken by the oral route was never restricted.

In 3 cases transient hyperglycaemia was seen during steroid treatment (more than 180 mg %). 2 of these patients received insulin, one of them for more than one week. In no instance a permanent deterioration of glucose tolerance was seen.

4 of the 6 patients who had a gastric hemorrhage, had a history of gastric ulcer. In 2 cases surgical intervention was needed.

We did not observe delay in wound-healing, nor an increased incidence of bacterial infection. We did not observe more masked hemorrhages in the post-operative phase.

We found a manifest decrease in the dislocation of the anatomical structures, when using steroids in many patients, as did Galicich and French. However, this was not the case in all patients that improved after steroid administration.

In our clinic it is customary to use cortisone-acetate in the prevention of cerebral edema. This steroid has apart from its anti-inflammatory effect also a mineralocorticoid effect, retaining NaCl and inducing potassium loss. However, this mineralocorticoid effect is clinically not important when no intravenous saline was given. Only when the sodium concentration fell below 125 mEq/l sodium chloride was given intravenously. The salt content of the food was never restricted.

Many neurosurgeons prefer dexamethasone in the prevention of cerebral edema. This steroid has no mineralo-corticoid effect, perhaps meticulous follow-up of the electrolyte concentrations in the blood is not necessary.

However, optimal postoperative management of dexamethasone treated patients should also include regular determination of serum electrolytes since this steroid may have a diuretic action. Its diabetogenic effect is comparable to that of cortisone-acetate. The mineralo-corticoid action of cortisone-acetate gives this steroid an advantage above dexamethasone in patients rendered adrenally insufficient by impaired secretion of ACTH following the neurosurgical procedure. When sodium depletion occurs, the adrenals will still be able to increase the production of the mineralocorticoid aldosterone. However, before aldosterone production is stimulated, some degrees of water and salt depletion will have to be present.

For the reasons mentioned above, we are of the opinion that mineralocorticoid inactive steroid dexamethasone offers no advantage above the natural hormon cortisone that does have mineralocorticoid activity.

In addition the lower potency per milligram of cortisone makes it possible to dose the anti-inflammatory effect of steroid-treatment better than with the highly potent dexamethasone. This last argument is mainly theoretical.

Summary and Conclusions

Cortisone-acetate administered to patients undergoing craniotomy for brain tumors or subarachnoid hemorrhage has favourable effect on the post-operative course.

In the patients operated upon without pre-operative cortisone administration 25.5 % had symptoms and signs of increased intracranial pressure due to postoperative cerebral edema. In the other group this was 4.25 %.

The only serious complications from the prophylactic cortisone regime we observed, were gastro-intestinal bleedings in 6 patients.

The actual mechanism of steroid action is still unknown. This is again emphasized by some observations we did in patients who had an impressive improvement in the neurological status, but in which we could not show any reduction in the pretreatment displacement of the cerebral vasculature.

It is concluded that the prevention of the development of postoperative cerebral edema is highly effective and safe, but with Rasmussen and Gulati, we agree that prophylactic cortisone is not a panacea, that it does not prevent cerebral edema completely and it is not a substitute for gentle manipulation of the brain. It must be regarded as an aid in increasing the safety of craniotomies for lesions in which postoperative cerebral edema may be a significant factor.

References

French, L. A., Galicich, J. H.: The use of steroids for control of cerebral edema. Clin. Neurosurg. **10**, 212–223 (1964).

Galicich, J. H., French, L. A.: Use of dexamethasone in the treatment of cerebral edema resulting from brain tumors and brain surgery. Amer. Practit. **12**, 169–174 (1961).

Rasmussen, T., Gulati, D. R.: Cortisone in the treatment of postoperative cerebral edema. J. Neurosurg. **19**, 535–544 (1962).

The Effect of Dexamethasone on Water and Electrolyte Content and on rCBF in Perifocal Brain Edema in Man*

Hans J. Reulen, Alexander Hadjidimos, and Kurt Schürmann

Department of Neurosurgery, University of Mainz, Mainz, W. Germany

With 4 Figures

Summary. The results of clinical studies are reported dealing with the relationship between cerebral edema and regional cerebral blood flow in patients with brain tumor as well as with the effect of dexamethasone on this relationship. rCBF is found to be significantly reduced in brain tissue surrounding brain tumors. Autoregulation as well as cerebrovascular reactivity to $PaCO_2$ is focally or generally impaired. Water content of perifocal white matter is markedly increased. The combination of tissue lactacidosis, low regional blood flow and vasoparalysis seems to be a characteristic finding in this type of *local* brain edema. The increased local tissue pressure, due to the increased tissue water content, is a main factor responsible for the local flow decrease. A locally elevated tissue pressure will tend to collapse the capillaries and the venules, raise the local cerebrovascular resistance and counteract the vasodilating effect of a low tissue pH.

Administration of dexamethasone (16 mg or 24 mg daily during 4–6 days) reduces the water and sodium content in edematous white matter surrounding a brain tumor but does not influence the potassium content. Measurements of rCBF before and after dexamethasone treatment (24 mg daily during 5–7 days) discloses a significant increase in mean rCBF. Impaired vasomotor response to changes in arterial PCO_2 as well as to changes in arterial blood pressure is markedly improved. The beneficial effect of this drug could be locally demonstrated even in absence of marked signs of increased ICP (case report).

Introduction

Brain tumors are often associated with perifocal or generalized brain edema and increased intracranial pressure. The extent of brain edema and the related intracranial dynamics may determine the final outcome of patients undergoing craniotomy. Therefore, the main interest of clinicians has long been directed towards the control of brain edema and increased intracranial pressure (ICP).

The following report is concerned with findings in patients with brain tumors. The report summarizes 3 series of studies dealing with the relationship between cerebral edema and cerebral blood flow and the effect of dexamethasone on this relationship.

---

* Supported by a grant of the Volkswagen-Foundation.

1. rCBF in Brain Edema

Global and regional cerebral blood flow in patients with brain tumors was found to be diminished by 30–40% [7, 13, 17, 18, 31, 33]. Regions corresponding to the tumor location frequently show an absolute or relative hyperaemia and in a few cases a relative hypoaemia. However, rCBF is always found to be markedly decreased in the surrounding brain tissue, particularly in the immediate neighbourhood [17, 18]. In most instances, the mechanisms regulating the cerebral blood flow are *focally* impaired. Autoregulation of cerebral blood flow to blood pressure changes is impaired or lost in the majority of cases, especially in and around the tumor region [7, 18, 33]. As a result the blood flow follows passively the blood pressure changes. Additionally, the vasomotor response to changes in $PaCO_2$ – increase in flow with hypercapnia and decrease in flow with hypocapnia – is abolished in these areas [7, 18, 24, 33]. Sometimes even unexpected changes were observed in the opposite direction. A focal rise in flow following hyperventilation indicates a shifting of the blood flow from the "healthy" towards the involved areas and has been called "intracerebral inverse steal syndrome" [24, 33].

What are the factors responsible for the depression in tissue flow as well as the defect in vasomotor response? Classically it is considered that *local* circulation is determined by the effective perfusion pressure, the cerebrovascular resistance and the blood viscosity. Various experimental findings presented evidence that brain edema and tissue acidosis, both present in brain tissue surrounding tumors interfere with these determinants and are responsible for most of the described changes.

The Role of Brain Edema

How does edema influence local blood flow? In edematous brain tissue surrounding human brain tumors an increase in water and sodium content has been observed, especially in the white matter. Potassium content is lowered in the cortex and remains unchanged in the white matter as compared to normal values [10, 11, 35, 39]. A local increase of the water content of the white matter from 70 to 80% necessarily increases the volume of this tissue area by about 50%. That means that the *local tissue pressure* in edematous brain should be expected to be markedly elevated. Brock *et al.* [8] recently have provided evidence that pressure gradients exist within the skull between the normal and the edematous hemisphere. They have proposed that these pressure gradients between the edematous and normal hemisphere are the reason for the displacement of cerebral structures. A rising extravascular pressure due to pathological accumulation of edema fluid in the extracellular space may approach the intravascular pressure in the downstream end of a capillary and tend to collapse this capillary. In order to maintain blood flow the intracapillary pressure must be as high – in fact a little higher. The decrease in arteriovenous pressure difference in association with the decrease of capillary radius increases the resistance and drops the flow [19, 26, 37]. It has been shown that the "critical closing pressure" – the arterial pressure at which flow stops – increases when extracapillary pressure is raised by accumulation of edema fluid [4, 38].

Our data suggest that this relationship can also be attributed to the depression in flow in brain edema in man (Fig. 1). Measurements of rCBF and brain biopsies were performed in 14 patients with brain tumors and brain lesions at the time of craniotomy. Following opening of the dura, rCBF was measured over the brain tissue adjacent to the tumor using the [133]-Xe-clearance method [20]. Following the rCBF measurement one or two tissue samples including both grey and subcortical white matter for the determination of water content were removed corresponding to the location of the respective scintillation probe in an area which later had to be extirpated [19, 37].

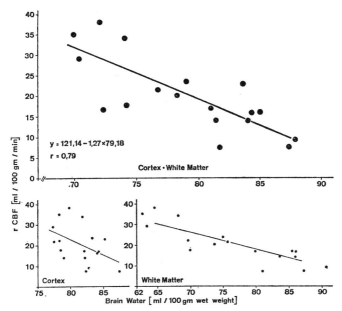

Fig. 1. Relation between regional water content (abscissa) and regional cerebral blood flow (ordinate) in cerebral edema adjacent to brain tumors and brain lesions. Each circle represents the values of one tissue area.

Upper panel: Data of regional brain water content represent the mean of the individual values of water content of cortex and of subjacent white matter.

Lower panel: Data of regional brain water content represent the individual values of water content of cortex (left panel) and of white matter (right panel). All rCBF values were corrected to a standard $PaCO_2$ of 40 mmHg

Figure 1 indicates that with increasing local tissue water content the local tissue flow of the respective tissue area decreases. Recent observations in experimentally induced brain edema following a water intoxication or a local cold injury are in agreement with these findings [12, 28]. It may therefore be concluded from these data that *increased local tissue pressure due to brain edema is a main factor responsible for the depression in flow* observed in patients with brain tumors. The interpretation of the results would have been probably more convincing if direct measurements of local interstitial fluid pressure could be obtained. Unfortunately the methods for the measurement of tissue pressure are still a matter of discussion.

The Role of Tissue Acidosis

In edematous tissue surrounding brain tumors an accumulation of lactate and an increase in lactate/pyruvate-ratio has been found concomitant with a breakdown of the

241

labile energy-rich phosphate compounds CrP and ATP [32, 35, 36], indicating an underoxygenation of this tissue areas. This has been confirmed in experimentally induced cerebral edema following water intoxication [28], local cold injury [12, 36] and occlusion of the middle cerebral artery [3]. Correspondingly Pampus [34] has found a variety of different tissue pH adjacent to brain tumors, the average of which is markedly reduced. In CSF a comparable increase of lactate, of lactate/pyruvate-ratio and a simultaneous decrease of pH and of bicarbonate has been observed [15]. It is generally accepted that brain tissue acidosis is reflected by similar changes in CSF and brain extracellular fluid.

It is evident from various studies that the brain extracellular pH is a main factor controlling CBF in normal brain by regulating cerebral *arteriolar* resistance [25, 40]. A local acidosis increases the diameter of the arterioles and subsequently the blood flow while a local alkalosis acts in the opposite direction. With this in mind it may be conceived that a tissue acidosis induced by cerebral hypoxia is followed by a hyperaemia [42]. A longlasting tissue acidosis may lead to a state of extreme vasodilatation which causes an impairment or a loss of normal arteriolar response to changes in arterial blood pressure and in arterial PCO_2. This hypothesis was postulated by Lassen [25] in 1966. Such vasoparalysis has commonly been found experimentally and clinically in brain tumors, head injuries and vascular lesions [7, 12, 26, 33]. *As a consequence of the loss of autoregulation* (passive pressure – flow relationship) *the local tissue flow becomes dependent from the local tissue perfusion pressure,* i. e. the difference between arteriolar blood pressure and local tissue pressure. The latter may be conditioned by both, the ICP as well as the local edema. It seems obvious that with a given level of ICP different local tissue pressures may be encountered around a brain tumor.

In edematous tissue the effect of the vasodilatation is locally counteracted by the increased tissue pressure. That may further explain the concomitant occurrence of *low tissue flow, vasoparalysis* and *low CSF pH*. Hence, this combination may be used to characterize severe brain edema. Consequently we assume that in less edematous areas and borderline regions local tissue pressure is not high enough to counteract the effect of a slight tissue acidosis so that hyperaemia will occur in such regions [19, 37]. The experiments of Frei *et al.* [12] as well as Bartko *et al.* [3] support this assumption.

The CSF-acidosis may also explain another event occuring in brain edema. In the state of loss of arteriolar tonus the arterial pressure head should be transmitted to the capillary level with subsequent transcapillary transudation of fluid into the surrounding brain tissue. This *"break-through"* of pressure may be the explanation of the findings of Klatzo *et al.* [22] that in blood-brain barrier damage associated with cold injury edema an elevation of the systolic blood pressure to 200 mmHg produces a conspicuous acceleration in the spreading of the edema as well as the protein tracers used. When hypertension is accompanied by severe hypercapnia (CSFpH = 7.0), Meinig *et al.* [29] found that even in normal brain acute hypertension above 180 mmHg (MABP) is followed by a significant increase of water content of the white matter.

II. Effect of Dexamethasone on Perifocal Brain Edema

In agreement with previous reports [9, 14, 27] the administration of large doses of dexamethasone in patients undergoing craniotomy and removal of brain tumors resulted in a significant improvement of the immediate postoperative course and a decrease of mortality. The operative mortality dropped from 29 % before to 15 % after the introduction of dexamethasone. This includes all deaths occurring postoperatively during the hospitalization. Similar figures have been published by Bucy and Jelsma [9].

Don Long *et al.* [27] provided electron microscopic evidence of marked reduction of ultrastructural characteristics of perifocal edema following dexamethasone treatment. Astrocytic swelling in the cortex was less apparent and the enlargement of the extracellular space in the white matter, filled with plasmalike fluid, was remarkably diminished. An attempt was made to estimate whether this effect of dexamethasone, demonstrated by ultrastructural observation, can be assessed by a more quantitative method. The effect of dexamethasone was compared with the effect of two different diuretics, ethacrynic acid and spirolactone.

42 patients undergoing craniotomy due to brain tumors or brain lesions were pretreated with either dexamethasone (4 mg every 6 h, intramuscularly), with ethacrynic acid (75 mg daily) or with spirolactone (600 mg daily). All patients were treated with the uniform dosage of the respective drugs during 4 to 6 days before the operation. 18 untreated patients served as controls. In order to avoid subjective selection of patients, the patients were alternatively classified in one of the 4 groups according to the day of their hospitalization.

At the time of craniotomy tissue samples of grey and subjacent white matter were obtained from areas which had to be operatively removed. No hypertonic solutions were administered and care was taken to avoid tissue damage before sampling. Care was also exercised in sampling deep white matter, since the water content of the arcuate zone, the corpus callosum and the deep white matter differs significantly in normal human brain [10, 11]. However, in some instances samples were contaminated with arcuate zone.

Samples used for measurement of water and electrolyte content were excised from one or two areas adjacent to the tumor. Samples used for the analysis of metabolites were removed by the use of a rongeur precooled in liquid nitrogen and immediately transferred into liquid nitrogen. Procedures for the determination of water, electrolytes and metabolites in brain tissue have been described previously [35].

18 patients were not pretreated with either dexamethasone or a diuretic. The changes in the perifocal brain tissue consisted in a marked increase of the water and sodium content of the white matter as compared to values obtained from morphologically normal areas during lobectomy [35] or from normal human brain at autopsy [10, 11, 39]. Potassium content of the white matter was not significantly altered. In the cortex a slight increase of sodium was observed in comparison to the values found distant to brain tumors (Table 1).

When dexamethasone treatment was started 4–6 days prior to the craniotomy the water and sodium content of the perifocal white matter was significantly reduced (Fig. 2). Although the diminution of water content amounted to about 3,5 %, the value of 75.7 % is still considerably higher than the value of normal human white matter (centrum ovale) which was reported as 69–71 % at autopsy [10, 11]. In the cortex a moderate decrease in sodium content was observed. It should be mentioned that in a recent series, consisting of 10 patients pretreated with 24 mg of dexamethasone (8 mg at 8 h intervals intramuscularly for 4 days) similar results have been obtained.

For comparison the results obtained after the use of ethacrynic acid and spirolactone are illustrated in Figure 2. Diuretics have sometimes been used in combination with other drugs in the treatment of brain edema. However, few studies have been carried out to prove their effectiveness or to compare their effect with corticosteroids.

Table 1. Effect of dexamethasone and of diuretics on the water, sodium and potassium content of edematous brain tissue surrounding brain tumors and brain lesions

	n	Cerebral Cortex			White Matter		
		Water	Sodium	Potassium	Water	Sodium	Potassium
Untreated	18	81.0±0.7	39.9±2.0	43.0±2.6	79.0±1.3	42.0±2.6	28.6±1.8
Dexamethasone 16 mg/day	16	80.3±0.9	30.5±1.1[a]	46.7±2.8	75.7±1.2[a]	31.0±2.3[b]	27.8±2.1
Dexamethasone 24 mg/day	10	81.5±0.5	37.5±2.6	52.0±1.6	75.4±0.9[a]	36.8±2.7[a]	25.3±1.9
Dexamethasone 16 + 24 mg pooled	26	80.8±0.6	33.1±1.4	48.3±2.0	75.6±0.9[a]	32.8±1.9[c]	27.1±1.5
Ethacrynic acid	13	81.6±0.5	31.5±1.6	44.9±1.5	77.3±1.7	34.0±1.2[a]	26.8±3.3
Spirolactone	13	83.9±0.8	32.2±2.0	43.4±2.0	78.4±1.8	33.4±3.0[a]	28.6±3.5

[a, b, c] = significantly different from untreated; [a] = $P < 0.05$; [b] = $P < 0.01$; [c] = $P < 0.001$
$\bar{x} \pm s\bar{x}$ are given. Water content is expressed as g/100 g fresh weight of tissue.
Electrolyte content is expressed as mEq/kg dry weight of tissue.
n = Total number of patients in each group.

In studying the ICP Miyazaki et al. [30] noted a decrease of intracranial pressure below the initial value in 23 of 37 patients with brain tumors and head injuries following the administration of ethacrynic acid. Wilkinson et al. [41], however, showed that in dogs a single dose of ethacrynic acid caused no significant drop in increased ICP due to edema (induced by the intracarotid injection of sodium lauryl sulfate). More recently spirolactone has been found to be effective in experimentally induced brain edema [2]. Although a small diminution of the water and sodium content of white matter was stated following the use of ethacrynic acid or spirolactone they were not as effective as dexamethasone. These findings correlate well with the clinical response of the patients to the different drugs. A dramatic alleviation of symptoms routinely followed the administration of dexamethasone, particularly in patients with symptoms of increased intracranial pressure. Conversely this relief was not observed following the use of the diuretics.

The current study is open to some reasonable criticisms. The method of randomly sampling tissue specimens at various distances from the tumor, the different histology, weight and location of the tumors may influence the results. However, when the results of the two groups of dexamethasone-treated patients are pooled (group I = 16 mg daily; group II = 24 mg daily; n = 26) and are compared with the present untreated group (n = 18) or with a previously examined group of 13 untreated patients [35] the differences in the white matter are even more significant (Table 1). This study therefore certainly substantiates the previous electron microscopic observations of Long et al. concerning the effect of dexamethasone on human brain edema adjacent to brain tumors. It also agrees with a recent study showing an anti-edema effect of corticosteroids in an experimentally induced primary brain tumor [16]. Additionally corticosteroids seem to exert an effect on tumor growth [16, 23], but this in our opinion cannot explain the rapid alleviation of symptoms in steroid-treated patients.

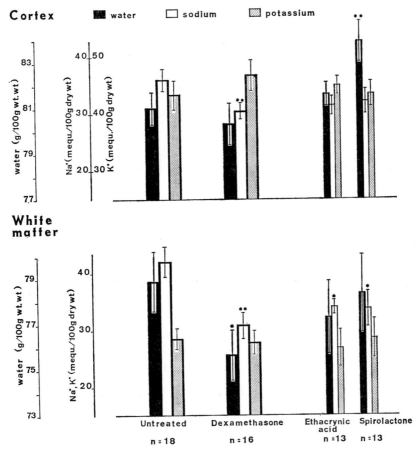

Fig. 2. Effect of dexamethasone and of diuretics on water and electrolyte content of edematous grey and white matter surrounding brain tumors and brain lesions

There is a certain discrepancy between the often remarkable neurological improvement and the only partial reduction of brain edema. These findings suggest that the improvement of patients following steroid therapy may not be due only to the diminution of edema. Other, as yet unknown, effects may be involved. However, the present study provides no further evidence concerning the mechanisms of action of dexamethasone on brain edema. The question still remains open whether dexamethasone counteracts the mechanism responsible for the rate of formation of edema or supports the rate of resolution of edema.

III. Changes of rCBF in Patients with Brain Tumors Receiving Dexamethasone

According to the introductory hypothesis cerebral blood flow in brain edema is mainly influenced by an increased tissue pressure and a metabolic tissue acidosis. If dexamethasone decreases the amount of brain edema an increase in rCBF should be expected.

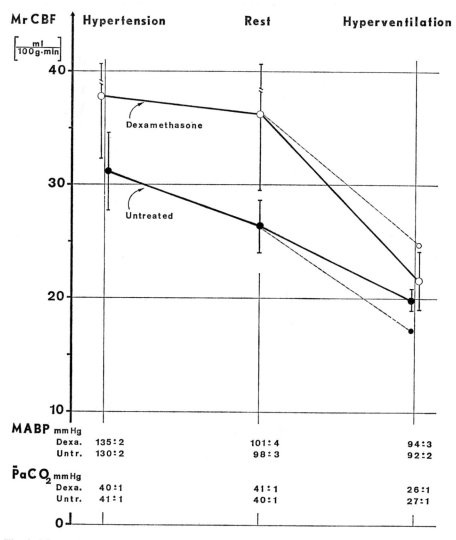

Fig. 3. Mean rCBF and vasomotor response in 6 patients with brain tumor before and after 5–7 days of dexamethasone administration (24 mg/day). Values are illustrated at:
a) the resting state,
b) during hyperventilation and
c) during hypertension.

Values at rest and during hypertension are corrected to a standard $PaCO_2$ of 40 mmHg (1). The broken line shows the expected change of MrCBF following hyperventilation

In a presently continuing study, 6 patients with brain tumors (2 meningiomas, 1 metastasis, 1 glioma, 1 glioma recurrency, 1 large partially thrombosed (ca. 60 g) aneurysm, acting as a space-occupying lesion) were submitted to rCBF measurements

246

before and after 5–7 days of dexamathasone administration (24 mg daily). Global and regional vascular regulating mechanisms were investigated by means of functional tests. All rCBF studies were performed under general neurolept-anaesthesia. After endotracheal intubation patients were relaxed with flaxedil and mechanically ventilated. For rCBF measurements the intraarterial ^{133}Xe-clearance technique [20] was used with a modified 16-channel scintillation probe equipment previously described [6]. In all patients determinations of rCBF were made at a) the resting state; b) during hyperventilation and c) during hypertension. Hypertension was induced by infusion of a pressure substance (Akrinor). Arterial pH, PCO_2 and PO_2 were determined using microelectrodes (Radiometer Copenhagen). rCBF values were calculated according to the "two-minutes-flow-index" [21]. Values obtained during the resting state and during hypertension were corrected to a standard PCO_2 of 40 mmHg by the formula of Alexander et al. [1].

The findings are summarized in Figure 3. In agreement with previous results mean rCBF in the resting state was found to be significantly reduced to 26.3 ± 2.2 ml/100 g min as compared to normal values (50 ± 5 ml/100 g min). Following the first rCBF study all patients received dexamethasone (3 × 8 mg/daily i.m.) during 5–7 days and thereafter the study was repeated. The most striking observation was that the mean hemispheric blood flow was increased by about 38% to 36.3 ± 6.6 ml/100 g min. Except one patient (glioma recurrency) all others showed individual increases in flow rate between 23 and 90% following the treatment.

This favourable effect of dexamethasone becomes even more obvious when the results of the functional tests are regarded. Hyperventilation in untreated patients discloses a clearly diminished vascular response to CO_2. The global decrease in flow of the tumor bearing hemisphere was less than should be expected from the respective $PaCO_2$ reduction. The expected flow diminution as derived from the ▲$PaCO_2$ is illustrated in Figure 3 by the broken line. The difference between the measured and the expected value may be expressed as "CO_2 regulation defect" (Table 2). In addition an induced rise of blood pressure was followed by an increase in blood flow indicating an abolition of autoregulation of cerebral blood flow. Thus a state of vasoparalysis was present.

After 5–7 days of treatment the mean hemispheric flow showed a markedly improved response to blood pressure changes as well as to changes in arterial PCO_2. It may be concluded that *dexamethasone increases the reduced blood flow* in patients with brain tumors *and restores the state of vasomotor paralysis* so far as normal vasomotor response can be revealed. The regional alterations before and after the treatment will be emphasized by the report of one of the 6 cases.

B.A., a 57 years old male, was admitted because of a shortlasting unconsciousness. There was no papilledema. The EEG showed a focal slow-wave pattern fronto-temporal on the left side. Brain scan revealed a well circumscribed hot spot parasagittal frontal left. (Fig. 4). Left sided carotid arteriogram indicated a typical falx meningioma. An abnormally dilated branch of the pericallosa artery was feeding a focal capillary blush.

The first rCBF investigation was performed under general neurolept-anaesthesia while the patient was untreated. Following a treatment with dexamethasone (3 × 8 mg daily intramuscularly) during 6 days the rCBF investigation was repeated under identical conditions (Table 2).

A. *In the resting state :* During the first study mean hemispheric rCBF was found to be 28.6 ± 1.4 ml/100 g min. As seen in Figure 4 regional flow measurements disclosed a rela-

Table 2. rCBF in a 57 year old man before and after 6 days of dexamethasone treatment (24 mg/day). Values are given for the explanation of Figure 4

	Untreated	Dexamethasone
	Rest	
MABP (mmHg)	90	95
$PaCO_2$ (mmHg)	40	43.8
PaO_2	140	122
MrCBF (ml/100 g min)	28.6 $\pm$ 1.4	38.5 $\pm$ 1.5
MrCBF$_{std.}$ (ml/100 g min)[a]	28.6 $\pm$ 1.4	35.3 $\pm$ 1.4
		% change: $+23.4$
	Hyperventilation	
MABP (mmHg)	90	90
$PaCO_2$ (mmHg)	25	22
PaO_2 (mmHg)	123	110
$\blacktriangle$ $PaCO_2$ (mmHg)	15	22
MrCBF (ml/100 g min)[b]	22.3 $\pm$ 1.88 (-22%)	18.9 $\pm$ 2.0 (-51%)
MrCBF$_{exp.}$ (ml/100 g min)[b]	17.9 (-37.4%)	19.1 (-50.3%)
CO_2-regulation defect[c]	-41%	$+1\%$
	Hypertension	
MABP (mmHg)	135	140
$\blacktriangle$ MABP (mmHg)	45	45
$PaCO_2$ (mmHg)	39	42.8
PaO_2 (mmHg)	164	160
MrCBF (ml/100 g min)	28.1 $\pm$ 2.3	34.4 $\pm$ 2.3
MrCBF$_{std.}$ (ml/100 g min)	28.8 $\pm$ 2.3	32.1 $\pm$ 2.1

[a] $MrCBF_{standard} = \dfrac{MrCBF_{measured}}{1 + 0.25\,(PaCO_2 - 40)}$ ml/100 g min

[b] $MrCBF_{expected} = MrCBF(rest)_{measured} - (\blacktriangle\,PaCO_2 \times 2.5\% \text{ of } MrCBF_{standard})$

[c] $\blacktriangle\,MrCBF_{expected} - \blacktriangle\,MrCBF_{measured} = CO_2\text{-regulation defect (in ml/100 g min)}$

$100 - \dfrac{\blacktriangle\,MrCBF_{measured} \times 100}{\blacktriangle\,MrCBF_{expected}} = CO_2\text{-regulation defect (in \%)}$

[a, b, c] are derived from the principles of Alexander *et al.* 1964, Høedt-Rasmussen 1967.

tive hyperaemia in the area corresponding to the tumor site in contrast to an absolute hypoaemia of the peripheral brain tissue. Following dexamethasone treatment, mean hemispheric rCBF was found to be increased to 35.3 $\pm$ 1.5 ml/100 g min (by 23.4%). Values are corrected to $PaCO_2 = 40$ mm Hg. The improvement affected much more the surrounding tissue than the tumor region. The relative focal hyperaemia seemed less pronounced.

B. *During hyperventilation*, global blood flow decreased in the untreated patient. However the vasomotor response to the CO_2 change was reduced in the perifocal tissue and completely abolished at the tumor site. A pathological "inverse steal effect" is also evident in this area. Following dexamethasone the global vasomotor response to CO_2 shows no significant abnormality, and no CO_2 regulation defect can be detected. The focal response of the surrounding brain tissue seemed completely restored, only a slight remaining defect of CO_2 reactivity was seen at the tumor site.

C. *During hypertension:* In the untreated patient there was no marked defect of auto-regulation regarding the mean rCBF (% changes = +0.67). However, the regional measurements disclosed a lack of cerebral autoregulation over the tumor region and to a less degree over some regions in the surrounding brain tissue. Following dexamethasone partial improvement of the autoregulation defect over the tumor regions and the adjacent areas could be observed.

UNTREATED   **DEXAMETHASONE**

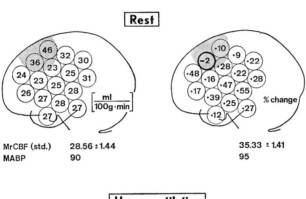

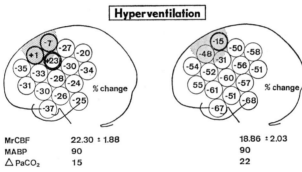

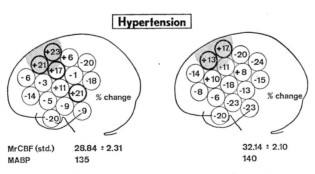

Fig. 4. Case report. rCBF and vasomotor response before and after dexamethasone treatment

The results of the present series confirm previous findings that rCBF is decreased in patients with brain tumor, mainly at the edematous tissue surrounding the tumor, and that vasomotor response to changes in blood pressure and in $PaCO_2$ is focally or generally disturbed [7, 18]. They provide evidence that the extent of local brain edema is a main factor responsible for the regional reduction in flow. In edematous areas tissue perfusion seems to depend on the tissue pressure, which may be conditioned by both, the ICP as well as the local brain water content.

This studies strongly suggest that dexamethasone exerts a favourable effect on the pathological status of the brain tissue surrounding brain tumors. That consists in a reduction of perifocal brain edema, particularly in the white matter and in an increase in flow rate at the non-tumoral brain tissue. Moreover cerebrovascular regulation mechanisms are more or less completely restored after dexamethasone treatment. We consequently believe that the reduction of perifocal edema and the amelioration of cerebral blood flow may account for the rapid clinical improvement of these patients.

References

1. Alexander, S. C., Wollman, H., Cohen, P. J., Chase, P. E., Behar, M.: Cerebrovascular response to $PaCO_2$ during halothane anaesthesia in man. J. appl. Physiol. **19**, 561–565 (1964).
2. Baethmann, A., Koczorek, K. R., Reulen, H. J., Wesemann, W., Hofmann, H. F., Angstwurm, A., Brendel, W.: Die Beeinflussung des traumatischen Hirnödems durch Aldosteron, Aldosteron-Antagonisten und Dexamethasone im Tierexperiment. In: Postop. Störungen des Elektrolyt- und Wasserhaushaltes, p. 163. Schattauer 1967.
3. Bartko, D., Reulen, H. J., Koch, H., Schürmann, K.: Changes in rCBF, cerebral water and metabolite content following occlusion of middle cerebral artery in cats. In: Reulen, H. J., Schürmann, K. (Eds.): Steroids and Brain Edema. Berlin-Heidelberg-New York: Springer 1972.
4. Beer, G.: Role of tissue fluid in blood flow regulation. Circulat. Res. Suppl. **29**, 154 (1971).
5. Betz, E., Heuser, D.: Cerebral cortical blood flow during changes of acid-base equilibrium of the brain. J. appl. Physiol. **23**, 726–733 (1967).
6. Brock, M., Hadjidimos, A., Schürmann, K., Ellger, M., Fischer, F.: Zur klinischen Messung der örtlichen Hirndurchblutung nach der intraarteriellen Isotopen-clearance-Methode. Dtsch. med. Wschr. **94**, 1377–1381 (1969).
7. — — Deruaz, J. P., Schürmann, K.: Regional cerebral blood flow and vascular reactivity in cases of brain tumor. In: Brain and Blood Flow, pp. 281–284. London: Pitmann Medical and Scientific Publishing Co. 1971.
8. — Beck, J., Markakis, E., Dietz, H.: The importance of intracranial pressure gradients for regional cerebral blood flow. Minerva med. **13**, 194 (1971).
9. Bucy, T. C., Jelsma, P. K.: The treatment of glioblastoma multiforme. Exerpta Medica Int. Congr. Series No. 193 (1969).
10. Feigin, J., Adachi, M.: Cerebral oedema and the water content of normal white matter. J. Neurol. Neurosurg. Psychiat. **29**, 446–450 (1966).
11. — Budzilovich, G., Ogata, J.: Edema of the grey matter of the human brain. J. Neuropath. exp. Neurol. **30**, 206–215 (1971).
12. Frei, H. J., Pöll, W., Reulen, H. J., Brock, M., Schürmann, K.: Regional energy metabolism, tissue lactate content and rCBF in cold injury edema. In: Brain and Blood Flow, pp. 125–129. London: Pitman Medical and Sientific Publishing Co. 1971.
13. Gänshirt, H.: Die Sauerstoffversorgung des Gehirns und ihre Störung bei der Liquordrucksteigerung und beim Hirnödem. Berlin-Heidelberg-New York: Springer 1957.
14. Galicich, J. G., French, L. A.: Use of dexamethasone in the treatment of cerebral edema resulting from brain tumors and brain surgery. Amer. Practit. **12**, 169 (1961).
15. Gordon, E., Rossanda, M.: The importance of the cerebrospinal fluid acid-base status in the treatment of unconscious patients with brain lesions. Acta anaesth. scand. **12**, 51 (1968).
16. Gurcay, O., Wilson, Ch., Barker, M., Eliason, J.: Corticosteroid Effect on Transplantable Rat Glioma. Arch. Neurol. **24**, 266–269 (1971).

17. Hadjidimos, A. A., Brock, M., Haas, J. P., Dietz, H., Wolf, R., Ellger, M., Fischer, F., Schürmann, K.: Correlation between rCBF, angiography, EEG and Scanning in brain tumors. In: Cerebral Blood Flow, pp. 190–193. Berlin-Heidelberg-New York: Springer 1969.

18. — — Hadjidimos, M., Deruaz, J. P., Schürmann, K.: Die fokale und perifokale örtliche Hirndurchblutung bei zerebralen Tumoren. Prognostische Möglichkeiten durch Vergleich prä- und postoperativer Befunde im extratumoralen Hirngewebe. In: Ergebnisse der klinischen Nuklearmedizin, pp. 1020–1029. Stuttgart-New York: Schattauer 1971.

19. — Reulen, H. J., Brock, M., Deruaz, J. P., Brost, E., Fischer, F., Samii, M., Schürmann, K.: rCBF, tissue water content and tissue lactate in brain tumors. Relation to preoperative and postoperative rCBF measurements. In: Brain and Blood Flow, pp. 378–385. London: Pitman Medical and Scientific Publishing Co. 1971.

20. Høedt-Rasmussen, K.: Regional Cerebral Blood Flow. The Intraarterial Injection Method. Copenhagen: Munksgaard 1967.

21. Hutten, H., Brock, M.: The Two-Minutes-Flow-Index (TMFI). In: Cerebral Blood Flow, pp. 19–23. Berlin-Heidelberg-New York: Springer 1969.

22. Klatzo, J., Wisniewski, H., Steinwall, O., Streicher, E.: Dynamics of cold injury edema. In: Klatzo, J., Seitelberger, F. (Eds.): Brain Edema. Wien-New York: Springer 1967.

23. Kotsilimbas, D. G., Meyer, L., Berson, M., Taylor, J. M., Scheinberg, L. C.: Corticosteroid effect on intracerebral melanomata and associated cerebral edema. Neurology 17, 223–227 (1967).

24. Lassen, N. A., Palvölgyi, R.: Cerebral steal during hypercapnia and the inverse reaction during hypocapnia observed by the 133-Xenon technique in man. Scand. J. Lab. clin. Invest., Supp. 102, XIII-D (1968).

25. — The luxury perfusion syndrome and its possible relation to acute metabolic acidosis localized within the brain. Lancet 2, 1113–1115 (1966).

26. Langfitt, T. W., Weinstein, J. D., Kassel, N. F., Gagliardi, L. J., Shapiro, H. M.: Compression of cerebral vessels by intracranial hypertension. 1. Dural Sinus pressure. Acta neurochir. 15, 212 (1966).

27. Long, D. M., Hartmann, J. F., French, L. A.: The response of human cerebral edema to glucosteroid administration. Neurology 16, 521–528 (1966).

28. Meinig, G., Reulen, H. J., Magavly, Chr., Bartko, D., Schürmann, K.: Der Einfluß des lokalen und generalisierten Hirnödems auf die regionale Hirndurchblutung. Donau-Symposium für Neurologie, Wien 1971.

29. — — Hadjidimos, A., Siemon, Chr., Bartko, D.: Induction of filtration edema by extreme reduction of CVR associated with hypertension. Minerva med. 13, 196 (1971).

30. Miyazaki, Y., Suematsu, K., Nakamura, J.: Effect of ethacrynic acid on lowering of intracranial pressure. Arzneimittel-Forsch. 19, 1961–1965 (1965).

31. Oeconomos, D., Kosmaoglu, B., Prossalentis, A.: rCBF studies in intracranial tumors. In: Cerebral Blood Flow, pp. 172–175. Berlin-Heidelberg-New York: Springer 1969.

32. Olesen, J.: Total CO_2, lactate and pyruvate in brain biopsies taken after freezing the tissue in situ. Acta Neurol. scand. 46, 141–148 (1970).

33. Palvölgyi, R.: Regional cerebral blood flow in patients with intracranial tumors. J. Neurosurg. 31, 149–163 (1969).

34. Pampus, F.: Die Wasserstoffionenkonzentration des Hirngewebes bei raumfordernden intracraniellen Prozessen. Acta neurochir. 11, 305–318 (1963).

35. Reulen, H. J., Medzihradsky, F., Enzenbach, R., Marguth, F., Brendel, W.: Electrolytes, fluids and energy metabolism in cerebral edema in man. Arch. Neurol. 21, 517–525 (1969).

36. — Hey, O., Fenske, A., Schürmann, K.: Alterations of energy-rich phosphates in brain tissue and of glucose, lactate and pyruvate in blood, CSF and brain tissue following a cold induced edema. (In preparation.)

37. — Hadjidimos, A., Brock, M., Deruaz, J. P., Schürmann, K.: Regional cerebral blood flow and cerebral edema in man. I. Influence of local tissue water and local tissue lactate. Acta neurochir. (In Press.)

251

38. Rodbard, S.: Capillary control of blood flow and fluid exchange: Circulat. Res. Suppl. **28**, 51 (1971).
39. Stewart-Wallace, A. M.: A biochemical study of cerebral tissue and of the changes in cerebral oedema. Brain **62**, 426–438 (1939).
40. Wahl, M., Deetjen, P., Thurau, K., Ingvar, D. H., Lassen, N. A.: Micropuncture evaluation of the importance of perivascular pH for the arteriolar diameter on the brain surface. Pflügers Arch. ges. Physiol. **316**, 152–163 (1970).
41. Wilkinson, H. A., Wepsic, J. G., Austin, G.: Diuretic synergy in the treatment of acute experimental cerebral edema. J. Neurosurg. **34**, 203–208 (1971).
42. Zwetnow, N., Kjällquist, A., Siesjö, B.: Cerebral blood flow during intracranial hypertension related to tissue hypoxia and to acidosis in cerebral extracellular fluids. Progr. in Brain Res. **30**, 91 (1968).

Clinical Studies on the Effect of Corticosteroids on the Ventricular Fluid Pressure

GUNVOR KULLBERG

Neurosurgical Department B., University Hospital, Lund, Sweden

With 6 Figures

If corticosteroids reduce cerebral edema they should also reduce the raised intra-cranial pressure associated with edema. A study of the steroid effect from this angle has the advantage that the intracranial pressure can be measured continuously, even in a clinical context. Furthermore, the raised intracranial pressure is from the clinical point of view one of the most important consequences of cerebral edema.

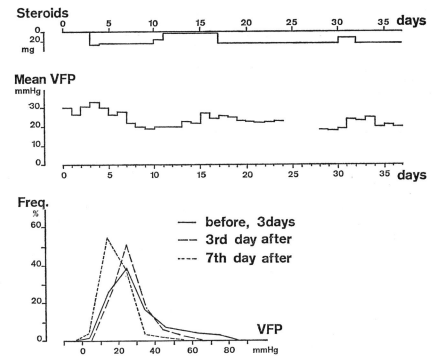

Fig. 1. Case of malignant glioma. Moderate reduction of mean pressure in relation to steroid treatment. Three pressure distribution diagrams have been selected to demonstrate the change in pressure pattern: first reduction of high pressure episodes, later decrease of basal pressure

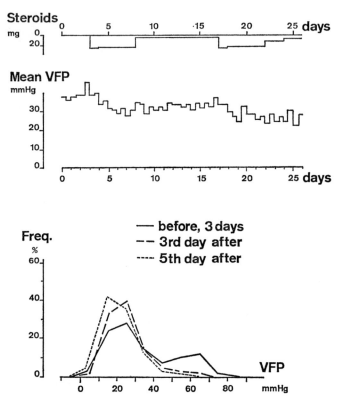

Fig. 2. Case of malignant glioma. Moderate reduction of mean pressure in relation to steroid treatment. Pressure distribution diagrams show reduction of high pressure episodes, little change in basal pressure

Monitoring of the intracranial pressure, i.e. the ventricular fluid pressure (VFP), according to the method of Lundberg [1] has been used in our department for several years as a routine procedure in certain cases of intracranial lesions. Many of these patients received treatment with corticosteroids for the purpose of reducing cerebral edema. The majority were subjected to other therapeutic or diagnostic procedures affecting the VFP but some cases appeared reasonably free from such interfering factors and were selected for a more detailed study of the influence of the corticosteroids on the VFP.

The evaluation of slowly occurring changes in the VFP required a condensation of the information contained in the lengthy VFP curves, which were difficult to review by mere inspection. In addition to calculating mean pressure values, we have chosen to represent curve sections of suitable length, usually 24-h-periods, as diagrams showing the frequency distribution of pressure classes.

Pressure observations at short regular intervals were grouped into pressure classes of 10 mm width (0–10, 10–20 etc., mmHg); the number of observations, expressed as percent of total, was plotted against the pressure classes. Such diagrams demonstrate the extent of the pressure variations, as well as the predominant level of the pressure, the basal pressure, which is usually different from the mean pressure.

254

The corticosteroids used were dexamethasone or betamethasone, as a rule in a dose of 16–24 mg daily, given intramuscularly in divided doses, sometimes with an initial intravenous injection of 10 mg at the start of the treatment.

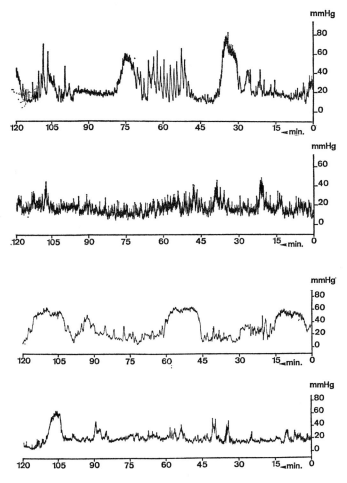

Fig. 3. VFP curves, each representing a 2-h-period of recording, exemplifying pre- and post-treatment pressures. The two upper curves illustrate the case described in Figure 1, prior to treatment and on 7th day of treatment. The two lower curves illustrate the case described in Figure 2, prior to treatment and on 5th day of treatment

In a previous publication [2] we reported on five cases of malignant brain tumor, where corticosteroid treatment was found to have a pressure-reducing effect. Some of the data are shown in Figures 1–3. A beginning decrease of the pressure could be discerned one to several days after the start of the treatment. When a distinct pressure reduction had occurred, the steroid dose was abruptly reduced and again increased in order to check the causal relationship between treatment and pressure reduction. These changes in dosage were followed by corresponding alterations in the VFB.

255

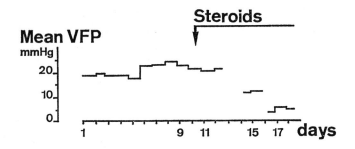

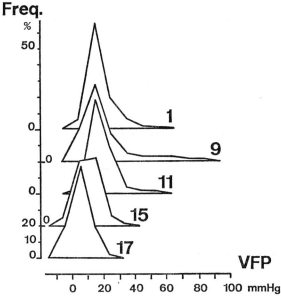

Fig. 4. Case of head injury with increasing VFP and development of plateau waves. Steroid treatment begun on 10th day. Pressure distribution diagrams, representing days 1 and 9 prior to treatment, days 11, 15 and 17 with treatment, demonstrate the changes in pressure pattern.

Note that the frequency scale has been moved two intervals for each diagram in order to simplify identification

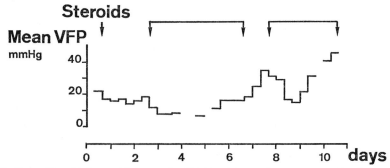

Fig. 5. Case of head injury with increasing VFP, without plateau waves. Single injection of steroids on day 1, later two separate periods of treatment. Only temporary effect of steroid treatment.

256

The pressure reduction as reflected in the mean pressure values was rather modest, amounting to some 5–10 mmHg. More striking was a change in the pattern of pressure fluctuations in cases with plateau waves. A comparison of consecutive pressure diagrams indicated that the first change that occurred during steroid treatment was a reduction of the high pressure episodes, while the basal pressure decreased only later, if at all.

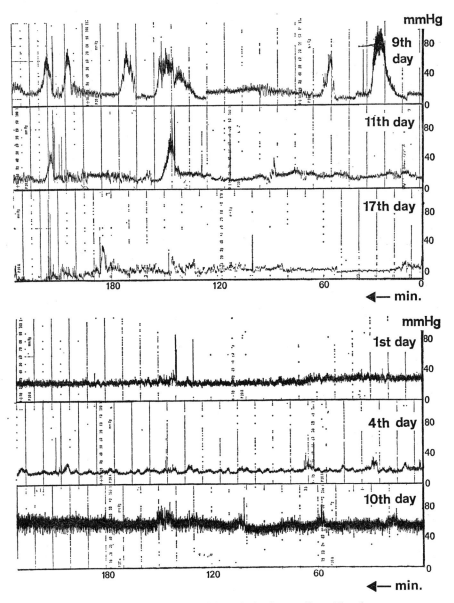

Fig. 6. VFP curves each representing a 4-h-period of recording. The three upper curves illustrate the case described in Figure 4, days 9, 11 and 17. The three lower curves illustrate the case described in Figure 5, days 1, 4 and 10

Improvement of the clinical picture seemed related to the pressure changes, the relation being particularly evident in the reduction of the intermittent symptoms accompanying plateau waves. In one case, however, a marked improvement of the level of consciousness preceded any detectable change in the level or pattern of the pressure.

Similar studies on patients with cerebral edema of other origin such as head injuries seemed desirable, but the common use of osmotherapy and the unpredictable spontaneous course made evaluation difficult in these acute conditions. In some cases however, the findings suggested a causal relationship between steroid treatment and reduction of pressure.

Figures 4 and 6 illustrate such a case. This patient was admitted unconscious with a closed head injury. Angiograms showed no dislocation of cerebral vessels. The VFP was initially moderately elevated with some fluctuations but during the following 10 days it took a progressive course with development of plateau waves of increasing height and frequency. New angiograms showed diffuse swelling of the left hemisphere. Steroid treatment was started on the tenth day. The following day the plateau waves began to subside and later there was a gradual return to practically normal pressure. The patient improved simultaneously and regained full consciousness.

Another case of head injury is illustrated in Figures 5 and 6. Recording of the VFP disclosed a progressively increasing pressure with irregular fluctuations but no plateau waves (Fig. 6). When corticosteroids were given the pressure decreased but only temporarily. The steroid therapy was discontinued as it was thought to have no effect. However, following this the pressure rose rapidly to a high level (Fig. 5). Steroid treatment was therefore restarted. Again there was a temporary pressure decrease but in spite of continued therapy the pressure soon rose to very high levels and the patient finally died. It seemed likely that the steroids did have an effect on cerebral edema in this case, although not great enough to overcome the spontaneous tendency to progression.

Recording of the VFP verified that corticosteroids can reduce a raised intracranial pressure under certain circumstances. Our general impression is that the steroids have little or no effect on the type of pressure which is characterized by continuous elevation to a high level. The pressure pattern with plateau waves seems to represent a condition where the corticosteroids can exert their influence more efficiently. Clinical improvement seemed on the whole related to the changes in pressure and thus probably to a reduction of cerebral edema. However, one exception was noted, indicating that other actions of the steroids may be partly responsible for the therapeutic effect.

References

1. Lundberg, N.: Continuous recording and control of ventricular fluid pressure in neurosurgical practice. Acta Psychiat. Neurol. Scand. Suppl. No. 149. Copenhagen: Munksgaard 1960.
2. Kullberg, G., West, K. A.: Influence of corticosteroids on the ventricular fluid pressure. Acta Neurol. Scand. Suppl. 13, 41, 445–452 (1965).

Double Blind Study of the Effects of Dexamethasone on Acute Stroke

Bernard M. Patten, Jerry Mendell, Bertel Bruun, William Curtin, and
Sidney Carter

Neurological Institute, 710 West 168th Street, New York, NY. 10032, USA.

Summary. A double blind study of the effects of dexamethasone on acute stroke was
conducted at the Neurological Institute of New York. At the end of the study, it was found
that 17 patients had been treated with placebo and 14 patients had been treated with dexamethasone. The dose of steroid was 16 mg daily for 10 days followed by tapering doses from
12 mg to zero over the ensuing 7 days.

The patient's functional capacity was appraised by the use of a scoring system similar to
the system used by the Parkinson Disease Research Foundation for the evaluation of parkinsonism, but adapted for use in stroke. On the basis of the scoring system, patients treated
with steroid improved their functional status during the treatment period an average of 12%,
while those treated with placebo got worse by 12%. In reviewing the results on the 15 patients most severely affected by their stroke, the benefit with steroid was even more clearly
demonstrated because the treated group improved 23% while the placebo group got worse
by 14%. These latter results were statistically significant at the $P = 0.02$ level.

We conclude that dexamethasone can be a useful adjunct to the therapy of the patient
with a severe stroke. The suggestion is that the beneficial effects of steroid are in part due to
their ability to decrease brain edema secondary to massive brain infarction.

Introduction

In 1970, cerebral vascular disease was the third most frequent cause of death in the
United States, and the disability of those surviving a stroke constituted a major reha-
bilitation and public health problem. Despite recent advances, the therapy of stroke
remains unsatisfactory. Consequently, there is a search for any agent which improves
the patient during the acute phase of the illness in the hope of decreasing the morbidity
and mortality of this disease.

For many years corticosteroids have been alternately condemned and praised in
the acute phase of therapy of stroke. The condemnation has come from conclusions
drawn from a clinical study in which the investigators themselves indicated that their
data were not statistically significant [1]. Plum's observation of potentially unfavor-
able effects of dexamethasone on ischemic-hypoxic rats has also discouraged general
use of corticosteroid in patients with stroke [2].

Two favorable reports conclude that these agents are useful in the therapy of
acute stroke, especially in patients with lethargy and other signs of cerebral edema
[3, 4]. It should be noted that one of these studies is not controlled and the other fails
to report any statistical analysis of its data.

In view of the importance of stroke as a national health problem, and the conflicting opinions on the use of steroids, there was need of a strictly controlled, double blind, statistically significant study of the effect of a glucocorticoid on stroke. The results of such an investigation, recently concluded at the Neurological Institute of New York, are reported here.

Materials and Methods

Plan of Study:

A. Selection of Patients

All patients with the sudden onset of a focal neurological deficit within 24 h prior to admission were included, provided they or a close relative gave written, informed consent.

B. Patient Exclusions

Patients were excluded if they had subarachnoid hemorrhage from a ruptured aneurysm or arteriovenous malformation. The clinical course and cerebral angiography were used to make this distinction. Seven patients were exluded at the conclusion of the study, but before statistical analysis, for reasons outlined in Table 1.

Table 1. Patients excluded from statistical analysis

Patient's Number	Age	Treatment	Diagnosis	Reasons for Exclusion
10	64	Placebo	Subdural Hematoma	Autopsy showed patient herniated from subdural hematoma.
12	43	Steroid	Cerebral Infarction	Diabetes got worse and steroid was stopped in 12 h.
14	65	Steroid	Subarachnoid Hemorrhage	Patient had aneurysm that ruptured. Remarkable improvement occurred during therapy, but aneurysm rebled and patient died.
17	68	Placebo	Brain Stem Infarction	Patient was moribund on admission. Died within 24 h. Autopsy showed ruptured aortic aneurysm.
34	80	Nothing	Cerebral Infarction	Study solution was not given due to nursing error.
35	72	Steroid	Cerebral Infarction	Remarkable improvement could have been due to anticoagulant therapy given with steroid.
37	61	Placebo	Cerebral Infarction	Remarkable improvement could have been due to Rheomacrodex given with placebo.

C. Drug Administration

Within 24 h of admission, patients were assigned to receive either dexamethasone or placebo allocated according to random number. The material was supplied in identical appearing vials which bore the patient's number in the study. Neither the patients nor the professional staff were aware of which material was being used. Each vial contained a special label which provided for emergency identification of the material without breaking the code for the entire study. Patients received 10 mg of dexamethasone (or equivalent of placebo solution) intravenously at the time of initial treatment followed by 4 mg intramuscularly every 6 h for 10 days. Doses were then tapered to zero over the ensuing 7 days.

Table 2. Neurologic status evaluation stroke study

Mental Function	Motor Function (Score each extremity separately)
A. *Orientation*	0. Normal
_____ 0. Fully	1. Useful but not normal
X 1. Slight impairment	2. Semiuseful
2. Mild impairment	3. Moves against gravity
3. Moderate impairment	4. Feeble non-useful movements only
4. Severe impairment	5. Plegic
5. Complete disorientation	
6. Can not appraise	

Motor Function extremity scores:

Score	Extremity
3	RUE
0	LUE
2	RLE
0	LLE
5	Total

B. *Recent Recall*

_____ 0. Normal
_____ 1. Slight impairment
X 2. Mild impairment
_____ 3. Moderate impairment
_____ 4. Severe impairment
_____ 5. Completely impaired

Aphasia

_____ 0. Normal
_____ 1. Slight
_____ 2. Mild
_____ 3. Moderate
X 4. Severe
_____ 5. Complete

C. *Digit Span*

_____ 0–6 Backward
_____ 1–5 Backward
_____ 2–4 Backward
_____ 3–3 Backward
X 4–2 Backward
_____ 5–1 Backward

Apraxia

_____ 0. Normal
_____ 1. Slight
_____ 2. Mild
X 3. Moderate
_____ 4. Severe
_____ 5. Complete

D. *Remote Memory*
one pt. for each incorrect

0 1. Year of Birth
0 2. Place of Birth
0 3. Parents' names
0 4. Occupation
0 5. Size, composition of family

Total disability scale :
Circle: 1 2 3 4 5 6 7 8 9 10

Overall Clinical Impression of Current status

Mild stroke _____
Moderate stroke _____ X _____
Severe stroke _____

Totals: 1
         2
         4
         5
         3
         ─────
         19 pts.

All patients received a prophylactic regimen of oral antacid with each injection. The usual attention to hydration, bowel and bladder care, control of infection, and frequent turning was provided.

D. Evaluation of Patients

Patient evaluation included a history, physical examination, complete blood count, sedimentation rate, blood urea nitrogen, VDRL, plasma electrophoresis, LE prep, serum Na, K, CO_2, Cl, prothrombin time, urinalysis, electrocardiogram, electroencephalogram, brain scan and lumbar puncture. On admission and on days 3, 6, 10, and 17 patients were scored by a team of neurologists using a patient evaluation sheet patterned after the evaluation form of the Parkinson Disease Research Foundation, but adapted for use in stroke. The scoring system concentrated on functional status and correlated closely with the general clinical impression of the severity of the stroke. Changes in average scores adequately reflected changes in the patients' clinical status.

Table 3

II. Disability status scale

Score **8**

0 = normal neurologic examination (all grade 0 in functional systems)

1 = no disability, minimal signs, e. g. Babinski sign, vibratory decrease (grade 1 in functional systems)

2 = minimal disability – e.g. slight weakness; mild gait, sensory visuomotor disturbance (1 or 2 functional systems grade 2)

3 = moderate disability though fully ambulatory – e.g. monoparesis, moderate ataxia, or combinations of lesser dysfunctions (1 or 2 functional systems grade 3 or several grade 2)

4 = relatively severe disability though fully ambulatory and able to be self-sufficient and up and about for some 12 h a day (1 functional system grade 4 or several grade 3 or less)

5 = disability severe enough to preclude ability to work a full day without special provisions; maximal motor function walking unaided no more than several blocks (1 functional system grade 5 alone, or combination or lesser grades)

6 = assistance (canes, crutches, braces) required for walking (combinations with more that 1 system grade 3 or worse)

7 = restricted to wheel chari – able to wheel self and enter and leave chair alone (combinations with more that 1 system grade 4 or worse; very rarely pyramidal system grade 5 alone)

8 = restricted to bed but with effective use of arms (combinations usually grade 4 or above in several functional systems)

9 = totally helpless bed patients (combinations usually functional grade 4 or above in most functional systems)

10 = death due to stroke

For example: patient No. 1, as illustrated in table 2, entered the study with a right hemiparesis, severe aphasia, apraxia, and mild impairment of recent memory with poor backward digit span giving him a total score of 19. After treatment, he had a mild hemiparesis, slight aphasia, moderate apraxia, and no change in memory or digit span giving a total score of 12. His total disability scale (Table 3) also improved from 8 to 4 and serves as a cross check of the numbered score. Angiography was done when indicated to rule out aneurysm or arteriovenous malformation or to evaluate extra-cranial vessels as the source of the patient's difficulty. A large amount of epidemiologic data was also collected but will not be discussed or reported here.

Table 4. Results of therapy

A. Complete series   n = 31

Treatment	Number of patients	Average age	Average initial score	Diagnosis	Percent of patients im-proved	Percent change in average score of all patients
Steroid	14	69	25	12 cerebral infarcts 2 brain stem infarcts	64 %	12% better
Placebo	17	70	25	14 cerebral infarcts 3 cerebral hemorrhage	41 %	12% worse

B. Severely ill patients with initial score > 25   n = 15

Treatment	Number of patients	Average age	Average initial score	Diagnosis	Percent of patients im-proved	Percent change in average score of all patients
Steroid	7	69	39	6 cerebral infarcts 1 brain stem infarct	71 %	23% better
Placebo	8	69	37	7 cerebral infarcts 1 cerebral hemorrhage	25 %	14% worse

Results

There were 31 patients in this study, 16 men and 15 women. The average age was 69 and the average initial score was 25. 14 patients were treated with steroid and 17 were treated with placebo. A comparison of the treated with the control group (Table 4) shows that on the basis of the change in the average score, the treated group improved 12% and the untreated group got worse by 12% ($0.1 > p > 0.05$). Analysis of the change in average score of the 15 patients most severely affected by their stroke (initial score 25 or greater) indicates the treated group improved 23% whereas the untreated group got worse by 14%. These results for the most severely ill patients are statistically significant using the Wilcoxon Rank Order test with $P = 0.02$, double tail rule included.

In the whole series, using the scoring system as the measure of clinical change, $7/17$ or 41% of the patients on placebo were better, at the end of the treatment period, than they had been on admission, whereas $^9/_{14}$ or 64 % of the patients on steroid were better than they had been on admission. The results for the severely ill patients (admission score > 25) indicated that $^2/_8$ or 25 % of the patients on placebo were better than they had been on admission, whereas $^5/_7$ or 71 % of the steroid treated were better than they had been on admission. Table 5 lists all of the patients in the study, their ages, initial and final scores and their clinical course.

We conclude that dexamethasone was more effective than placebo in the treatment of acute stroke, and that the drug had its greatest beneficial effect in patients with the most severe disease. In this study, short term, high dose steroid therapy was remarkably free of significant side effects, a finding noted by others [5]. One patient's diabetes was exacerbated, and the steroid had to be stopped in her case. Otherwise, we saw none of the signs and symptoms usually considered to be steroid side effects such as moon face, edema, weight gain, muscle cramps, anxiety, depression, psychosis, peptic ulcer, purpura, infection, catabolic and antifibroplastic activities, or hypertension.

Comment

Edema, sometimes accompanied by herniation, is a well recognized complication of brain infarction [6]. Careful pathological studies indicate that the swelling of necrotic brain develops regularly and rapidly over the first 5 days after insult. Thereafter, it gradually subsides, and disappears in about 2 weeks. Papilledema and elevated cerebrospinal fluid pressure are not seen even in the most severe infarctions [7]. Presumably, the major adverse effects of cerebral edema secondary to infarction are due to local expansion with compression and displacement of neighboring structures without generalized increase in intracranial pressure. The abnormal amount of fluid results in tissue disruption, ischemia due to compression, and perpetuation of cell death [8]. During the acute phase of illness, a vicious cycle of edema producing necrosis and necrosis producing edema causes a build-up of local swelling and consequent clinical deterioration. Most deaths during the first week after stroke are, in fact, related to edema [7]. The prevention or amelioration of edema is, therefore, a logical approach to therapy.

Corticosteroids have been recognized for a long time as powerful agents useful in reducing the cerebral edema associated with surgical lesions [9], head trauma [10], and primary or metastatic cerebral tumor [8, 11]. Experimental edema induced by various methods is unequivocally reduced by these agents [12, 13]. Clinically, the improvement in patients is often dramatic, long lasting, and of value in the management of the underlying brain disease. Dexamethasone, of all the corticosteroids, appears to be clinically the most useful because of its potency and low salt retaining properties [5].

The pharmacodynamic mechanism by which steroids work is unknown. Studies with the amphibian bladder show that the function of the sodium-potassium pump is augmented by corticosteroids so that it is possible that correction of edema is closely related to improved ionic gradients due to more normal operation of the sodium pump [14]. Kullberg's interesting patient with metastatic carcinoma had a steroid-induced clinical improvement before a reduction of ventricular pressure, an observation suggesting that steroids may function by altering a process more fundamental than edema itself [15].

264

Table 5. Total series   n = 31

Placebo   n = 17

Age	Sex	Initial	–	Final score	Diagnosis	Result
82	F	23	–	15	CI	Improved
78	M	10	–	12	CI	Worse
85	F	40	–	40	CI	Same
68	M	26	–	50	CI	Worse
88	M	27	–	43	CI	Worse
63	M	15	–	11	CI	Improved
80	M	18	–	21	CI	Worse
58	M	8	–	1	CI	Improved
48	M	44	–	37	CI	Improved
52	M	11	–	11	CI	Same
77	F	16	–	47	CH	Worse
40	M	42	–	48	CH	Worse
79	F	20	–	14	CI	Improved
82	F	47	–	48	CI	Worse
62	F	31	–	25	CI	Improved
70	M	14	–	6	CH	Improved
81	M	37	–	42	CI	Worse

Steroid   n = 14

Age	Sex	Initial	–	Final score	Diagnosis	Result
70	M	16	–	8	CI	Improved
65	F	36	–	40	CI	Worse
68	F	11	–	6	CI	Improved
78	M	5	–	16	CI	Worse
88	F	17	–	49	CI	Worse
65	F	40	–	23	CI	Improved
60	F	43	–	37	Brain stem infarction	Improved
63	M	33	–	29	CI	Improved
66	M	50	–	50	CI	Same
71	F	31	–	13	CI	Improved
70	F	11	–	5	CI	Improved
79	M	39	–	16	CI	Improved
66	F	5	–	9	Brain stem infarction	Worse
57	F	11	–	9	CI	Improved

CI = Cerebral infarction
CH = Cerebral hemorrhage

Whatever their fundamental action, these potent agents deserve further controlled clinical studies. Since dose has been found to be of such crucial importance in the therapy of other nervous system diseases [16], dexamethasone should be tried in very high doses in the hope that further benefit may result.

265

References

1. Dyken, M., White, P. T.: Evaluation of Cortisone in the Treatment of Cerebral Infarction. J. Amer. med. Ass. **162**, 1531–1534 (1959).
2. Plum, F., Alvord, E. C., Posner, J. B.: Effect of Steroids on Experimental Cerebral Infarction. Arch. Neurol **9**, 571–573 (1963).
3. Russek, H. I., Russek, A. S., Zohman, B. L.: Cortisone in Immediate Therapy of Apoplectic Stroke. J. Amer. med. Ass. **159**, 102–105 (1955).
4. Rubenstein, M. K.: The Influence of Adrenocortical Steroids on Severe Cerebrovascular Accidents. J. nerv. ment. Dis. **141**, 291–299 (1965).
5. French, L. A.: The Use of Steroids in the Treatment of Cerebral Edema. Bull. N. Y. Acad. Med. **42**, 301–311 (1966).
6. Berry, R. G., Alpers, B. J.: Occlusion of the Carotid Circulation. Neurology **7**, 223–237 (1957).
7. Shaw, C., Alvord, E. C., Berry, R. G.: Swelling of the Brain Following Ischemic Infarction with Arterial Occlusion. Arch. Neurol. **1**, 161–177 (1959).
8. Long, D. M., Hartmann, J. F., French, L. A.: The Response of Human Cerebral Edema to Glucosteroid Administration. Neurology **16**, 521–528 (1968).
9. Rasmussen, T., Gulati, D. R.: Cortisone in the Treatment of Postoperative Cerebral Edema. J. Neurosurg. **19**, 535–544 (1962).
10. Gurdjian, E. S., Webster, J. E.: Head Injuries. Mechanisms, Diagnosis and Management, pp. 482. Boston: Little, Brown & Co. 1958.
11. Gårde, A.: Experiences with Dexamethasone Treatment of Intracranial Pressure Caused by Brain Tumors. Acta Neurol. Scand. Suppl. **13**, 439–441 (1965).
12. Prados, M., Strowger, B., Feindel, W. H.: Studies on Cerebral Edema. Arch. Neurol. Psych. **54**, 163–174 (1945).
13. Rovit, R. L., Hagan, R.: Steroids and Cerebral Edema: The effect of glucocorticoids on abnormal capillary permeability following cerebral injury in cats. J. Neuropath. Exp. Neurol. **27**, 277–299 (1968).
14. Long, D. M., Hartmann, J. F., French, L. A.: The Response of Experimental Cerebral Edema to Glucosteroid Administration. J. Neurosurg. **24**, 843–854 (1966).
15. Kullberg, G., West, K. A.: Influence of Corticosteroid on Ventricular Fluid Pressure. Acta neurol. Scand. Suppl. **13**, 445–452 (1965).
16. Cotzias, G. C., Papavisiliou, P. S., Gallene, R.: Modification of Parkinsonism: Chronic Treatment with L-DOPA. NEJM **280**, 337–345 (1969).

Discussion to Chapter IV see page 282

Experimental Aspects of Brain Edema
and Therapeutic Approach

Moderator: I. KLATZO

BARLOW (to Dr. Hossmann): This was a fascinating presentation. I would ask Dr. Hossmann the question as to whether we are really looking at the correct place. The authors have paid particular attention to the intercellular junctions. These were tight in complete ischemia. The results imply that there is a dynamic process involved, something that is affected by the lack of oxygen. I would like to know if the pinocytotic activity of the capillaries was different In the ischemic lesion as opposed to the lesser lesion. Could Dr. Hossmann answer the question as to what happens to pinocytotic activity of cerebral vessels in the various grades and the various groups?

HOSSMANN: In cerebral ischemia, after the pyramidal response was suppressed, we did not see pinocytotic activity in the endothelium of the cerebral capillaries. There were pinocytotic vesicles in groups 2 and 4, i.e. in those groups in which some kind of function was preserved, but the vesicles were not very frequent. We do not believe that the mode of protein exudation in the mercury lesion is the pinocytotic transport. Of course, as long as we do not see a breakdown of the tight junctions more frequently, we have to consider it as one of the possibilities. If there is an active transport of proteins across the blood-brain barrier ischemia certainly would inhibit such transport, but this should be confirmed by other means, e.g. by cyanide poisoning.

KLATZO: I would like to comment on the role of pinocytosis in endothelial cells with regard to the transport of various substances across the blood-brain barrier. Some investigators feel that pinocytotic transport is important and extremely active pinocytosis is observed in endothelium of some of the brain tumors. On the other hand, Drs. Brightman and Reese, from our laboratory, are sceptical about the role of pinocytosis in transporting substances across the endothelium. They see very little of pinocytosis under the normal conditions and they are inclined to relate the abnormal permeability of the barrier as occuring primarily due to endothelial damage or due to opening of the tight junctions between the adjacent endothelial cells.

CLASEN: I would like to question the interpretation that ischemia causes tightening of the endothelial junctions. The failure to demonstrate extravasation of the tracer could be due to too diminished blood flow developing as the result of the intracellular swelling which was so beautifully shown. Dr. Hossmann demonstrated Evans blue in the blood vessels with the skull closed. Do you have any blood flow data from animals with open skulls?

HOSSMANN: I do not think there is an impairment of cerebral blood flow. We have done blood flow measurements after ischemia, and we found that ischemia is followed by a period of hyperemia with a more than 100 % increase in flow. The tracer is injected during hyperemia; therefore the failure of protein exudation can not be attributed to a decrease in cerebral blood flow. The reason that we did not observe the no-reflow phenomenon after ischemia is probably due to the fact that we interrupted only the arterial blood supply to the brain but not the venous drainage. rCBF was only measured with closed skull using ^{133}Xe.

BROCK (to Dr. Spatz): I would like to know what was the duration, the rate and the pressure you employed for the perfusion. How much of your lesions could be accounted for by the ischemia which you probably induce when you perfuse those brains.

SPATZ: We perfused the rabbits for 20 sec using the eye blanching as indicator of functioning perfusion within internal carotid area of blood supply. In a separate pilot experiment, we perfused a series of animals under the same conditions and measured the intracarotic arterial pressure. In all animals showing hyperemia, the pressure in the initial 5 sec went up above 700 mmHg. When the blood pressure remained above 400 mmHg for the remaining time of perfusion, we were sure of producing brain hyperemia. In the non-hyperemic rabbits, the initial pressure went up above 500 mmHg and then fluctuated between 100 to 200 mmHg during the perfusion. Discrete areas of ischemia were present in otherwise hyperemic brains, but such areas were absent in the non-hyperemic group of animals.

LASSEN: I did not quite get the difference between those two groups. What is hyperemia in your definition? Does it mean increase in circulation or what does it mean?

SPATZ: Our definition of hyperemia was based on gross observation of increased blood content in distended cerebral blood vessels of the hemisphere ipsilateral to the side of perfusion as was illustrated in Figure 1. These findings were confirmed by the microscopical appearance of the brain capillaries shown in Figure 6c. We had not measured the blood flow but intend to do it in the future.

REULEN: In what kind of edema, do you believe, Dr. Demopoulos, do the free radicals play an important role? Is it the vasogenic or cytotoxic type of brain edema?

DEMOPOULOS: They can be involved in both. We are talking about all membrane systems, the opening of tight junctions or other specialized areas of membrane. A tight junction is really at the mercy of the surrounding phosphate lipids and how well packed they may be. Any pertubation in the surrounding phosphate lipid may alter the tightness of the tight junction. The molecules right around tight junction areas are constantly changing and any loosening or tightening of the surrounding molecules will perturb a tight junction. This is what I mean by moleculare mechanisms being able to disect through controversis. All that we are explaining are some broad basic mechanisms for damaging membranes. I think that this occurs in both kinds of edema, as well as in several other pathological processes.

268

Discussion to Chapter II

Effects of Steroids on Experimental Brain Edema

Moderator: H. M. PAPPIUS

CLASEN (to Dr. Pappius): The albumin concentration in the edema fluid associated with these lesions in the dog is about 10 % less than that of serum [Clasen et al. In: Klatzo, Seitelberger (Ed.): Brain Edema, p. 536–553 (1967)]. If this also applies to the cat, it could easily explain the fact that the serum equivalents calculated from tissue RISA are less than the measured weight increases. Uptake of iodinated serum albumin by glia has been demonstrated for the edema associated with extradural balloon placement [Cutler et al., Arch Neurol. 11, 225–238 (1964)] and uptake of fluorescein isothiocyanate-labeled albumin by glia has been shown for cold-injury edema [Klatzo and Miguel, J. Neuropath. exp. Neurol. 19, 475–487 (1960)]. This must be considered in any interpretation of serum equivalents in relation to weight or water increments.

PAPPIUS: In our experiments the agreement between RISA content and increase in weight is very close 3 and 7 h after the lesion is made. The discrepancy develops later and I feel that the protein content of the extravasated fluid is, in fact, close to that of the whole serum. With time, either the protein content of the fluid or the amount of the label is diminished. The protein appears to be removed faster than the water.

ZWETNOW: Dr. Pappius, how can you correct for any possible increase in the brain blood volume, which was shown to be detrimental by several investigators, Langfitt for one. We have shown, by quantitative measurements of brain blood volume, that it can increase up to 8 %, almost all the extracerebral volume of the intracranial cavity.

PAPPIUS: We kill our anaesthetized animals by exsanguination. By taking the difference between the RISA count of the experimental and the control hemisphere, we hope to correct for most of the blood. In the control hemisphere we have volume of blood of between 1 and 2 %. I think if there is any increase in the experimental hemisphere it would not be very great.

CLASEN: In the monkey with these lesions, the undamaged hemisphere has a blood volume of 1.5 %. The grossly normal portion of the damaged hemisphere shows a 40 % increase in albumin without an accompanying change in tissue iron. This was, therefore, interpreted as indicating exudation rather than an increase in blood volume [Clasen et al., Arch. Neurol. 19, 472–486 (1968)].

LASSEN: Corticosteroids can be compared with alpha-adrenergic-blocking agents. I just ask if you consider the effect of dexamethasone could be related to blood pressure changes (a reduction of pressure?) rather than to specific effects on edema. This would be very interesting for the whole meeting we are here for these days.

PAPPIUS: We have measured blood pressure of our animals at the time of the lesion and before we killed them, at the end of the experiment. We have never monitored the blood pressure during the 24 or 48 h period. Therefore I cannot answer your question, but I think that is something, that we must consider.

LONG: Perhaps I can answer Dr. Lassen's question in the presentation this afternoon. All of our animals treated with a variety of drugs had continuous blood pressure monitoring throughout the period of treatment.

WITHROW (to Dr. Long): Dr. Long, would you care to elaborate on what you mean by stabilization of sodium-potassium membrane pumps since the glucocorticoids are notoriously ineffective on sodium pumps throughout the body.

LONG: The information on which I base this comment are the data from the laboratories from the Department of Medicine at the University of Minneapolis. The sodium-potassium transport in isolated toad and frog bladder was poisoned with endotoxin. The addition of glucosteroids in large doses to this artificial system restored the sodium-potassium flux. I agree with you fully that most other information indicates that glucosteroids are not effective on cellular ion transport.

KLATZO: There is something that interested me very much in Dr. Long's presentation. I am referring to the photograph showing the difference between treated and untreated animals injected with Evans blue as a tracer and sacrificed 72 h after the injury. There was not much difference in the extent of the edema, but there was a striking difference in intensity of the blue staining. This to me indicates the difference in the rate of disappearence of the indicator and I am inclined to conclude from this photograph that dexamethasone has effect not so much on the rate of edema progression as on its resolution.

LONG: The changes in the resolution of brain edema are quite striking on a gross morphological basis. However, we do not have any quantitative information to indicate whether or not this is because there was less edema at first or whether the resolution had been positively accelerated.

CLASEN: Dr. Herrmann, you stated that you measured the blood volume in the cortex adjacent to the lesion with chromated red cells but you did not give us this data in your presentation. Was the amount of blood significant or was it very little?

HERRMANN: We used the blood content of the slices to determine the net BBB indicator concentration. Since, in our experiments animals were killed by air embolism the amount of blood remaining within the samples was very small.

LASSEN (to Dr. Long): Dr. Long, I will comply to your wish and commenting upon the importance of the blood pressure. It is a new recognation that the cerebral circulation is influenced very much by the damage of the brain tissue. In the normal brain the autoregulation guarantees a constant, normal blood flow down to a blood pressure of 40–50 mmHg. At high arterial pressure there is a break-through point where the blood flow increases. In acidotic brain tissue the flow response to blood pressure changes is changed. The break-through point creeps down when the tissue is damaged and acidotic, and it is currently felt, that even moderate hypertension will be able to increase the blood flow and enhance edema production. How far one can lower the blood pressure in hypertensive states is yet undetermined. I think the focus of attention for clinical management of a patient is certainly on what blood pressure level can we advocate; should it be moderately reduced, left unchanged or increased? One cannot in a general way come closer than to advance the question. In your lecture you commented on Dibenzylin – it is a drug of so great interest in this frame of reference. Did you or did you not feel that Dibenzylin did anything but change the blood pressure in a hypertensive direction.

LONG: Under the drug dosage which we have employed the blood pressure remained within the range of 80–140 mmHg unless I had indicated that the animal was hypertensive or hypotensive. What we are trying currently to do is to discover the effect on edema, when the blood pressure is allowed to fall in these animals.

REULEN: Dr. Lassen mentioned that autoregulation of blood flow is defective in damaged brain which results in a pressure-passive flow. I would therefore be careful in lowering the blood pressure below 100 mmHg until we do not know the intracranial pressure of a patient. The reduction of edema formation is one point and the possible hypoxic damage of the edematous tissue with defective autoregulation is the other point in arterial hypotension. Therefore, I would prefer a normal blood pressure.

270

BROCK: I agree that looking at blood pressure alone is only half of the problem. You should also record the intracranial pressure and if you want to be more precise, the tissue pressure in the brain. This certainly does play a very important role.

RANSOHOFF (to Dr. Hansebout): We have produced spinal cord injury by the same system but with a far greater force of 400 CGF. This results in a total paraplegia irreversible without therapy. 2 min after the injury initial hemorrhage occurs in the grey matter. 3 h after the injury edema is spreading into the white matter with further dissolution of the central grey matter. At 24 h complete dissolution of the central grey and the entire spinal cord has occured. By this time the spinal cord is simply a mass of necrotic tissue. If animals with this lesion are treated with 125 mg of methylprednisolone given 1 h after the injury, one sees in a 6 h animal some central hemorrhage and some edema, but preservation of most structures of the spinal cord. 24 h after the administration of steroids one has a spinal cord with a structure still presentable, the long tracts are preserved and these animals showed a return of function and walked. There is no question, if you examine a small section of this spinal cord, the edema would still be there. On the other hand, however, the total dissolution of the cord is prevented by the application of steroids. The question is, treating these animals with steroids results in a preservation of the cord, both anatomically and physiologically, with return of function, and when the major process which occurs here is a process of edema, then, to my simple mind it helps edema. Our best experimental results occur with the use of both steroids and EACA (epsilone aminocaproic acid).

PAPPIUS: You have been using a much greater force. Therefore it is possible that the development of edema with your model is more extensive and more rapid and in 24 h you would be able to show changes in water content which we did not because our lesion was much smaller. In our model the effects of steroids on brain edema where there, but they were minimal as far as total water content of the spinal cord is concerned. The edematous changes were always slightly less, but the difference was not statistically significant.

BAETHMANN: Dr. Hansebout, how do you explain the development of the edema distant to the lesion. Is it the same mechanism as in the cold injury model or is it different?

HANSEBOUT: I am not sure if the edema is actually spreading from the site of injury to distant segments of the cord or if it is developing in those distant segments or if both phenomena are occuring at the same time.

BRENDEL (to Dr. Barker): Tumor growth does not only depend on the kinetics of the tumor cells itself but also on immunological reactions of the host against the tumor. There are antibodies which may destroy tumor cells but also blocking antibodies which can protect the tumor. Since the antibody production is influenced by steroids your results may be explained by assuming that either the production of cytotoxic or of protective antibodies is modified by corticosteroids.

BARKER: We are presently investigating the immunological properties of brain tumors using the same animal model. We have not, as yet, determined the effect of steroids on the imunological response of the rat to its brain tumor.

KLATZO (to Dr. Siegel): I would have some hesitation to consider this kind of micro-embolisation as a proper model for cerebral ischemia or brain edema. I had a chance to study many histological sections from similar experiments. The picture is very heterogenous and you can see intermingled areas of complete necrosis, ischemia, hyperemia, etc. It would be very difficult to interpret the lack of effect of steroids in such a model.

LASSEN: I want to comment that this model is called ischemic to invoke a reduction of blood flow. As Dr. Klatzo just commented, ischemia is certainly found in small focal areas. The blood flow of the brain in these conditions was studied by P. Prosenz (The cerebral hyperperfusion syndrome, Verlag Brüder Hollinek, Wien 1970) and it was found to be about double the normal level, probably due to accumulation of lactic acid enhancing blood flow in all these regions. So we should be a little reserved about what is ischemia. Here we have inhomogenous circulation.

HOSSMANN: I also wonder if the term ischemic edema is appropriate in this particular type of lesion. Zülch and Tzonos (Naturwissenschaften **51**, 539–540, 1964), using micro-emboli with a diameter of 30–37 microns, showed that there was an extravasation of protein rich fluid around the veins in the white matter. This type of edema therefore is probably a vasogenic one, and in view of this observation I am a little bit surprised that dexamethasone did not help.

HARRISON (to Dr. Pappius and Dr. Bartko): I will briefly describe some preliminary results obtained by Dr. Ross Russell, Dr. Drownbill, and myself on the effects of large doses of dexamethasone on the cerebral swelling associated with cerebral infarction in the gerbil. The Mongolian gerbil (Meriones unguiculatus) has an incomplete circle of Willis with no major posterior communicating arteries. Unilateral ligation of the common carotid artery in the neck under barbiturate anaesthesia produces fatal cerebral infarction in approximately 60 % of animals. Large doses of dexamethasone (5 mg/intraperitoneally) given immediately after operation, and again at 24 h reduce this mortality (Table 1; Group B). The difference in mortality is significant at the 1 % level. Other dosage schedules (Groups C and D) are less effective (5 mg/kg each dose).

Table 1. Mortality Following Unilateral Carotid Ligation in the Gerbil

Treatment schedule		n	Mortality	
A	None	26	17	(65 %)
B	Dexamethasone 5 mg/kg Immediately post-op and 24 h later	16	3	(19 %)
C	Dexamethasone 8 h and 24 h post-op	16	5	(31 %)
D	Dexamethasone 8 h post-op	16	9	(56 %)

Table 2. Water Content of Cerebral Hemispheres 8 h after Ligation of the Right Carotid Artery in the Gerbil

Group	n	Water Content % Right	Left	
Carotid ligation, no steroid	20	78.8 ± 1.8	77.2 ± 1.2	$p < .01$
Carotid ligation, dexamethasone	20	77.9 ± 1.5	77.2 ± 0.7	$p < .05$
No operation	10	77.3 ± 0.8	76.9 ± 0.9	N.S.

Statistical significance: right hemisphere versus left.

The water content of the two cerebral hemispheres is shown in Table 2. Thus, 8 h after ligation of the right common carotid artery the water content of the ipsilateral hemisphere is significantly increased. In animals given a single intraperitoneal injection of dexamethasone (5 mg/kg) immediately after surgery the right hemisphere still shows evidence of brain edema but it is less marked. The contralateral hemisphere shows no evidence of edema. These figures for the different groups of animals obscure the fact that not all animals show swelling of the right hemisphere.

The degree of swelling of the right hemisphere in the individual animal can be estimated as a "swelling percentage" [Plum, F. *et al.*, Arch. Neurol. **9**, 563–570 (1963)]. This refers the excess water content of the right hemisphere over that of the left, to the percentage dry weight of the right hemisphere. 14 of 20 animals showed more than $+6\%$ swelling so calculated after carotid ligation (Table 3). With dexamethasone administration only 6 of 20 animals showed this degree of swelling ($p < 0.05$). In parallel with these changes, the proportion of animals showing clinical abnormality was also reduced. All animals showing circling movements or seizures had more than 6 % swelling of the right hemisphere.

Table 3. Effect of Dexamethasone on the Swelling Percentage of the Cerebral Hemisphere Ipsilateral to the Ligated Carotid Artery and on Behaviour Changes

Group	n	More than 6 % swelling percentage	Circling and/or seizures
Untreated	20	14 (70 %)	12 (60 %)
Dexamethasone	20	6 (30 %)	5 (25 %)

There is thus evidence in this model that dexamethasone in large doses reduces the morbidity and mortality following cerebral infarction and that this is accompanied by a reduction in the frequency and degree of brain edema.

Discussion to Chapter III

Mechanisms of Action of Steroids on Brain Edema

Moderator: D. M. LONG

LONG: I have some findings in human brain tumors and human brain edema which touch Dr. Barlow's topic directly. We heard yesterday from Dr. Klatzo about tight junctions and their importance in protein permeability. We know that human brain tumors are permeable to all types of proteins and are often associated with brain edema. It was our feeling that the human brain tumor represented a perfect model to discover the importance of the capillary structure in increased permeability and development of brain edema. Our first step in studying this problem was to discover if tight junctions occurred in normal human brain. Here you see an example of a typical tight junction, very similar to those demonstrated by Brightman and Reese in a variety of experimental animals. The now classic pentalaminar configuration is obvious at these two points in the course of the junction. We then studied a series of over 150 brain tumors. These tumors cover the entire gamut of human brain neoplastic disease, ranging from meningiomas and schwannomas through malignant gliomas and metastatic tumors. There are many abnormalities of the capillaries within these tumors, and I simply wish to illustrate those that I think are related to protein permeability.

Here you see a fenestrated membrane with small islands of cytoplasm connected by individual strands of plasma membrane. The second type of abnormality is illustrated here. There are simply large gaps between individual and endothelial cell cytoplasm. These gaps are quite large without any sign of junctional substructure and quite obviously should be permeable to water and to protein. The third type of junctional abnormality is a typical junction without fusions of membranes along its length. These junctions are the rule in meningiomas and schwannomas. They occur less commonly in malignant gliomas. Fenestrated membranes and gap junctions, on the other hand, are routinely found in metastatic tumors and in gliomas.

In the benign gliomas, we have yet to find capillary abnormalities which obviously can be related to the increased protein permeability.

HAGER: Dr. Barlow, your findings in the thalamus are not surprising. Spielmeyer has shown 45 years ago alterations of the nerve cells in the thalamus, after severe epileptic seizures. After cardiazole convulsions Siemann in 1947 has demonstrated cutted nerve cell loss also in the thalamus. These changes may be reversible and it may be conceived that you find also such reversible alterations of the blood-brain barrier.

BARLOW: I would like to thank Dr. Hager for his interesting comment on this problem.

SCHÜRMANN: Dr. Barlow, I was very impressed by the case that you have demonstrated which developed a midline displacement due to hemispheral edema after a series of seizures. I would like to add an occasional observation that we have made. A brain tumor patient without a displacement of the midline developed a series of unilateral seizures. Thereafter we observed a increase of the volume of the tumor-bearing hemisphere with a midline displacement. I wonder whether the volume increase (brain edema) might be caused by the same mechanism as you have described in your experiments.

BARLOW: This is an interesting comment. A tumor is a setting for abnormal blood-brain barrier permeability of low degree. With the added pathophysiologic insult of the seizure, and the hypertension that accompanies most seizures, it would seem that this could easily raise the water content of the tissue, giving rise to hemispheral edema.

REULEN: Dr. Barlow, in your seizure experiments you demonstrated that epinephrine infusion increased albumin entry into the thalamus. Did it also increase the water content of the thalamus?

BARLOW: That particular series of animals did not have water content determinations done.

REULEN: That leads to my second question regarding the relation between protein entry and edema formation. We know circumstances where brain water and electrolyte content rises and cerebral edema develops without an increased protein permeability, for instance in TET edema, after water intoxication, early ischemic edema etc. I would like to know if, on the other hand, an increased protein permeability with leakage of plasma protein into brain tissue is always accompanied by an increased leakage of water and electrolytes. This combination is usually seen in vasogenic edema. Do you know circumstances with markedly increased protein permeability without edema formation?

BARLOW: I do not think I can answer that question exactly. Under ordinary circumstances when great quantities of albumin enter the brain, it is generally accompanied by water. With a minor degree of albumin entry, it may or may not be accompanied by water. The curious situation expressed by stroke is interesting in this regard. A stroke immediately and at the time of infarction leads to some protein permeability and occasionally some increase in tissue water. However, the protein permeability of an infarct is greatest long after the edema has subsided, something like 7 or 14 days, when the abnormal isotope brain scans are seen. At this point the lesion is not occupying an expanded volume, but actually a smaller volume within the nervous system. There is a discrepancy between the increase in water and the protein permeability and I believe they are separate phenomena.

BRODERSEN: I would like to add information on the pathophysiology of cerebral circulation during seizures. Even in paralyzed, ventilated animals cerebral blood flow is increased 2–3 fold, arterial blood pressure increases and the autoregulation is lost during seizures [Plum et al., Arch. Neurol. 18, 1–13 (1968)]. We have in anaesthetized, paralyzed and ventilated humans recently observed, that during electrically induced seizures cerebral blood flow and oxygen uptake increased about 100 % [Brodersen et al., submitted to Arch. Neurol. (1972)]. You found an increased albumin uptake, when you increased the blood pressure after convulsions. This situation is comparable with what happens, when the arterial blood pressure is increased above the upper limit of cerebral autoregulation, the breakthrough of autoregulation (Ekstrøm-Jodal et al. In: Fieschi, C. (Ed.): Cerebral blood flow regulation, acid-base energy metabolism in acute brain injuries. Basel: Karger 1972).

BARLOW: We have measured cerebral blood flow by the indicator fractionation technique on a regional basis and have also found a flow increase in cortex and thalamus amounting to 50–100 %. I doubt, however, that the flow increase itself is responsible for the albumin entry. Something must open the gate and then increased blood flow and hypertension will increase the influx of proteins.

BARLOW (to Dr. Pappius): I would like to ask Dr. Pappius a question of interpretation. You have measured specific activities at one point of time and described the phenomenon in terms of the rate. It seems to me that the higher levels of relative specific activity could equally well mean the opening of a new compartment of sodium which would be an alternative and equally interesting interpretation of Katzman's data and your data. There may be a relatively protected, perhaps intracellular compartment of sodium that is opened up in the edema and you might be showing it.

PAPPIUS: I am fully aware of this problem. These are preliminary data and, as a matter of fact, the plans for next year are to do kinetic studies, e. g. doing these analyses at different time intervals. By this way we hope to gain information on whether it is influx or efflux of sodium that is affected.

BAETHMANN: Dr. Pappius, an involvement of active transport mechanism in the production and resolution of edema is a very attractive hypothesis. You suggest that active transport

275

mechanisms are involved in the resolution of edema, and they may even be enhanced by the application of furosemide. I think, one should just expect the contrary since this drug is inhibiting active transport mechanisms but not enhancing them.

PAPPIUS: Our results with furosemide show that this drug has a direct effect on the brain. We were studying the distribution of sodium between blood and brain and this was affected by furosemide even in the normal brain. I am fully aware that furosemide is said to inhibit active transport in the kidney. The interpretation of the effect of furosemide on the brain depends on how you place your sodium pump, in which direction. I would like to invoke active transport mechanisms in formation of vasogenic edema, but I feel that there is really no basis for it in this type of edema.

BARLOW (to Dr. Clasen): I would like to rise the question as to the extent that the tumors were searched histologically.

CLASEN: We prepared about 6 slides from large tumor nodules. With smaller multiple lesions, fewer slides were prepared from individual nodules but each nodule was examined.

RANSOHOFF: In the human model that you utilized here, these were single intracranial metastases with edema. In human cerebral metastatic diseases, it is very frequent that one lesion will show a great deal of edema and similar lesions in the same or the opposite hemisphere will not show any edema.

CLASEN: Cases with single metastatic nodules were used in evaluating edema by means of hemispheric weights. The histologic studies included these as well as cases with multiple metastases. All slides were graded blindly so that we did not know whether we were looking at the same or different cases. The results for individual cases were astonishingly homogeneous but not completely so. The judgement that the edema is reduced in cases responding to steroids is based on the hemispheric weight data. In the histologic studies we were more interested in the character of the edema fluid as reflected by PAS staining which is related to an increased concentration of alpha 2 globulins [Clasen et al. In: Klatzo, Seitelberger (Ed.): Brain Edema, p. 536–553 (1967)].

HAGER: I think there exists an effect of corticosteroids on the glia reaction of proliferation. We could prove this in chronic lesions. The peritraumatic lesion is influenced by corticosteroids in terms of the number of proliferated astrocytes especially in the quantity of the formation of glia phenomens as well as in the texture of the cells. It is not a condensed scar formation but almost always a spongy state. I think that your human model is a little problematic. You can have metastatic tumors in which you have only a mild microglia reaction and you can have metastatic tumors in which you have a proliferation of all glia components.

CLASEN: The favorable clinical response in most patients with metastatic brain disease to steroid therapy, as well as the diminution of the cerebral edema associated with this disease by the drug is in no way problematic. The same may not be said about the cerebral edema associated with head trauma either clinically or experimentally. We choose to study metastatic edema both because of morphologic and pathogenic similarities to the edema associated with cold injury. We were, of course, aware of the fact that there are differences in the reaction of the brain to metastatic lesions. The question which we posed was whether these differences could be related to the clinical response of the patient to steroid therapy. The answer which we have given I leave you to evaluate from your own material.

PATTEN: I disagree with Dr. Clasen's interpretation of his results. He showed that patients treated with, and responding to steroids, have less inflammation at autopsy than those not responding to therapy. An alternative explanation is that the responders actually had their inflammation erased by the steroids with resultant reduction of edema and clinical improvement. The so called paradoxical case shown at the end of his paper, in which Dr. Clasen predicted no response to steroids because the brain biopsy showed metastatic tumor surrounded with inflammation, is certainly more easily understood in terms of this alternative explanation. Steroids have been known for many years as profoundly effective anti-inflammatory agents. I bet the more inflammation surrounding the tumor the greater would be the relief of symptoms. Similarly, in muscle disease, the more the disease resembles polymyositis, on the biopsy, the greater the chances that the patient will respond to steroid therapy.

CLASEN: In the case of the monkeys, as I indicated, there was no demonstrable anti-inflammatory effect of the steroid in the brain. Nor can suppression of exudative inflammation have played a role in the steroid effect observed with the Klatzo lesions since such changes are essentially absent in these lesions. Dr. Patten's remarks, therefore, apply solely to the metastatic disease data. Part of our data, which I did not present, included 8 cases not treated with steroids. Of these, 4 showed significant inflammation. Dr. Patten's explanation could, therefore, apply in only about half of the cases responding to steroids. On the other hand, his interpretation, it seems to me, leaves completely unexplained the finding that significant inflammation is present in patients not responding to steroids, as well as the experimental data. I do not think that our conclusions that the presence of inflammation adversely affects the response of cerebral edema to steroids is a misinterpretation of these data. The effect, however, may be quantitative in nature. In any case, we have a testable hypothesis, which God and the National Institute of Neurologic Diseases and Stroke willing, I hope to pursue.

LASSEN (to Dr. Demopoulos): We have heard from Dr. Klatzo and also from Dr. Long about the importance of the blood pressure during the formation of edema. Could the effect of the antioxidants probably be due to a blood pressure change.

DEMOPOULOS: Not all of our animals were monitored throughout the 24, 48 or 72 h intervals. Each group was checked initially, midway and towards the end. We did not note that the DPPD or the EOP had any measurable effects on the blood pressure.

TAYLOR: You were hinting, Dr. Demopoulos, that you might be using DPPD clinically. I would therefore like to ask you a little more about its toxic effects, because it seems to be ineffective at 100 mg, effective at 500 mg, and lethal at 1,000 mg/kg. It is obviously going to be very difficult to handle clinically. I should like to have your comments about that.

DEMOPOULOS: We are really not intending to use them. We were saying that from the point of view of antioxidants it is possible to pick several of them that have the same mode of action. In this way they might be used in combination, so that the toxicity of each might be different and might be minimized. DPPD as a matter of fact, for a time has been on the approved list of the food and drug administration and has been taken off that approved list, and with good reason.

BARLOW (to Dr. Bouzarth): May I ask Dr. Bouzarth if he has looked at the plasma cortisol level in subjects with pseudotumor. Also, a second, broader question, which Dr. Ransohoff and I were discussing, and that is an inquiry regarding the problem of dependence on corticosteroids in these neurosurgical patients. How long may one go on corticosteroids before the depression of cortisol level is a serious and significant problem? Is there a place in neurosurgical care of these patients for the alternate day schedule which medical people frequently are adopting when they plan in terms of long duration of corticosteroid use?

BOUZARTH: These few cases with pseudotumor we have had, seemed to have a normal or slighty above normal plasma cortisol level, from what you could expect for patients hospitalized without brain disease. In terms of long term steroid therapy we keep our patients on it for 5–7 days and then wear them off so that by 9th day patients are not getting steroids any more. This has created somewhat of a problem because many of these patients are doing so well on steroids that they want to get out of the hospital. Patients who have a metastatic disease are kept on daily doses of dexamethasone as an outpatient. Only about 5–10 % of the patients showed signs of significant toxicity. The most recent one was the development of a peptic ulcer.

LANDOLT: I would like to go further into the problems concerning the effects of the corticosteroids in the immediate postoperative period. It is generally said that in a prolonged treatment with dexamethasone effects on the serum electrolytes should not be expected. This is not true in the early postoperative period. Any type of surgery causes a typical metabolic response called the mild sodium-potassium shift. The sodium is dropping on the first or second day after surgery below the normal limit but does not fall under 130 meq/l. There is a concomitant increase of the potassium level above 4.5 meq/l. I examined the occurence of this mild sodium-potassium shift in 126 patients operated because of intracranial aneurysms by the same surgeon. This electrolyte shift could be observed in 32 patients among the 126 (Table 1). It was definitely more frequent in patients receiving a prophylactic dexamethasone treatment. The difference is statistically significant. There exists a second group of patients with a severe electrolyte shift, showing a sodium drop below 130 meq/l. This is a very dangerous complication which is not influenced by dexamethasone.

Table 1. Frequency of sodium-potassium shift after dexamethasone treatment

Medication	Aneurysms operated	Mild shift	Severe shift
With dexamethasone	50	11 = 36 %[a]	4 = 8 %[b]
Without dexamethasone	76	14 = 18 %[a]	5 = 7 %[b]
Total	126	32 = 25 %	9 = 8 %

[a] Significant difference in Student test ($p < 0.05$).
[b] No significant difference in Student test.

The gross fluid balance (fluid intake minus urine volume) occurring 24 h before establishment of the hyponatremia was checked in 25 of the 32 patients who showed the mild sodium-potassium shift and in which enough data were available. The values range from minus 800 to plus 2400 cc with an average of plus 810 cc. Three groups of patients can be pointed out if the extrarenal water loss is estimated to amount to 800–1200 cc (Table 2). The first

Table 2. Fluid balance occurring 24 h before establishment of hyponatremia

Number of patients	Range of gross fluid balance (fluid intake minus urine volume) cc	Estimated total fluid balance after deduction of extrarenal loss
5	below 0	
1	0– 250	negative
3	250– 500	
1	500– 750	
1	750–1000	positive or negative
7	1000–1250	
4	1250–1500	
1	1500–1750	positive
2	above 1750	

one will end up in a total fluid balance which will be negative. The second one can have either a positive or a negative balance if the extrarenal losses are taken into account. Only the third one will have a positive fluid balance and therefore show some fluid retention. About 50 % of our patients have probably a negative total fluid balance. Dexamethasone does not show any influence on the total fluid balance if 1000 cc is considered to be the mean value of a l extrarenal water loss (Table 3). The specific gravity of the urine voided in the phase of establishment of the hyponatremia was always above 1.010. We therefore suggest that dexamethasone can cause a sodium loss if applied in the postoperative stress situation, probably by either affecting the glomerular filtration or by interference with production or action of aldosterone. The latter would very well fit with the observation of Dr. Bouzarth.

Table 3. Influence of dexamethasone treatment on fluid balance

Fluid balance	Treatment with dexamethasone	Treatment without dexamethasone	Total
More than 1000 cc positive	6	8	14
Less than 1000 cc positive	7	4	11

No significant differences in four fold chi square test ($p > 0.2$).

KRÜCK: Dr. Landolt, the drop in serum sodium concentration and the increase in potassium concentration, you referred to, is very surprising to me. In most of the cases, we find the opposite changes with a decreasing potassium concentration and a rise of sodium concentration. We believe this is due to an overproduction of aldosterone after operation. Do you have any information on changes in ADH activity in those patients with very low serum sodium concentration? Your findings are very similar to water intoxication, for instance to the state of inappropriate secretion of ADH in the Schwartz-Bartter-syndrom.

LANDOLT: No, sorry I don't have. I do not think that this is so in the patients showing the mild sodium-potassium shift, which is actually nothing extraordinary. Moore (Moore, F. D.: Metabolic care of the surgical patient. Philadelphia: Saunders 1960) wrote that the bigger the operation the more often you can observe the drop in sodium. I cannot explain the difference in behaviour of your and our patients. I do not think that we are dealing with inappropriate ADH secretion since potassium shows a tendency to fall in this condition whereas it rose in our cases.

ZWETNOW: My question would be concerning the same point of water intoxication in those cases you gave dexamethasone and saw a drop in serum sodium concentration. Did you see any clinical symptoms that could sustain the clinical diagnosis of water intoxication?

LANDOLT: No, with this mild sodium-potassium shift you don't see any clinical effects. But a sodium drop below 130 meq/l brings you in the dangerous region. This has to be watched very carefully.

KRÜCK: Did you measure the renal sodium loss or do you have any other explanation for this very low serum sodium concentration?

LANDOLT: I have not measured the 24 h urine excretion of sodium. So I cannot answer your question.

BOUZARTH: I would like to add some observations related to Dr. Landolt's studies. We have studied in detail fluid balance in three groups of patients. One group did not receive any medication undergoing craniotomy. A second group received mannitol as a single dose preoperatively and the third group, dexamethasone. We have found as much as Dr. Landolt reported in the nontreated group. In the mannitol group we have found that the normal, expected increase in extracellular fluid volume, occuring on the 2nd post-operative day, is abolished by a single dose of mannitol. The same is true in the group given steroids before and after surgery. In fact, in this group the extracellular fluid volume was diminished over what normally would be expected. There was an increased renal excretion of sodium and potassium and there was a larger volume of urine in the dexamethasone group, when compared to the controls. It is our feeling that one of the mechanisms of action of dexamethasone in the total organism is this diuretic effect, both of water and of electrolytes.

HERRMANN (to Dr. Baethmann): I have some questions concerning the electric resistance or impedance measurements. What size of the electrodes did you use? Where did you place the electrodes and what frequency did you use for the measurement?

BAETHMANN: The size of the electrodes was approximately 2–2.5 mm in diameter and they were placed ca. 6–10 mm apart on the exposed cortical surface after the removal of the dura. Care was taken to avoid any damage of the tissue which usally could be achieved without greater problems. The frequency used to measure the impedence was 1000 cycles/sec.

HERRMANN: With this set-up you intended to measure the extracellular space of the unterlying brain tissue. Using a bipolar measuring system we always get an error caused by the electrode-electrolyte interface impedance which depends on measuring frequency, geometric factors, size and surface characteristics of the electrodes, and on the specific impedance of the tissue. This systemic error makes an absolute measurement of the tissue impossible if it is not taken absolutely in account. The values you obtained can therefore not be considered as specific impedance with the dimension $\Omega \cdot$ cm. Your surface electrodes may easily be short circuited by a film of CSF, so that your results can be influenced to an unknown extent by the electrolyte content of this fluid. Measuring the specific impedance of brain cortex one has to consider that it decreases with increasing frequency starting at approximately 5 cycles/sec [Ranck, J. B., Exp. Neurol. 7, 144–152 (1963)]. There is no unique interpretation of this low frequency dispersion range (5 c.p.s. – 50 k.c.p.s.). However, using 1 kcps the current must penetrate part of the cells, so that a specific impedance measured at this frequency does not represent the extracellular space. Ranck [Exp. Neurol. 7, 153–174 (1963)] has analyzed this problem and states: "... the analysis shows that the specific impedance of the cerebral cortex gives little information relative to the size of the interstitial spaces."

BAETHMANN: One has to be aware that one is measuring only an electrical parameter. However, under appropriate experimental conditions, the tissue conductivity for a given current can be considered as a measure of the extracellular ion concentration. This is very well documented by Van Harreveld, concerning studies of chloride movements and electron-microscopy in brain tissue done in parallel to impedance measurements. (Van Harreveld, A.: In: The Structure and Function of Nervous Tissue, Vol. IV, 447, New York and London: Academic Press 1972). Also Cole, whose fundamental doubts you were referring to, even more recently provided additional justification for the validity of the tissue impedance as a parameter of the extracellular ion concentration also in tissue with high cellular density as, e.g., the brain. [Cole, K. S. et al., Exp. Neurol 24, 459 (1969).] If we were only measuring the conductivity of an electrolyte fluid-layer around the electrodes and nothing else, as you are suggesting, we should not find the precipitous drop in conductivity after circulatory arrest as has been demonstrated.

WITHROW: As Dr. Baethmann has demonstrated in the first slide he could not find any difference in the electrolyte effects between dexamethasone, aldosterone and desoxycorticosterone. Do you have any explanation for this. Dexamethasone is used because it has no salt retaining properties. Aldosterone and DOCA both cause salt retention. Have you tried to maintain an adrenalectomized animal on dexamethasone alone? What kind of electrolyte problems does he get into?

BAETHMANN: The more or less identical effects of the gluco- or mineralotropic steroids on the cerebral electrolytes in adrenalectomized animals surprised us as well, and we have no conclusive explanation yet for this observation. One may suspect that in the case of aldosterone or DOCA glucotropic "side-effects" are involved. The characterization of the corticosteroids as gluco- or mineralotropic is derived from their metabolic activity or their action on target organs as, e.g., the kidney. This does, however, not necessarily mean that the steroid action on other tissues, as e.g., the brain is identical with their effects heretofore known. I am not aware of any studies proving convincingly that e.g. aldosterone affects active transport mechanisms in the brain.

WITHROW: It has been studied in the CNS [Woodbury, D. M., Koch, A., Proc. Soc. exp. Biol. Med. 94, 120–123 (1957)]. I think they showed a decrease in cellular sodium.

BAETHMANN: I know these results, however, the conclusions drawn from these studies were based on the use of the chloride space as a measure of the extracellular compartment.

HAGER: Dr. Baethmann, do you think the compartments which you demonstrate with the freeze substitution method are close to the intravital compartments? Why did you not use the planimetric method for analyzing your electron micrographs?

BAETHMANN: Yes, Dr. Hager, I think so, because the results obtained from freeze substituted electron-microscopical preparations are more or less in agreement with data obtained from impedance studies, two methods which are independent from each other. I doubt, whether a planimetric approach is feasible in freeze substituted material, because the preparation is not a homogenous one, i.e., the quality of the electron-microscopical section deteriorates with increasing distance from the tissue surface due to the decreasing velocity in freezing which finally results in ice crystal formation. I think, however, the differences of the experimental group, when compared to controls, were quite obvious.

KRÜCK: Dr. Schmiedek, how often could you observe an escape phenomen during treatment of your patients with aldosterone? Did the patients develop signs of hypokalemia? Did you find blood pressure changes, especially hypertension, in the aldosterone treated patients?

SCMIEDEK: To your last question: We don't have any evidence in our series for the development of hypertension as a result of aldosterone administration. Probably, because the few days we give aldosterone, is a too short period of time. With regard to your first question, which I did expect, actually, I have to admit, that I did not yet go through all the clinical data of these patients. But as far as I remember there were only two instances of escape phenomenon during the course of the treatment.

REULEN: I would like to comment on the method of tissue sampling. Where did you remove the samples of the white matter? There is a paper published by Adachi and Feigin [J. Neurol. Psychiat. 29, 446–450 (1966)] demonstrating great variations in the water content of the white matter. According to these studies water content of the arcuate white matter amounts to 79%, of corpus callosum to 73% and of deep white matter to 71%. Therefore, when studing the effect of a drug on the water content of the brain – and the changes found beeing less than the normal differences in the white matter – care must be taken, that white matter specimens are removed exactly from the same depth.

SCHMIEDEK: First of all, don't worry, our methods for tissue sampling are very much alike those proposed by Dr. Reulen [Reulen, H. J. et al., Arch. Neurol. 21, 517 (1969)]. On the other hand, it should be kept in mind, that the data of the study you are referring to were derived from autopsy material. But, of course we are quite aware of the possible errors and pitfalls being necessarily involved in an investigation like this.

REULEN: What was the clinical response of your patients pretrated with aldosterone. Did you notice a marked relief of symptoms and did they as well as with pretreatment with glucosteroids.

SCHMIEDEK: I think, I did go into this, though very briefly, in my presentation. As I mentioned, by far the most of the patients were doing surprisingly well, postoperatively. But we certainly do need some more patients pretreated with aldosterone, before we can make any definite statement. Since we did not yet pretreat patients with glucosteroids, I cannot comment on this part of your question.

Discussion to Chapter IV

Effects of Steroids on Brain Edema in Man
(Head injury, brain tumors, inflammation, stroke)

Moderators: J. W. F. BEKS and J. RANSOHOFF

RANSOHOFF: Dr. Beks, would you again tell us how the choice of these patients was made. Was this a random choice, made all at one time, or was this a retrospective study? In other words, did you take 400 patients before steroids and 400 patients after steroids?

BEKS: It was a retrospective study. We took the patients in a certain period from 1961 until 1963 and a same period from 1968 until 1970.

SIEGEL: I have several questions for Dr. Maxwell, concerning the brain scan response following dexamethasone. Could you please tell me the total number of patients that had serial scans, the number out of this total that had positive responses, whether the response correlated with the clinical response of the patient and finally the shortest time interval in which he saw a decrease in brain scan activity.

MAXWELL: It is not our usual policy to delay surgery after making the diagnosis of brain tumor and so our experience in this regard is relatively limited. Among a group of 15 patients with brain tumors and positive scans, 3 showed unequivocal improvement on the scan after 72 h of steroid therapy. This correlated well with their clinical improvement. There was a larger group, however, where clinical improvement occured and no change was noted on the repeated scan. I cannot comment on the time one can expect to see maximum improvement on the scan after steroid therapy when such improvement does occur since we do not have a series where scans were repeated at frequent and varied intervals.

LONG: We have a study currently under way utilizing a human choriocarcinoma in primate brain. This tumor grows very predictively, presenting symptoms within a 24 h period and causes death again within a 24 h predictable period. We have studied these tumors with and without steroids by serial angiography and by serial brain scans. The aim of this study is to be able to predict the effect of chemotherapeutic agents upon this tumor model. Brain scanning has proven ineffective in predicting the response to steroid, which is dramatic in these animals, as it is in patients with metastatic tumors.

MÜKE: We examined 200 patients undergoing surgery to study the effect of dexamethasone on brain edema. The diagnosis indicated the presence of meningeomas, gliomas, metastatic tumors, craniopharyngeomas, acustic neurinomas, spongioblastomas and aneurysms. The first group of one hundred patients received dexamethasone, the other one (untreated group) did not. Each group of patients was formed over a time period of about one year. Operation technique, anaesthesia and other basic treatment were not varied during this period. The average age in both groups was about 43–45 years. The number of men and women was in both groups about the same. Dexamethasone was administered in a dosage of 4 mg, 4 times daily. Treatment was started one day prior to the craniotomy and was continued 3–7 days after the operation. Side effects and complications were controlled.

The severity of brain edema was evaluated by clinical methods, taking into account the following examinations: 1. level of consciousness; 2. breathing; 3. pupil reaction; 4. blood pressure; 5. cerebrospinal fluid pressure; 6. angiography; 7. EEG examination; 8. pathological examination.

In the untreated group 26 patients were found with brain edema, 19 of these died, but only 11 patients died from brain edema. In 8 patients with brain edema death was primarily not due to brain edema; 3 of them died from postoperative intracranial bleedings, 4 of them from pulmonary complications and one from liver cirrhosis. In the dexamethasone treated group only 16 patients were found having brain edema; 11 of these died, but only 5 from brain edema. The death of two resulted primarily from postoperative bleedings, the death of another four from pulmonary complications.

The differences between the steroid treated group and the untreated group are most impressive if the glioblastomas are compared in both groups. In the untreated group 9 out of 17 patients developed brain edema, 6 died. In the dexamethasone group only 2 out of 15 patients developed brain edema, 1 died. The effects were also seen during operation. In the group without dexamethasone 4 cases had a brain swelling during operation, in the group with dexamethasone only one.

Plasma sodium-concentration was lower and plasma potassium-concentration was higher in the untreated group as compared to the steroid-treated group. Electrolytes were measured over a period of seven days. The sodium/potassium ratio was higher in the dexamethasone group through this period than in the group without dexamethasone. Postoperative complications due to dexamethasone were rare. In the dexamethasone treated group wound healing seemed more impeded (1:4), hyperglycaemia (1:4), and gastrointestinal hemorrhage (1:4) were seen more frequently. In contrast, brain prolapse (3:1), pulmonary complications (8:4) were not as frequent as in the untreated group. Meningitis, thrombosis and urinary infections occured in both groups with about the same frequency (3:3, 2:3, 4:5).

HERRMANN (to Dr. Reulen): Did you measure the concentration of lactic acid and of high-energy phosphate compounds in the brain tissue samples in untreated and dexamethasone-treated patients. Was there any change following dexamethasone treatment? I am asking this, because it might give some hint to your interesting autoregulation studies.

REULEN: Tissue metabolite concentrations could be determined in perifocal edematous tissue of some untreated as well as some dexamethasone-treated patients. Mean concentration of PCr and ATP was increased in dexamethasone-treated patients, while lactate concentration and the lactate/pyruvate ratio were not significantly reduced after steroid treatment. It would be, however, hardly possible to draw conclusions regarding restoration of autoregulation from small changes in *tissue* lactate concentration, since the extracellular lactate concentration is not known. Lactate concentration in ventricular CSF, which would be probably more reliable, was not measured.

MILLER: I have two comments. The first is about your definition of intact autoregulation and the second about the role of increased tissue pressure in explaining your results. We should be very cautious before saying that failure of cerebral blood flow to increase following a rise in arterial pressure always means that autoregulation is intact. In both patient and animals studies done with Dr. Langfitt we found that this could be present when there was known to be considerable brain damage; in the animals this followed a stage in the experiment where autoregulation had been shown to be impaired, further brain compression had been carried out and intracranial pressure was now increasing spontaneously (after deflation of the epidural balloon) signifying to us that brain swelling was present. Constant, but low, CBF during an increase in blood pressure under these circumstances is not intact autoregulation.

I find it hard to explain low CBF in cerebral edema purely on the basis of increased tissue pressure, because of two observations. The first is that in our experiments during brain swelling there was not even a transient increase in CBF despite increases of arterial intravascular pressure. The second observation was that in some comatose patients with brain swelling, intravenous mannitol produced remarkable increases in CBF without significantly reducing intracranial pressure. It may well be that we have to think of purely mechanical, obstructive factors affecting the capillary wall or the smaller intracerebral veins during cerebral edema, rather than trying to invoke pressure changes in order to explain low cerebral blood flow.

REULEN: I do not think that we are dealing in our studies with "false autoregulation". As you mentioned, false autoregulation occurs in severley damaged brain or during final stages. The patients which we examined only showed slight or moderate signs of intracranial pressure and a clear impairment of autoregulation before steroid treatment, which was definitely improved following dexamethasone. A prerequisite of false autoregulation to occur is the increase of ICP during hypertension. In 5 out of the six patients lumbar CSF pressure was monitored during both CBF measurements and was found to remain unchanged or decreased following dexamethasone treatment.

Concerning your second remark I am not sure, whether our results can be compared with your findings and therefore I can not give an exact answer. You have been working with very severe brain swelling, which was not defined as brain edema and might be of other origin. I might add, that it is known from well defined models of brain edema that hypertonic solutions cause a definite reduction in intracranial pressure. This, however, is due to a diminution of the water content of normal brain areas, whereas edematous brain is not influenced [Pappius, H. M. et al., Arch. Neurol. 13, 395 (1965); Clasen, R. A. et al., Arch. Neurol. 12, 424 (1965)]. Therefore an increase of CBF following mannitol seems to be related to the decrease in ICP (increase of cerebral perfusion pressure in a brain with loss of autoregulation) rather than to a direct effect on brain edema. The finding, therefore, speaks in favor of the importance of local tissue perfusion pressure.

LASSEN: I have some comments to this very nice demonstration. It is true what we just heard from the Glasgow group that autoregulation can falsely appear to be regained, but these are extreme conditions with a very high intracranial pressure and does not pertain to Reulen's studies and I think that when he interprets the results with a return of autoregulation he certainly is on safe ground. What I would comment on is that for good reasons you have discussed your dexamethasone effects in relation to brain edema. Some effects you have noted, however, are probably unrelated thereto, because we noted that some of the flow increases were in remote areas far from the lesion. I would like to have your comment on the possibility of an improvement of metabolism and function of the brain influencing also the blood flow in the more remote regions.

REULEN: In general the most pronounced flow increases following steroid-treatment appeared in the areas neighbouring the lesions. I do agree that the flow increase recorded in some remote areas might be explained by an improvement of cerebral metabolism and function.

TAYLOR: Three slides where shown to illustrate the effect of dexamethasone given to neurosurgical patients. Serial observations were made as often as necessary using an intravenous method to label a length of the general circulation about 12 sec long, and observing its first passage through the head. The most pronounced, beneficial effects were seen in patients with cerebral tumors awaiting operation. Similar control was achieved over the edema which followed operation and cerebral vascular accident and the edema surrounding abscesses. Clinically it has been impossible to assess accurately the influence of dexamethasone on brain swelling after trauma because the administration of steroids is never the only therapeutic measure in use at one time. Serial observations have shown that angiography greatly reduces the cerebral circulation, particularly in patients who have a radiologically demonstrable aneurysm with hemorrhage. It is suggested that these patients may be protected against endothelial and membrane damage with resultant edema, if dexamethasone is given before the injection of contrast media. Investigations are proceeding.

PATTEN (to Dr. Kullberg): Was your impression that the clinical improvement preceded the pressure changes or did the improvement occur coincident with the pressure changes?

KULLBERG: During recording of the ventricular fluid pressure we have noticed at least one patient, who definitely improved clinically before there was any change in the ventricular fluid pressure. The patient woke up from a drowsy state and we could at that stage not see any changes in the ventricular fluid pressure. So apparently no improvement of the edema or brain swelling had occured when she got better. Most of the patients had intermittent episodes of various kinds; headache, lowering of consciousness and so on, in association with high

284

pressure waves. Particularly these symptoms and attacks disappeared soon after the start of the treatment in relation to the improvement of pressure.

BEKS: I would like to confirm that with a clinical experience. In our series we have a patient with a brain tumor who was clinically much improved following steroids. In angiograms, done before and after steroids, however, no reduction of the midline displacement could be seen. In other words there was a definite functional improvement without a change in edema.

LUNDBERG: I would like to make a short comment on the effect of steroids on the plateau waves which was demonstrated in Dr. Kullberg's paper. This effect may evoke speculation about the origin of the plateau wave phenomenon. For instance, one might assume that the plateau waves are some kind of acute attacks of brain edema. However, from the very beginning there was strong evidence that the plateau waves phenomenon primarily is of hemodynamic origin. We have lately been able to confirm this view and I think that there is a much simpler explanation. A prerequisite for the plateau waves to occur is a tight intracranial situation, in other words, a situation where the capacity for buffering intracranial pressure/volume variations is reduced. By reducing brain edema and thus the brain volume steroid therapy may to some extent restore this capacity so that volume/pressure variations in the intracranial blood compartment are better compensated for.

ZWETNOW: Your pressure waves are easily interpreted in terms of what we call the elastance of the intracranial space. We borrowed the elastance term from lung physiology. We have defined it as the ratio between the increase between the cerebrospinal fluid pressure and the increase of the volume of the cerebrospinal fluid space ($\Delta Pcsf/\Delta Vcsf$). During your pressure waves the intracranial situation would be characterized by the steep part of the elastance curve.

What I do not understand, is why the steroid treatment reduced the frequency and height of the plateau wave but fails to influence a progressively increasing intracranial tension. Have you tested the autoregulation of the cerebral blood flow in the cases with the progressively increasing intracranial tension? One wonders why these bad cases exhibit a completely pressure-passive vascular bed without any spontaneous hemodynamics and thus no pressure waves.

BOUZARTH (to Dr. Patten): I noted in the placebo group there are 3 patients diagnosed having cerebral hemorrhage and none in the treated group. On the other hand in the treated group 2 patients had brain stem infarction, where in the control group there were none. Now, if we are going to talk about herniation of the brain it is my feeling that it is the cerebrum that herniates against the brain stem rather than the brain stem herniates against the cerebrum. Therefore I have to come to the conclusion with a small group of patients that it is really not correct that dexamethasone is of benefit on the acute stroke. I would hope that you would continue your studies with a larger number of patients who have an exact diagnose based both on arteriography and clinical picture and then compare patients with the same disease process. I can guarantee that the occlusion of middle cerebral artery on the nondominant hemisphere is completely different from occlusion of the middle cerebral artery on the dominant hemisphere.

PATTEN: Well, I think that is an important point. We thought that the common denominator of all our cases was that they were diagnosed as having a stroke and that they did have injured nervous tissue. In the statistical analysis we did exclude patients with cerebral hemorrhage to see, what the results would be after their exclusion. We still came up with the significant statistical improvement in the steroid treated group. Brain stem infarction and cerebral hemorrhage, both of these types of stroke are what we are dealing with clinically. All these patients have injured brain tissue which, I think, can be improved by the administration of steroids. I agree with you that a more complete and detailed study should be done. At the time we concluded the study a nursing strike took place in our institute. We were not able to admit any further strokes. So we stopped the study at that point.

BARLOW: I hope that this study can be done again since the numbers of patients are too small to make a clinical conclusion, whatever the statistics show. Although it was a double blind study and properly conceived, you had a distribution of patients that was really quite dissimilar in your different groups. For example, most of the brain stem infarcts fell into the steroid treated group. On the other hand, the hemorrhages all fell into the untreated group. If you do it again, a better patient selection device should be organized. It is the group of massive hemispheral vascular accidents, which undoubtedly do have edema, which I should think should be concentrated upon, individually studying infarct and hemorrhage.

May I make one other comment in relation to the permeability change that takes place late (7–14 days) in cerebrovascular accidents. I think that this is not an expression of an edematous process but more likely a result of new capillary growth in the infarcted area and the leakage of those capillaries. Heymans and the group at Duke had studied this problem in the experimental animal, but as far as I know, have not published it yet.

PATTEN: Dr. Barlow said that brain stem infarction is a less serious disease than cerebral infarction and that the patients in the steroid group had two patients with brain stem infarction whereas there were no brain stem infarctions in the placebo group. I might question whether brain stem infarction is a less serious disease. Posterior inferior cerebellar artery syndrome is relatively benign causing a lateral medullary infarction. I think some of the brain stem infarctions can be quite serious being so close to the respiratory center and blood pressure center and so forth. Those two patients with the brain stem infarctions in the treated group, one of them was worse by 80 % after treatment than she was on admission and the other one was better by only 12 %. So the net result of including the brain stem infarctions in the steroid group actually decreased the average performance of that group. Therefore, if we were to exclude the cerebral hemorrhage and the brain stem infarcts we would still have a statistically significant benefit to the patients treated with steroids.

Round Table Discussion

Moderators: J. W. F. BEKS, I. KLATZO, D. M. LONG, H. M. PAPPIUS, K. SCHÜRMANN

KLATZO: I don't know if I share your optimism as to whether we will find solutions to problems of brain edema at the end of this session.

I would like to preface my remarks with a plea. Let us have all experimental models well-defined, both morphologically as to the nature of the pathological changes, and biochemically as to the type of edema. Otherwise, we will be handicapped by confusion and uncertainty in attempting to interpret the findings.

Cold lesion seems to be best defined as the model for the vasogenic type of brain edema. Hexachlorophene intoxication can be used as a clear-cut model for the cytotoxic type. Experimental production of cerebral ischemia either by occlusion of major arteries or by embolisation is rather a confusing model for brain edema. The pathology of cerebral infarction is simply too heterogenous and therefore this model is rather unsuitable for evaluation of various therapeutic measures which may be beneficial for brain edema.

With regard to the role of tight interendothelial junctions in vasogenic edema, I believe, we have clarified certain points. It is now beyond any doubt that these junctions can temporarily open allowing passage of serum contents and their spreading via the intercellular spaces of brain parenchyma. A further study of the tight junctions should be directed especially to the factors which can alter their alignment and thus affect the permeability of the endothelial barrier. We have demonstrated a direct effect on the junctions by application of hyperosmotic solutions. But our observations on serotonin indicate that besides being affected *directly* the endothelial barrier can be also altered *secondarily* by some action of cellular elements in the vascular walls other than endothelium. This brings up the problem of the vascular spasm and its relationship to the permeability of the blood-brain barrier. It would be important to elucidate the nature of the blood-brain barrier changes observed in conditions such as an acute hypertension, air embolism, electric stimulation, etc., in which the presence of the vasospasm has been implied.

Now, moving from the endothelium into the brain parenchyma, I was interested to hear Dr. Pappius' remark concerning the astrocytes. They remain mysterious as far as their function is concerned. Our previous studies have shown that astrocytes react very promptly in vasogenic type of edema showing a vigorous pinocytotic uptake of serum proteins and production of glial fibrils. Whether protein uptake and formation of glial fibrils are related remains not clear. The fact, however, that the astrocytes are in the stage of intense metabolic activity is supported by histochemical observations on various respiratory enzymes. Astrocytes have also been implicated in transport of glucose between the blood and the neurons. Strongly supporting this contention are observations on abnormal accumulation of glycogen in astrocytes in various pathological conditions associated with neuronal injury. Astrocytic involvement in electrolyte transport and ionic homeostasis has been suggested from many sources. The intriguing possibility mentioned by Dr. Pappius that the resolution of edema may be related to outward transport of electrolytes from the astrocytes must remain at the moment a matter of conjecture. We must remember that in vasogenic edema there are wide open extracellular spaces which would allow for unrestricted movement of electrolytes. There is also an indication of certain directional "currents" as can be conjectured from a gradual accumulation of serum proteins and waste products from areas of edema around the blood vessels and pial and ependymal surfaces.

As far as the dynamics of edema are concerned, this symposium has brought to light very clearly the significance of hemodynamic forces involved in vasogenic type of edema. Some years ago we reported a strikingly straightforward relationship between the systolic blood pressure and the extension of edema. This close relationship has been also mentioned by several investigators at our symposium. I would like again to caution that any evaluation of therapeutic measures should be undertaken always with thorough recording of the systolic blood pressure.

I enjoyed the excellent paper by Dr. Reulen and we should be grateful to him for bringing up the important problem of *tissue pressure* in brain edema. In this respect I have the following comments. It is a well recognized fact that in vasogenic type of edema, in addition to extracellular accumulation of the fluid, swelling of the astrocytes is also common. The most likely explanation for this would be a certain degree of hypoxia as the astrocytes are known to react with swelling in improper fixation procedures or in other experimentally produced hypoxic conditions. The hypoxia itself could be related to increased tissue pressure. Some electron micrographs in such conditions indicate that intensely swollen astrocytic vascular processes can considerably narrow or obstruct the vascular lumen. Thus, we may have a full vicious circle: hypoxia – swelling of astrocytes – interference with circulation – hypoxia. This reminds me another vicious circle sometimes operative in brain edema i.e. tentorial herniation interfering locally with circulation, increasing swelling of the brain tissue – and further herniation.

Since brain tissue hypoxia seems to be involved in these situations, a clinical management of hypoxia might be a very important aspect to be considered in therapeutic measures.

SCHÜRMANN: We have to thank you for this clarifying synopsis of the various processes involved in the formation and resolution of brain edema. I enjoyed particularly your comment on the tissue pressure as well as the tissue perfusion pressure, and I would agree that they are playing an important role in this context. Dr. Klatzo, before we go into the details of pathophysiology of brain edema, I would like to ask you a methodological question. Most experiments, dealing with brain edema, especially with the cold injury edema, are performed in animals with open skull. In the clinical situation, the skull is usually closed. May this difference exert an influence on the dynamics of the edematous process?

KLATZO: I think this point is clearly exemplified in the difference between Dr. Clasen's and our model of cold injury edema. In Dr. Clasen's preparation, the skull remains closed and this results in greatly increased intracranial pressure which influences the extent and intensity of necrosis and hemorrhage shown by the lesion. In our preparation the skull is open and the necrotic or hemorrhagic region is limited to the injured cortex. Although this preparation may be further removed from clinical situations, we consider an advantage to have a well defined area of "pure" vasogenic edema not contaminated by necrosis or hemorrhage, especially for biochemical assays. Basically, the models are similar, i.e., both produce vasogenic type of brain edema.

CLASEN: The degree of necrosis and hemorrhage seen in our lesions is not the result of the skull being closed. By reducing the contact surface of the freezing instrument and the time of application, smaller lesions can be produced. I thought I had made this clear in my presentation.

BROCK: I propose that the lesion produced by the Clasen-method and the one induced by the method of Klatzo are different from the pathophysiological point of view. While in the presence of an open skull an increase of tissue pressure is less liable to develop (the increase in the tissue fluid content leading to tissue herniation through the craniotomy hole), the lesion produced with a closed skull invariably leads to a marked increase in tissue pressure and to a corresponding decrease in tissue perfusion pressure. The secondary circulatory alterations in this latter case can be expected to be more profound and to spread faster. These facts have been well demonstrated by Heipertz and by Christ of our group. Heipertz found that a marked hyperemia develops around a cryogenic lesion induced with the skull open, while Christ has shown that this reactive hyperemia can not take place when the skull remains closed and intracranial pressure increases.

288

KLATZO: I concur to great extent with what you said; but I would like to point out that also in our model of cold injury edema, i.e., with the open skull, we have a considerable widening of the edematous white matter which strongly suggests that there must be also greatly increased tissue pressure in such areas. Thus, I would not be inclined to consider Dr. Clasen's model with closed skull and ours with open skull as of fundamentally different nature.

SCHÜRMANN: Perhaps we might leave this topic for a moment and turn back to our basic question concerning the formation of edema. We have heard a lot of testimony on the importance of the blood pressure as the driving force of fluid extravasation in the vasogenic type of edema. I suppose that we should devote a part of this discussion to the question as to whether the absolute blood pressure is the main factor, and to what extent changes in intracranial pressure influence this mechanism. I wonder, whether Dr. Reulen could give us a little more precise data. Apart from this question we should try to elaborate in general terms, what to me, as a clinician, seems to be an important point. Arterial hypotension seems to reduce the spreading of the edema, but is there a lower limit of blood pressure where trouble can be expected with underperfusion and especially underoxygenation of the brain, especially the damaged brain. Dr. Clasen would you first care to comment on the latter subject?

CLASEN: The edema associated with cold induced lesions in the monkey can be diminished by reducing the aortic systolic pressure to 70 mm for a 9 h period. This, however, is associated with an increase in the water content of the undamaged hemisphere suggesting an untoward effect [Clasen, R. A. *et al.*, Arch. Neurol. **19**, 472–486 (1968)]. Intracranial pressure was not measured in these experiments but it has been shown that the increased intracranial pressure associated with these lesions is diminished in the hypothermic dog. [Rosomoff, H. L., Surg. Gynec. Obstet. **110**, 27–32 (1960).] Systemic hypothermia diminishes the edema without causing any increase in water content of the undamaged hemisphere.

REULEN: I think, we have forgotten for a long time the importance of the intracranial pressure (ICP). The effective cerebral perfusion pressure (CPP) may be determined by the difference between the mean arterial blood pressure and the intracranial pressure; for instance, the ventricular fluid pressure. Thus, the cerebral perfusion pressure can be altered by lowering the arterial blood pressure and by a rise of the intracranial pressure as well. A lowering of CPP in arterial hypotension or during increased ICP due to an enlargement of CSF volume does not reduce cerebral blood flow until the CPP drops below the autoregulatory range of CBF, that is, about 40–50 mmHg. [Zwetnow, N. *et al.*, Acta Physiol. scand. Suppl. **339**, 1–31 (1970); Miller, D. *et al.*, Progr. Brain Res. **35**, 411–432 (1971).] The situation is quite different in edematous brain. Regional CBF is diminished with increasing tissue water content, even if ICP is not markedly increased. If, in addition, cerebrovascular autoregulation is lost in acidotic brain, which results in a pressure-passive flow, any drop in CPP will result in a conspicuous decrease in tissue perfusion and may lead to tissue hypoxia (Meinig, G. *et al.* In: Intracranial Pressure, Springer 1972).

I think, neither the mean arterial blood pressure nor the CPP is the real driving force of the extravasation of edema fluid. Under the circumstances of cerebral edema, the interstitial pressure of the edematous tissue area is expected to rise due to the volume increase of this area. Therefore the local tissue pressure in this area should be higher than the ventricular fluid pressure. We know from recent studies that we have a diminution of the perfusion of edematous areas probably due to a compression of capillaries and venules, on the one hand, and a reduction of the resistance of the arterioles due to the local lactacidosis, on the other hand. A CSF-lactacidosis and an increased brain lactate concentration is a common finding in severe cerebral edema (see Reulen, H. J., this meeting). That means that the arterial pressure head is partially transmitted to the capillary bed, and the real driving force of the vasogenic edema formation process therefore should be the difference between the tissue pressure and the intracapillary pressure. Both cannot be measured at the moment with accuracy, and therefore we can only speculate about these relationships.

There is some evidence that this pH-dependant transmission or *"break-through"* of pressure to the capillaries occurs also in the edema-adjacent brain tissue. Local flow has been found to be increased in the neighborhood of a cold lesion. It is a still open and classical question, whether a very high capillary pressure may induce a "filtration edema". Meinig, G. et al. [In: Cerebral Blood Flow and Intracranial Pressure. S. Karger 1972] in our laboratory have recently observed an increase in water and sodium content in the white matter, if hypertension has been induced simultaneously with a severe hypercapnia ($PaCO_2$ = 150–180 mmHg, CSFpH = 7.0). This has occured without evidence of Evans blue exudation. This clearly indicates the transcapillary filtration of a low-protein edema fluid in the white matter. We are now studying whether the break-through of the pressure can be restored and consequently edema formation diminished following hypocapnia induced by hyperventilation. It becomes evident from these examples that the fluid movement through a damaged cerebral capillary may be modified by various factors, not only by the condition of the tight juntions, but also by the local chemical and hemodynamical factors of a small tissue area.

BROCK: It should be born in mind that blood pressure within an arteriole of the brain is of the order of only 30–40 mmHg. Intracranial pressure is normally 10–15 mmHg. This leaves a pressure head of 15–30 mmHg as driving force for the circulation within the brain tissue. Small increases in intracranial pressure and/or local tissue pressure may cause marked decreases in this driving force ("tissue perfusion pressure") not detectable if "cerebral perfusion pressure" is measured. Even if one admits that cerebral lesions are accompanied by arteriolar dilatation, which tends to increase tissue perfusion pressure, the increase in extravascular (tissue) pressure due to fluid extravasation may eventually lead to a complete local circulatory arrest in the affected areas. The Hannover group [Pöll, W. et al. In: Brock, M., Dietz, H. (Eds.): Intracranial Pressure. Experimental and Clinical Aspects. Berlin-Heidelberg-New York: Springer 1972 (in press)] has found that brain tissue pressure is usually somewhat lower than cerebrospinal fluid pressure, and that the development of local brain edema is associated with the development of local tissue pressures higher than the pressure of the surrounding CSF pressure. The conclusion is that local changes in circulation and pressure within the tissue are prevalent for the development of brain edema and that the pathogenetic process involved should be studied under this aspect.

ZWETNOW: Tissue pressure is, of course, a paramount importance when we consider brain edema. I don't quite understand Dr. Brock's reasoning. A prerequisite for your hypothesis of a selective and critical decrease taking place in the tissue perfusion pressure when the intracranial pressure rises, would be that the pressure in the arterial end of the capillaries remains unchanged when the intracranial pressure is increased. I find it difficult to accept that the capillary pressure could remain constant under these circumstances. All available evidence would point towards the capillary pressure increasing concomitantly to the increase in the cerebrospinal fluid pressure. Consequently, the pressure difference – the tissue perfusion pressure – would be reduced in proportion to the decrease in the global cerebral perfusion pressure (P_a – P_{csf}), but hardly more.

SCHÜRMANN: I would like to come back to the effects of steroids on the brain. I would like to challenge Dr. Withrow and ask him if there is any evidence concerning the permeation of steroids, especially dexamethasone, into the brain tissue? What are the steroid concentrations in the CSF and brain tissue? How long are they maintained following a bolus injection?

WITHROW: As far as I know, no one has done the experiment. If one can relate dexamethasone distribution to cortisol and corticosterone distribution one would guess that when dexamethasone blood levels fall the free levels of steroids in tissue would decrease rapidly. We do have the phenomenon of tissue binding, and it is still to be resolved as to how fast the bound steroids come out. Now, whether the bound steroids are doing the work, or whether they are pharmacologically inactive, I am not prepared to say, and I don't think anyone else is either. Another point that should be raised is that we apparently have no reservoirs other than the tissue binding in the central nervous system to keep the steroids there, because it has been shown that CSF levels follow the blood levels very rapidly.

SCHÜRMANN: Unfortunately we did have not enough time to discuss the possible mechanisms underlying the resolution of edema. Dr. Klatzo, would you like to make your concluding remarks concerning this topic. Where are the obvious gaps, and where do you

290

believe are the most promising approaches to clarify the mechanisms of the formation and resolution of edema in the near future.

KLATZO: I would like to come back for a moment to the question of systolic blood pressure and to consider some therapeutic implications of this factor. First, a note of warning. I keep in mind the observations of Dr. Brierley from England whose experiments demonstrated extensive brain tissue damage by rapid lowering of the blood pressure. I have the impression that intolerance of brain tissue to lowering of blood pressure is not gradual but an abrupt phenomenon when a certain threshold is reached. This reminds me of some of my observations in tissue culture. Perfusing the cultures with hypotonic solutions under the direct optical observation one does not see a gradual distension of the cells proportionally to fall in osmolarity but there is a sudden "explosion" of the cells when certain osmotic values of medium are reached. It appears as if some cellular mechanism which has been compensating for maintenance of osmotic homeostasis suddenly stops. I wonder whether the similar all or nothing phenomenon could be operative with regard to effect of hypotension, and I would be very cautious in application of hypotension in clinical trials. On the other hand, control of hypertension seems to me important and advisable in vasogenic type of brain edema.

In this symposium several new therapeutic possibilities have been mentioned. One concerns the application of inhibitors of biogenic amines. There are forthcoming reports that biogenic amines may be involved in pathomechanism of brain edema. I have briefly presented our observations on serotonin. If biogenic amines can significantly contribute to the development of edema, it is clear that substances which inhibit their synthesis or cause their depletion might have an important therapeutic effect. This whole subject requires a thorough investigation and I suspect it will be extensively discussed during the next symposium on brain edema. Another possibility of therapeutic approach has been mentioned here, i.e., by application of free radical inhibitors. This subject is entirely new to me and I would be very interested in further developments in this area.

SCHÜRMANN: We come now to the next subject of our discussion. We were all challenged by the reports presented by Dr. Pappius and her group, that steroids may improve or restore a disturbed nervous function despite persistent brain or spinal cord edema. I should like to ask Dr. Pappius if she could elaborate on this a little bit in her summary.

PAPPIUS: I would like, first of all, to return to the problem of the definition of "cerebral edema". In my opinion it must be strictly limited to the "increased volume due to increased fluid content". And in the case of vasogenic edema, it is clearly a fluid containing sodium and protein. Any model of brain injury also consists of other components: changes in blood pressure, hemodynamics in general, effects on cerebral autoregulation, vascular permeability, tissue pressure, intracranial pressure, whatever as you wish to add. But these are not cerebral edema. If the experimental results that we obtain do not correlate with edematous changes, then clearly the other components must be investigated in greater detail and, as far as possible, separately. For the benefit of our clinically orientated colleagues, I am fully aware of all the difficulties that they have to face in establishing criteria for the causes of the neurological signs and symptoms which they generally ascribe to cerebral edema. But I think they should not dismiss the simpler, perhaps more precise experimental studies. We are in a position where we can more easily separate the various components involved. If we want to discuss the experimental work from the point of view of the clinician, we should restrict our considerations to the so-called vasogenic edema models. In this I am, of course, agreeing with Dr. Klatzo, who said, that we should define very clearly what models we are working with. For example, I think that the triethyltin model is not of general clinical interest. Secondly, at the moment, I am personally not happy with the models of ischemia that have been developed. I the case of our experiments, I think we have gross necrosis which probably is a complicating factor, and I also am not satisfied, at least in our hands, with the model referred to by Dr. Siegel, that of injecting microspheres. This produces very diffuse changes, so that one cannot separate the necrotic, the edematous and the normal tissue. So I do feel, that at the moment, one of the things we should look for in the future is the development of a better experimental model for the study of cerebral infarction. In this connection I want to mention the work reported by Dr. Bartko and Dr. Reulen. They are probably approaching the ideal of having a reasonable experimental model for cerebral ischemia.

When discussing the effects of steroids, it is very important to establish whether we are looking at the effects of steroids on edema only or whether these effects affect other components of the overall system, especially membrane integrity. I really don't think this is semantics. The lack of rigidity of criteria has given us a lot of trouble before; it is not so very long ago that we were told, mostly on the basis of clinical experience, that hypoxia always causes cerebral edema. Now we know that poor oxygenation plus hypercapnia causes extreme dilatation of the blood vessels which increases intracranial pressure, but which in actuality is not cerebral edema. It can clearly be corrected by maintaining an open airway. I think this is a good example of the consequence of lack of criteria for "edema". We were really led astray.

Thus, if we are to develop methods that are going to help to develop therapy which will be of benefit clinically, the basic processes involved in the therapy must be understood. If maintenance of membrane integrity is the most important aspect of steroid therapy, then we should concentrate on that aspect of the problem. We should look for other agents to maintain this membrane integrity. Conversely, if the control of edema is of benefit to the patient, then we should be studying other agents to control it. It is not sufficient to look just for drug effects on the edema. This applies to our own experiments with furosemide. We showed a diminution of edema. But by our standards the functional state of the animal was not improved. I would be very interested to hear of clinical experience with furosemide. For instance, does the patient do as well on furosemide as on dexamethasone. If edema is not the primary problem then we should test other drugs on things other than cerebral edema. I am aware of the problem of assessing the functional state in animals. We have had these problems and I have used the EEG assessment done by people not directly involved in our experiments, quite often not as enthusiastically accepted by our own EEG experts. So I fully appreciate that I am on rather shaky ground here. In this respect, I think the studies with spinal cord trauma are much more helpful. The ratings are less questionable and more clear-cut. I am really quite impressed by the ease with which spinal cord edema and the effects of this edema can be assessed. On the other hand, we must remember that spinal cord lesions are not exactly comparable to cerebral lesions. I think that the lack of a good method for testing cerebral function in animals should stimulate efforts to develop such methods rather than encouraging us to ignore effects on function in the experimental situations.

CLASEN: With respect to the definition of "cerebral edema" proposed by Dr. Pappius, I would like to add the adjectives "extravascular" and "intracellular" to the term "fluid" and also to emphasize the unit involved. If the first modifier is not added, then, since blood is "fluid", cerebral congestion would be included in the definition. With respect to the unit, if it is the cell, than a shift of water from the extracellular to the intracellular space would qualify as edema, although there be no increase in *tissue* fluid. The second modifier would also exclude this situation. I am also glad that Dr. Pappius chose the term "fluid" rather than "water". It is theoretically possible that edema fluid, by virtue of an increased protein content could have a dry weight equal to that of whole brain. In this situation, there would be no increase in tissue water normalized to a unit of dry or whole mass.

PAPPIUS: I would very much like to see the term brain edema restricted to extracellular accumulation of fluid and then restrict the term "cellular swelling" to the intracellular fluid accumulation. The shift of water from the extracellular to the intracellular compartment is really not of primary importance in studying cerebral edema associated with injury. It does occur in asphyxia. As far as measuring the swelling of astrocytes, I don't have a method. I wish I had. The definite demonstration of the role of astrocytes in resolution of edema is a problem that will keep some of us busy for many years.

LONG: A few hours ago I made a statement which was infinitely more inflammatory than I intended although I must say that I am glad that I made it, because the explanations of Dr. Pappius and Dr. Klatzo have been, I think, very worthwhile. If I remember correctly, I said that sodium is not edema, potassium, chloride and water are not edema and increased intracranial pressure is not necessarily edema. The definition of the model is an extremely important thing. Water may be increased in the cytotoxic model of edema as well as in vasogenic edema. The simple fact that water is increased or decreased is not adequate to characterize an edema model. We must know something about the dynamics and we certainly must know at least the histology, if not the ultrastructure of the process. Unless we do not know these basic histological and pathophysiological facts, it is not appropriate to simply describe our changes in water and electrolytes as edema. The histology of the cold lesion is very well known, and therefore, it is entirely appropriate to characterize changes in this or any well standardized lesion by the parameters of water and electrolytes.

I think that we made it clear in the experimental presentations, that we do not believe that there is a one to one ratio between removal of extracellular water from white matter and the beneficial effect of steroid in every experimental model that we have utilized and that includes four types of spinal cord injury. The steroids do bring about a definite decrease in cerebral or spinal cord water, wherever it is. I know nothing about the site of action. We do believe that *one* of the effects of the steroids is an actual reduction or prevention of the edema which develops following these various kinds of lesions. This does not exclude other possibilities. Indeed, Drs. French, Hartman, and I first suggested membrane effects in 1962 (presentation to the Society of Neurological Surgeons).

KLATZO: I have an impression that Dr. Pappius' remarks refer mostly to vasogenic type of edema and it appears that the study of cytotoxic edema has been generally neglected. I feel sorry about that since I believe that many mechanisms can be best elucidated by comparing these two different types.

OVERGAARD: I think we should for a moment try to reflect on the condition of the people who treat the patients. I was very amazed to hear Dr. Klatzo twice mention the action of hexachlorophene in the brain, if this substance is applied to the skin of monkeys. We start the day by washing our hands with hexachlorophene. I would ask you, should we stop using hexachlorophene for our hands or should we take a shot of dexamethasone before we go into the operation theatre?

KLATZO: We washed the whole monkey from feet to head twice a day. If you are prepared to do this with a patient you might be in trouble.

REULEN: I would like to add something to the definition of cerebral edema. I think it is correct if we define our models in terms of changes in the fluid compartments of the brain by chemical *and* histological or better ultrastructural methods. However, there are other changes, which may be of additional importance, especially in evaluating the effect of a certain drug. We know that rCBF is reduced in experimental and clinical brain edema. There is an impairment or a loss of the local regulation of cerebral blood flow, which may effect edema-formation by itself. The brain volume increase induces a rise in intracranial pressure. In some of the commonly used edema models a breakdown of the high-energy phosphates and an increase of lactate and of the lactate/pyruvate ratio has been found, indicating tissue underoxygenation. There is a CSF-acidosis in severe edema, which might reflect a brain extracellular acidosis, probably influencing enzymatic systems, etc. . . .

Most of these changes are secondary to brain edema and seem to be related to its local or global severity. Obviously, the increased fluid content in the extracellular space affects other systems. If steroids affect edema, they consequently also must affect cerebral blood flow, blood flow regulation, oxidative metabolism, intracranial dynamics etc. Therefore, before dismissing an effect of steroids on brain edema, we should keep in mind that we measure water, sodium, chloride and potassium as only part of our problem. In this context I would like to come back to an interesting aspect of Dr. Pappius' work. It was shown that dexamethasone in fact reduced the amount of edema in the injured hemisphere but not the local amount of water and sodium in the most affected area. That means that the surrounding areas contain less edema fluid. Dr. Pappius, is there any evidence whether this reduction of total edema in the injured hemisphere is due to a reduced rate of formation of edema, to an increased rate or resolution, or do steroids have a specific effect on the areas bordering the edema; for instance on cell membranes?

PAPPIUS: Our results agree with those of Hagan and Rovit. That is, the volume of tissue affected by edema is diminished in the steroid-treated animals. This can be demonstrated by the difference in weight. Further if you compare the total sodium of the affected hemispere in treated and untreated animals, the total sodium will be smaller in the treated animals. But if you sample the edematous tissue, whether it be in the small edematous area of a treated

animal or the larger edematous area of an untreated animal, you will find that the characteristics of the edema are the same. Now turning to the question regarding the steroid effect
on membrane integrity. I think Dr. Long has been one of the first ones to show with the
electronmicroscope that steroids preserve membrane or cell integrity. It is possible that because the membranes are better preserved the spread of edema is diminished purely on mechanical grounds. I really cannot answer the question regarding the resolution of edema. As
I said earlier, if steroids stimulate in some way the removal of sodium from the edematous
tissue, then the water would follow and the remaining edema fluid would have the same
ratio of sodium to water. With this idea, we started the work with sodium 24 which I have
described. From our very preliminary data (and I stress that they are preliminary), it seems to
us that the sodium 24-distribution is not affected by steroid treatment, and therefore at this
stage we do not think that this is the mechanism of action of steroids.

BARLOW: Americans are very poor linguists, but I attempt to speak two languages (the
language of the clinician and the language of the experimentalist). I am fond of both. First, as
a clinician. There is a clinical phenomenon that I won't attempt to define, that is called
"edema". It is often associated with a neoplasm, a big hemisphere, certain signs and a sick
patient. Dr. Pappius has valiantly tried to define edema from the scientist's point of view. In
so doing she would like to restrict the word edema to a measurable increase in water and the
sodium and chloride that go with it to keep the water in balance within and outside of the
brain. I would suggest, however, that the edema she describes probably does not exist in the
clinic. The only situation in which it may exist is in the problem of pseudotumor cerebri. If
this is the case, these patients are extraordinarily comfortable. In other words, it suggests to
me, if pure edema exists in the clinic, it probably has very little effect on the functional human
beeing. So it must be true that other elements of the pathologic physiology are more important, and perhaps they can be dissected and defined, too. It seems to me, one can speak of
membrane dysfunction, one can speak of protein transudation which certainly accompanies
the vasogenic variety of experimental edema, and one can certainly talk about necrosis of
tissue, and probably of a number of other things as well. We should attempt to dissect these
various phenomena, and examine them separately.

I think that an increase in the water content of the nervous system is likely to be relatively
asymptomatic. I think it is likely to be true that minor degrees of protein transudation
can be handled metabolically by the brain. I don't think we know whether an overload of
this system produces toxic metabolites of protein catabolism that lead to dysfunction or not.
This question is open and should be investigated. But the one thing that seems to me likely is
that the corticosteroids work on aspects of the problem that have been referred to as membrane integrity, well beyond their effect on protein transudation or on water accumulation.
Therefore it is the function of these membranes that attracts my interest. And I am not
certain that we are at this point able to deal with the issue of free radicals, but we can look at
certain aspects of membrane function that have not been tested, such as issues of transport
(movements of metabolites in, transport of catabolites out). Another aspect of membrane
function is to withhold certain perhaps toxic circulating factors. This I don't believe we have
examined. We know that such a large molecule as protein leaks in, but what of other circulating substances that may well be entering – including Dr. Klatzo's catecholamines which
really have a potent CSF effect. So I think the membrane is the key here. Corticosteroids do
something to that membrane, but what? I would like to suggest at this point that as well as
looking at the "free radical", we look at a number of the various functions of membranes.

PAPPIUS: Could we not, however, somehow join the two languages and talk about brain
injury instead insisting on calling it "edema"?

DEMOPOULOS: There are two aspects of membrane structure and function that have not
been discussed at all, nor mentioned, and this is surprising since we are concerned here with
neural elements. These are what we call the solid state functions of membranes. We consider
membrane transport and compartmentalization as important things; yet, there are two
aspects of solide state functions that are disordered and follow the presentation that we have
discussed here especially with some aspects of Dr. Pappius' work. One is electron transport
along mitochondria, a solid state function where electrons are transported right down the
surface of the membrane. The same is true in some current thinking regarding nerve con-

duction, that it is a solid state function of the membrane. Steroids obviously could have a phenomenal effect on the solid state conductivity of membranes. In some of the work that Dr. Pappius has done, there is not complete resolution of edema but there still seems to be improvement of the animal. This could easily be explained by improving solid state function of nerve conduction as well as solid state function of mitochondria to improve electron transport. With respect to the latter point: the mitochondria having the most unsaturated fatty acids are the most susceptible to radical damage and this would be one site where steroids and antioxidants might be expected to help the most. I don't think that it is coincidence that with the pathology that is produced, among the first biochemical deficits that we see are diminutions in oxidative respiration and diminution of the membrane bound enzymes involved in electron transport.

I would like to take serious objection to the concept that membrane effect of steroids are hypothetical or theoretical. There are literally thousands of papers going from physics all the way up to subcellular structures (like lysosomes and mitochondrial function) where steroids have unquestionable effects. If you know some of the chemistry of steroids, there is only one place where a poor steroid molecule can go, and this is into the cell membrane.

PAPPIUS: Let me say that when I talk in terms of function I assume that effects on conduction are involved.

SCHÜRMANN: I think we are right in the heart of the problem of the mechanism of action of steroids. The principle idea seems to be that they have a variety of effects on the brain rather than a specific point of action. Dr. Long was the first who has stressed this point in his publications. Most forms of edema that seem to respond to steroids belong to the vasogenic type, and I regret that we did not get an answer as to whether the cytotoxic type of edema responds as well. However, this type of edema is not as clear as the vasogenic type. Dr. Bartko's study, however, shows that the early edema following a focal cerebral ischemia can be influenced by dexamethasone. I should like to ask Dr. Long to comment in his session and to give his statements concerning this topic.

LONG: The third session was entitled "Mechanisms of Action of Steroids on Brain Edema" and I think in actual fact we have been discussing this since Dr. Klatzo first began his summary. I have only a few points that I believe effectively summarize the diverse data that we have heard presented in this session. Basically, we have seen several effects upon rather gross measures of edema. First, I think several investigators have demonstrated an effect upon what we have loosely termed over the years as the blood-brain barrier, and which we are now beginning to refine into the permeability of various substances. There are two presentations that demonstrate some decreased permeability for proteins with steroids, and in one paper for sodium.

Secondly, several investigators, Dr. Herrmann, Dr. Reulen, Dr. Ransohoff and his group and myself, all demonstrated a reduction in the volume abnormality, which primarily is the extracellular water in brain edema. There was an effect upon electrolyte content, though the location of these electrolytes remains unknown. Then Dr. Pappius showed very well there could be an effect upon function, both electrical activity of the nervous system and the functional gross neurological status of the animals without any marked reduction in the tissue water content of the CNS. This brought into focus the fact that a simple reduction in edema may not be enough to explain the beneficial effect of steroids in patients harboring all manner of brain injuries associated with brain edema. Dr. Sano has shown us very graphically that individual cells – astrocytes – can be profoundly affected in their function by steroids, and I think this returns us again to the underlying mechanisms of both the formation and the resolution of brain edema, and certainly the effects of steroids upon all of the aspects of the edema problem. At this point I have no better explanation for any of this variables than we have heard presented. I think it will be for each one of us to digest this material as we return home over the next days, months, and years, and to try to answer these questions more specifically. I hope the next time we join together, many of these problems which we now discuss, will be academic and we will peer into the free radicals of the membranes with Dr. Demopoulos.

BOUZARTH: I have to tell a joke. When I came to this workshop I felt like the little boy in a Playboy magazine cartoon around Christmas time. He was one of the three kings and said to the little virgin Mary: "Isn't life funny, they pick me to be one of the wise man, and I am the dumbest kid in the class". I am even going to be more stupid now by trying to give you a little theory about dexamethasone action. I am doing this late because I don't want to have to defend it. Let us look at the normal stress response and a few systemic parameters.

Blood glucose is increased in stress, as is well known.
Urinary potassium is increased.
Urinary sodium is decreased.
Body water which is retained and is increased in the extracellular space.

In damage, the extracellular space becomes the so-called "third space". It has been described by the surgeons, and this, in the brain, would be cerebral edema. This is what happens in injury. Now, if we give a drug like dexamethasone several things happen. Glucose still goes up, especially in patients who have a tendency for diabetes. The urinary potassium goes up, even more than in control series (this is work that has come out of our laboratories). So with dexamethasone, we have a greater increase in urinary water output and in urinary potassium excretion when compared to untreated patients. Body water is not retained when compared to the group not receiving the drug, and on the second post-operative day there is expansion of the extracellular space. With dexamethasone the extracellular space remains normal and is not expanded. The third space is not measured directly, but it is measured indirectly.

Why should a stress response increase glucose? Why does it block insulin? I have tried to figure this out, and I have found that insulin is not required for the metabolism of glucose by the brain. In fact, it does not cross the blood-brain barrier. But glucose does. So in stress, the hyperglycemia is to give the brain the food stuff it needs, and the brain, for all practical purposes, requires glucose 90 % of the time. I could not figure out potassium, except that every time a neuron works, potassium goes extracellular and energy is required to bring it back in. Potassium is very toxic in the extracellular space. In fact, the heart stops if potassium goes up in the blood. Therefore, every effort is made, to get potassium back into the cell. When the brain uses glucose, potassium is pulled back in. I submit to you one of the reasons that cortisol in the normal stress response works, and dexamethasone works a little better, it that it makes the main food stuff more available to the brain. Second, it pumps potassium out of the extracellular space by way of the kidneys, and perhaps it may do something locally. Finally, it prevents expansion of the extracellular space, which in brain damage is cerebral edema; it does this, in part, as a subtle diuretic.

SCHÜRMANN: We will switch now to the last part of our discussion and I shall forward several questions which are of clinical relevance. Everybody agrees that the experimental observations on steroid effects in brain edema can hardly be transmitted to patients. We are urgently needing a clinical available method of controlling the effect of steroids on brain edema in the patient. Since cerebral edema cannot be measured directly in our patients we can probably use the measurement of intracranial pressure as has been shown by Dr. Kullberg very excitingly. Another possibility occured during the presentation of Dr. Maxwell, when he showed that the activity of the brain scan of tumor patients often was markedly reduced following dexamethasone treatment. It is one of the main challenges to develop techniques to measure brain edema in the living patient. The next point I wish to raise concerns the dosage of dexamethasone in tumor patients and in acute head injury. How long must tumor patients be pretreated? Are 16 mg of dexamethasone preoperatively per day enough? One of the most interesting aspects is the efficacy of steroids in acute head injury. Although the results of the New York group are not very optimistic, I feel that our treatment in those patients often is delayed. If there are analogies between the closed head injury and the experimental cold lesion we must start the steroid treatment with the shortest possible delay following the impact. This was a very convincing result of the experimental work of Dr. Long and his coworkers.

BEKS: As we have heard in the papers about the clinical use of steroids by neurologists and neurosurgeons, a great step forward in the struggle to combat brain edema has been made. There are however many problems left. Physiologists, pharmacologists and neurochemists have not solved yet the problems about the working mechanisms of steroids on brain physiology and particular the action on the blood-brain barrier. Probably the alterations in the functions of the blood-brain barrier by pathological processes are responsible for the development of brain edema. The prophylactic administration of steroids in brain surgery has very much reduced the complications in the postoperative phase. Perhaps the prophylactic administration of steroids makes the blood-brain barrier less sensitive for injuries during surgery.

The idea, that steroids do not act alone on brain edema but on entire brain, as is stated by Hanna Pappius, is supported by the results of studies done with isotopes on patients with space-occupying lesions. After the administration of steroids the clinical condition of a number of patients improved very much and the neurological symptoms decreased while the size of the space-occupying lesions stayed the same.

About the kind of steroids, the dosage and the duration of application, there is no consensus of opinion. In general there is a preference for dexamethasone, but also by use of other forms of steroids the results are good. It is a pity that during this workshop so little attention was payed by the clinicians to the complications of steroid administration. It is possible that this is due to the fact that most of them are so enthusiastic about the results in general, while they have at least a remedy with which in many cases brain edema can be prevented in the postoperative phase and badly ill patients can be brought in a better condition, so that sometimes serious complications are taken into the bargain.

CLASEN: One of the points raised during the clinical discussion was the measurement of cerebral edema in the living patient. We have recently completed experiments on the distribution of technetium in the dog with cold-induced lesions. [Hindo, W. A. *et al.*, Arch. Neurol (in press).] In this paper we predicted that in the case of single metastatic brain tumors, a scan taken 4 h after injection of the isotope would be larger that one taken at 15 min and suggested that this difference could be used as a measure of the edema around the tumor. I would like to offer this to my clinical colleagues for evaluation.

MILLER: One of the problems that became all too clear in trying to assess the effect of steroids on the clinical outcome in patients was the great variability of response. I think Dr. Kullberg also showed this when looking at intracranial pressure. The widely varying response of intracranial pressure to steroid treatment may be explained by differing intracranial volume/pressure relationships. We have recently demonstrated an exponential relationship between intracranial volume changes and pressure in patients suffering from increased ICP from a wide variety of causes. In other words even if a fixed dose of steroids removes a uniform volume of edema fluid from brain the change in intracranial pressure will depend on whether the volume/pressure relationship is in the steep or lower part. There is, however, another aspect which has not yet been mentioned, and I put this up merely as speculation. It is in which way cerebral edema may change the deformability of the brain, in other words its capacity to shift in response to an expanding lesion, and how steroids influence this property of the brain. I think that most neurosurgeons would agree that many of the clinical signs are related more to the degree of shifting and herniation of the brain, than to the actual level of intracranial pressure.

SCHÜRMANN: The next topic, which I would like to discuss concerns the treatment of spinal cord lesions and the question of treatment of patients with spinal cord tumors or extramedullary compression lesions before operation. As a clinician I was surprised by the fascinating results of Dr. Hansebout, Dr. Long, as well as Dr. Ransohoff. Although these 3 groups used different types of lesions, they uniformly reported a reduction of spinal cord edema or an improvement of the functional state. We need an additional, properly conceived clinical study, but I think this will be a new and important indication for the steroids during the first hour or hours following a spinal cord injury. Many people have talked about steroid pretreatment of patients with brain tumors. I wonder whether there is some experience in pretreating patients with intramedullary tumors or extramedullary compression lesions. Dr. Maxwell has reported the case with a cervial compression, treated in 1930 with an adrenal cortical extract and showed an amelioration of symptoms. Shall we give dexamethasone and will this result in any benefit concerning function or neurological improvement?

LONG: This is only a partial answer. We ignored the spinal cord injury problem as well as the spinal cord tumor problem in our clinical paper because we have no really definitive data. We have used steroids almost routinely in our patients with spinal cord injuries for over 10 years, and this would probably be 300 patients. However, as you know, almost nothing does these people any good when they are quadriplegic from the time of injury, they remain so no matter what we have done. The steroids have not shown any appreciable benefits in this group of patients. It has also been our practice to use steroids routinely with all intramedullary tumors and arteriovenous malformations. We do not have definite data to show whether steroids are of value, but we do feel that it is. This a purely empirical observation. I have one other comment that I should make. Patients with metastatic lesions compressing the spinal cord, not progressing rapidly, and especially with lymphomatous lesions that you would expect to respond to X-ray therapy quickly are often treated with steroids during the period of radiation.

It has been our distinct impression that the symptomatology in these patients of spinal cord compression will improve with steroids, and that they can be maintained throughout a course of X-ray therapy or chemotherapy without a decompressive procedure. But the diseases are so variable that we have made no attempt to try to quantitate this.

SCHÜRMANN: We have to make an attempt to clarify the question of the dosage of steroids, as well as the question of combination therapy of steroids with other drugs as mentioned by Dr. Long, Dr. Reulen, what is your opinion about the dosage and the duration of the pretreatment before planed neurosurgical operations. As for the combination therapy, we use hypertonic solution very rarely and only in order to lower an acute increase in intracranial pressure.

REULEN: We have only small clinical and experimental experiences with different dosages of dexamethasone. In our clinical studies we compared the effect of pretreatment with 16 mg/day or 24 mg/day, for 4–5 days, on the perifocal brain edema in tumor patients. We could not find a further reduction in the local amount of edema (water and sodium content of grey and white matter) with the higher dosage. However, the method or randomly sampling tissue specimens may not be advantageous for that purpose. Also, we do not have statistical evidence whether these patients do better after brain surgery. In patients with brain tumors who are admitted unconscious to our hospital, we have increased the initial loading dose to 16 mg and the dose during the first day to 24–32 mg. We are planning a clinical study where we will compare 2 instead of 5 days of pretreatment with the same dosage of the steroid in patients with brain tumors. In acute head injury the question is still open whether a high initial dose, comparable to that used in shock, might improve our clinical results. I would like to hand over this question to Dr. Long.

LONG: We have tried to approach this from an experimental standpoint in the past year with the choriocarcinoma primate tumor model described earlier. Unfortunately, about half way through a double blind study with steroids we lost the tumor through some problems, and the study has been ruined. It will be restarted when the tumor is recovered. Initially Dr. French used 40 mg of steroid injected into the carotid artery and then 40 mg as a loading dose i.v. or i.m. The lower doses, published previously, were employed quite empirically, simply because they seemed to work as well as the higher doses. We still use the same 10 mg loading dose and 16 mg in 4–6 divided doses in our routine work. As to the minimum dose, we begin to decrease from 16 mg per day and at some critical level (it varies for each patient) symptoms will reoccur. This, in fact, is the way we decide what individual dose we use for long term maintenance of a patient with a metastatic tumor or with a glioblastoma when this is necessary. We actually use the osmotic diuretics very sparingly. We do not use them in most problems of brain edema except for head injuries. When there is a need for acute reduction in intracranial pressure the steroids do not work fast enough, and the osmotic diuretics are necessary to simply salvage a patient so that diagnostic and therapeutic procedures can continue.

TAYLOR: We have been impressed by the fact that under operative conditions (I am not advocating this as a routine measure), an i.v. dose of 60 mg of dexamethasone will visibly bring the pressure down in about 20 min. I don't know how this happens and it does not fit very well into the theory of dexamethasone affecting membrane transport. The edema subsides so fast under these conditions that the fluid would almost have to be reversing its direction of flow back into the vessels. I have a question to Dr. Ransohoff concerning the steroid dependent brain. What kind of patients develop steroid dependency and is the phenomenon related to the large steroid doses, which you use in your clinic?

RANSOHOFF: Steroid dependency can be seen both in patients on long term steroid therapy for the treatment of cerebral edema, as with brain tumors, or in patients beeing treated with steroids for non-CNS disease. The latter phenomenon has been well described in the pediatric literature. In patients with tumors we have had the experience of removing meningiomas in patients who had been carried on steroids for months with the diagnosis of glioma. After surgery if steroids are discontinued too quickly, severe increased intracranial pressure results which is controlled by re-institution of steroid therapy. A gradual taper over several months will then be required. It would appear therefore that this steroid dependency phenomenon is related to an alteration in CNS membrane function in which they function normally only in a milieu of enough steroid packing. We have never seen this situation in high dose, short term steroid therapy in preparation for surgery were the operative procedure is adequate to provide relief of the increased intracranial pressure.

DEMOPOULOS: Dr. Ransohoff mentioned steroid dependency and how membranes may be affected. I thought the kind of evidence should be covered in this symposium that leads us to make statements that steroids intercalate into membranes. The second concept that I would like to discuss will be the turn-over of membrane biomolecules. This may be relevant to tapering steroid therapy.

With respect to the intercalation of steroids, by use of the techniques of spinprobes with membranes, plus nuclear magnetic resonance spectroscopy we find that steroids do intercalate in the membranes and that they really pull the fatty acid of the phospholipid right up close to it. And if we look at molecular models of membranes, proteins are viewed as being present within the archways that have been created by the phospholipids. These proteins, as mentioned earlier, derive their configurational activity by their proximity in hydrophobic associations with fatty acid tails of the phospholipids. These proteins are viewed as a mechanism for transport across membranes. They provide an actual internal polar tunnel where water and ions can be transported through. Now, if you keep in mind that the acid tails of phospholipids associate with proteins it then becomes an interesting situation when we add cholesterol and other steroid molecules. It may be possible to alter or to dislocate fatty acid tails from a protein; it would depend on how strong the hydrophobic interactions are. It may be that we can rotate the fatty acid tail away from the protein and upon to the cholesterol or steroidal molecule. This is the molecular mechanism that we envision as being responsible for turning on and turning off certain membrane-bound enzymes.

The final thinking is that of studying turn-over of membrane molecules, and this relates to not only the steroids, but to our earlier statements regarding free radical damage to membranes. It does *not* have to be irreversible, because we do have a turn-over of membrane molecules. These can be removed individually and replaced like bricks in a wall or they can be removed in clump and cluster, and replaced by new membranes that are synthesized.

BARLOW: Steroid dependency has become common experience in those children treated for a prolonged time with an ordinary dose of corticosteroids, which is common in the treatment of asthma and nephrosis. Among these children it is only the infrequent child who develops "pseudotumor". He usually develops it at a time when the steroid is withdrawn. This may well relate to some alterations of the CNS membranes. There are other possibilities, however. One would wonder whether the chronic use of steroids has depressed adrenal cortical function. It certainly is not apparent in terms of major electrolyte disturbance of a kind that you would attribute to overt adrenal insuffiency, but more subtle depression is not impossible. I would add one further observation. On a recent occasion, we did an angiogram and a jugular venogram in a child with the steroid withdrawal pseudotumor syndrome. In this particular child we found a jugular venous thrombosis. I would wonder whether this may not be more common, because as we do more jugular venograms in our patients, we are finding that many of the idiopathic benign intracranial hypertension syndromes are related to jugular or venous outflow thrombosis, which we had really overlooked before. These patients did not have associated ear or other intracranial adjacent infections.

BAETHMANN: The development of benign intracranial hypertension despite continued corticosteroid administration as mentioned by Dr. Barlow needs to be emphasized. Clinical reports give the impression that the long-time glucocorticosteroid therapy in some cases may even be responsible for the occurrence of pseudotumor cerebri. [Cohn, S. A., J. Neurosurg. **20**, 784 (1963); Dees, S. C., McKay, A. W., jr., Pediatrics **23**, 1143 (1959).] It is conceivable that the long-time suppression of the ACTH-adrenal axis by exogenous steroids affects the mineralocorticosteroids, e. g., the aldosterone production is experimentally found to be considerably reduced after dexamethasone suppression of ACTH [Müller, J., Acta endocrin. **63**, 1 (1970)], and thus contributes substantially to the development of the cerebral fluid disturbances.

LONG: I have a comment in extension of Dr. Barlow's statement about venous trombosis. Our head and neck cancer surgeons do bilateral radical neck dissections with removal of the entire jugular venous system bilaterally and acutely. Prior to the institution of standard pretreatment with dexamethasone in these patients the incidence of acutely increased intracranial pressure with papilledema was quite high. The addition of steroid treatment for 48 h before surgery has essentially eliminated this complication; we did not include this information among our patients, because these patients were out of our control.

SCHÜRMANN: At the end of this workshop I think we all feel very strongly that our meeting has raised far more questions than could be answered. The workshop also clearly showed our as yet limited knowledge concerning the phenomena underlying the formation and resolution of brain edema as well as its treatment. Therefore I agree with Dr. Reulen's suggestion that the different groups should gather regularly at varying places and try to answer the remaining and newly appearing questions. Finally I want to express my special thanks to all participiants who have made this meeting so vivid.

Subject Index

302